# Problem Solving in **Oncology**

# Problem Solving in
# Oncology

Edited by

**DEARBHAILE O' DONNELL**, MD
Department of Medical Oncology, St James's Hospital, Dublin, Ireland

**MICHAEL LEAHY**, PhD, FRCP
Department of Medical Oncology, Christie Hospital NHS Trust, Manchester, UK

**MARIA MARPLES**, MD
Cancer Research UK Clinical Centre, St James's University Hospital, Leeds, UK

**ANDREW PROTHEROE**, MBBS, MRCP, PhD
Cancer Research UK, Department of Medical Oncology, Churchill Hospital, Oxford, UK

**PETER SELBY**, CBE, MA, MD, FRCP FRCR FMedSci
Cancer Research UK Clinical Centre, Leeds Institute of Molecular Medicine, St James's University Hospital, Leeds, UK

CLINICAL PUBLISHING
OXFORD

CLINICAL PUBLISHING
an imprint of Atlas Medical Publishing Ltd

Oxford Centre for Innovation
Mill Street, Oxford OX2 0JX, UK

Tel: +44 1865 811116
Fax: +44 1865 251550
E mail: info@clinicalpublishing.co.uk
Web: www.clinicalpublishing.co.uk

**Distributed in USA and Canada by:**
Clinical Publishing
30 Amberwood Parkway
Ashland OH 44805 USA

tel: 800-247-6553 (toll free within U.S. and Canada)
fax: 419-281-6883
email: order@bookmasters.com

**Distributed in UK and Rest of World by:**
Marston Book Services Ltd
PO Box 269
Abingdon
Oxon OX14 4YN UK

tel: +44 1235 465500
fax: +44 1235 465555
e mail: trade.orders@marston.co.uk

© Atlas Medical Publishing Ltd 2008

First published 2008

A catalogue record for this book is available from the British Library

ISBN 13   978 1 904392 84 2
ISBN 10   1 904392 84 9

The publisher makes no representation, express or implied, that the
dosages in this book are correct. Readers must therefore always check
the product information and clinical procedures with the most up-to-
date published product information and data sheets provided by the
manufacturers and the most recent codes of conduct and safety
regulations. The authors and the publisher do not accept any liability
for any errors in the text or for the misuse or misapplication of
material in this work

Project manager: Gavin Smith, GPS Publishing Solutions, Herts, UK
Typeset by Phoenix Photosetting, Chatham, UK
Printed by TG Hostench S. A., Barcelona

# Contents

### SECTION 9    Psychosocial Issues and Symptom Control

# Preface

It is not difficult to assemble facts and figures about any aspect of cancer care or science these days. Five minutes at a keyboard can produce notable abstracts concerning any topic. Some excellent textbooks, of intellectual and physical weight, are found on most oncologists' bookshelves. So why write a book on problem solving in oncology? The answer lies in the need for individuals to assimilate information quickly and easily synthesize in a form to make it relevant to the problems that they meet in their everyday professional clinical activities. Many electronic and textbook sources are excellent at providing a particular piece of information but may not set it in the context of real-life clinical cases.

*Problem Solving in Oncology* has been written to provide the current evidence on a topic, brought together in a clinically relevant real-life, case-based format. It has been developed to serve the needs of both trainees in oncology and practising consultants. Each chapter has been developed by an interplay between an oncology trainee and an established consultant and the breadth of the topics covers most, but not all, aspects of oncology. Each chapter relates to the sort of cases which oncology professionals see every day and brings recent evidence on management to bear upon that case. Individual chapters can be read quickly and easily and serve both for education and training and to update the reader. We have kept the book small enough and short enough to be carried around, recognizing that reading of this kind will often be done on trains and planes and at home.

The editorial team is drawn from leading cancer centres in the UK and Ireland which combine large clinical practices with internationally recognized expertise in both biomedical sciences and patient-centred research. We hope that readers will find this book a uniquely useful resource to support them in their training and professional development in an enjoyable and accessible way.

The Editors
*October 2007*

# Acknowledgements

The editors and authors warmly acknowledge the support they have received in preparing this book. Nicole Goldman collated and oversaw the book's preparation, organized and formatted it. Yvonne Doyle supported Dr O'Donnell in her work. Dr Fiona Hicks advised on the chapters on palliative care and Dr Louise Hanna on the brain tumour chapter. Finally, Jane Pennington and Clinical Publishing were patient and helpful publishers whose vision for the series of *Problem Solving* books guided and stimulated us and without whose help the book would never have been written.

# Contributors

Dr Joss Adams, Oxford
Dr Faisal Al-Terkait, Leeds
Dr Anne Armstrong, Manchester
Dr Sofia Baka, Manchester
Dr Mike Braun, Leeds
Dr Fiona Collinson, Leeds
Dr Sue Darby, Sheffield
Dr Emma Dean, Manchester
Dr Sheila Fraser, Leeds
Dr Sandeep Goyle, Leeds
Mr Mohammad Abu Hilal, Leeds
Dr Uschi Hofmann, Leeds
Dr Satinder Jagdev, Leeds
Dr Ioannis Karydis, Oxford
Dr Omar Khan, Oxford
Dr Matt Krebs, Manchester
Dr Claire Mitchell, Manchester
Dr Jay Naik, Leeds
Dr Lucy Nicholson, Leeds
Dr Roisin O'Cearbhaill, Dublin
Dr Anne Marie O'Dwyer, Dublin
Dr Derek Power, Dublin
Dr Robin Prestwich, Leeds
Dr Andrew Proctor, Leeds
Dr Andrew Protheroe, Oxford
Dr Nitesh Rohatgi, Leeds
Dr Jens Samol, Oxford
Dr Rachel Sheils, Leeds
Dr Catherine Siller, Leeds
Dr Sheryl Sim, Leeds
Dr Asha Siva, Leeds
Dr Elena Takeuchi, Leeds
Dr Nav Vasudev, Leeds
Dr Simon Waters, Leeds
Dr Penny Wright, Leeds
Dr Cheng Yeoh, Leeds
Dr Alison Young, Leeds

# Abbreviations

3D-CRT three-dimensional conformal radiotherapy
5-HIAA 5-hydroxyindoleacetic acid
5-HT$_3$ 5-hydroxytryptamine
AC Adriamycin and cyclophosphamide
ACC adrenal cortical carcinoma
ACIS automated cellular imaging system
ACTH adrenocorticotropic hormone
ADT androgen deprivation treatment
AFP α-fetoprotein
AJCC American Joint Committee on Cancer
ALPI Adjuvant Lung Cancer Project Italy
ANC absolute neutrophil count
ANITA Adjuvant Navelbine International Trialists Association
ASC active supportive care
ASCO American Society of Clinical Oncology
ASTRO American Society for Therapeutic Radiology and Oncology
AUC area under the curve
BEP bleomycin, etoposide and cisplatin
BSO Bilateral salpingo-oophorectomy
CAB complete androgen blockade
CALGB Cancer and Leukaemia Group B
CBOP carboplatin, bleomycin, vincristine and cisplatin
CBR clinical benefit response
CEA carcinoembryonic antigen
CF cisplatin and 5-fluorouracil
CGA comprehensive geriatric assessment
CHOP cyclophosphamide, hydroxydaunomycin [doxorubicin], Oncovin [vincristine], and prednisone
CHR carboplatin hypersensitivity reaction
CISCA cisplatin, cyclophosphamide and doxorubicin
CK cytokeratin
CMF cyclophosphamide, methotrexate and fluorouracil
CNS central nervous system
CSA cryosurgical ablation
CSF cerebrospinal fluid
CT computed tomography
CTZ chemoreceptor trigger zone

CVC central venous catheter
DMSO dimethylsulphoxide
DRE digital rectal examination
DTIC dacarbazine
EBRT external beam radiotherapy
ECF epirubicin, cisplatin and 5-fluorouracil
ECG electrocardiogram
ECOG PS Eastern Cooperative Oncology Group performance score
ECX epirubicin, cisplatin and capecitabine
EDTA ethylenediamine tetraacetic acid
EGFR epidermal growth factor receptor
ELND elective lymph node dissection
EMA/CO etoposide, methotrexate, dactinomycin, cyclophosphamide and vincristine
EOF epirubicin, oxaliplatin and 5-fluorouracil
EORTC European Organisation for Research and Treatment of Cancer
EOX epirubicin, oxaliplatin and capecitabine
EP/EMA etoposide, cisplatin, methotrexate and dactinomycin
ER oestrogen receptor
ERCP endoscopic retrograde cholangiopancreatography
FAC fluorouracil, doxorubicin and cyclophosphamide
FAMTX 5-fluorouracil, doxorubicin and methotrexate
FE(50)C fluorouracil, epirubicin and cyclophosphamide
FIGO International Federation of Gynecology and Obstetrics
FISH fluorescence *in-situ* hybridization
FNA fine needle aspiration
G-CSF granulocyte-colony stimulating factor
GFR glomerular filtration rate
GIST gastrointestinal stromal tumour
GITSG Gastrointestinal Tumor Study Group
GM-CSFs granulocyte macrophage-colony stimulating factors
GP general practitioner
GTN gestational trophoblastic neoplasia
Hb haemoglobin
hCG human chorionic gonadotrophin

hCSF  haemopoietic colony-stimulating factor
HD  high dose intensity
HGG  high-grade glioma
HIFU  high frequency ultrasound
HR  hazard ratio
IALT  International Adjuvant Lung Cancer Trial
ICC  interstitial cells of Cajal
IGCCC  International Germ Cell Consensus
  Classification
IGCCCG  International Germ Cell Cancer
  Collaborative Group
IL  interleukin
IMRT  intensity-modulated radiation therapy
IV  intravenous
LACE  Lung Adjuvant Cisplatin Evaluation
LDH  lactate dehydrogenase
LVEF  left ventricular ejection fraction
MASCC  Multinational Association of Supportive
  Care in Cancer
MEA  methotrexate, etoposide and dactinomycin
MRC  Medical Research Council
MRCP  magnetic resonance
  cholangiopancreatography
MRI  magnetic resonance imaging
MSCC  metastatic spinal cord compression
MVAC  methotrexate, vincristine, doxorubicin and
  cisplatin
MUGA  multiple gated acquisition scan
NCCN  National Comprehensive Cancer Network
NCIC  National Cancer Institute of Canada
NHS  National Health Service
NK-1  neurokinin-1
NPC  nasopharyngeal carcinoma
NSABP  National Surgical Adjuvant Breast and
  Bowel Project
NSAID  non-steroidal anti-inflammatory drug
NSCLC  non-small cell lung cancer
NSE  neurone-specific enolase

NSGCT  non-seminomatous germ cell tumour
OGD  oesophagogastroduodenoscopy
PCV  procarbazine, lomustine and vincristine
PD  progressive disease
PDGFR  platelet-derived growth factor receptor
PET  positron emission tomography
PFS  progression-free survival
PR  progesterone receptor
PSA  prostate-specific antigen
PSTT  placental site trophoblastic tumour
PTCA  percutaneous transhepatic
  cholangiography
RCC  renal cell carcinoma
RECIST  Response Evaluation Criteria in Solid
  Tumours
RFA  radiofrequency ablation
rHuEPO  recombinant human erythropoietin
RPLND  retroperitoneal lymph node dissection
RR  relative risk
RT  radiotherapy
RTOG  Radiation Therapy Oncology Group
SAGE  serial analysis of gene expression
SLN  sentinel lymph node
SMA  smooth muscle actin
SNB  sentinel node biopsy
SWOG  Southwest Oncology Group
TAC  docetaxel, doxorubicin and
  cyclophosphamide
TCC  transitional cell carcinoma
TIA  transient ischaemic attack
TIP  paclitaxel, ifosfamide and cisplatin
TNF  tumour necrosis factor
UFT  uracil and tegafur
UKP  unknown primary
VEGF  vascular endothelial growth factor
VIP  vinblastine, etoposide and cisplatin
WCC  white cell count
WLE  wide local excision

# Chemotherapy

## PROBLEM

# 1  Chemotherapy: Response Assessment

## Case History

A patient has completed a course of chemotherapy and attends for the results of their post-treatment computed tomography (CT) scan. The reports reads: In the thorax, both previously noted metastatic deposits have reduced in size. The right mid-zone lesion now measures 4.5 cm by 2 cm compared with 5 cm by 3.5 cm previously. The left apical nodule which was previously 7 mm by 5 mm is no longer seen. However, in the upper abdomen, a 2 cm lesion is now noted in the liver, which was not scanned in the previous investigation.

**How do you evaluate the patient's response to chemotherapy?**

**How do the methods apply to the patient?**

**What will you say to the patient?**

## Background

**How do you evaluate the patient's response to chemotherapy?**

Response to chemotherapy in a patient with metastatic disease can be assessed by several approaches. These include subjective and objective methods of assessing disease response. When a patient is started on treatment it is important at the outset to ascertain how their disease will be monitored, taking into consideration the method of monitoring (which may be a combination of methods), the frequency of monitoring, and the implication of the results for further management.

### Clinical assessment

Patients receiving chemotherapy will have regular clinical reviews prior to, during and following completion of their chemotherapy. These reviews provide an opportunity to assess clinically the patient's response to their treatment. The patient can be asked about symptomatic improvement which may have occurred following completion of chemotherapy, for example, pain, anorexia, breathlessness, fatigue. There is a possibility of bias in both the patient's reporting of their condition and the interpretation of the information by the physician.

Scoring systems have been developed to try to standardise assessment of clinical response. These were initially developed for use in clinical trial settings but are now commonly used in medical practice, for example, the scoring systems used to assess performance status of patients. Commonly used tools are the Karnofsky score and the World Health Organization (WHO)/Eastern Cooperative Oncology Group (ECOG) performance score (see Appendix 1.1).

In clinical studies, quality of life of patients has also been evaluated when determining response to treatment. Studies have shown that there is often a significant correlation between quality of life reported by the patient, symptom improvement and objective tumour regression.[1] Assessment with scoring systems can be a valuable means of monitoring patient response. Routine use in clinical practice may sometimes be difficult as time during a consultation is often limited, and patients may find it difficult to complete the sometimes complex questionnaires. Studies, however, have shown that the integration of quality-of-life questionnaires in routine practice is feasible, and has a positive impact on patient–doctor communication and the patient's functional and emotional wellbeing.[2]

Clinical examination also may provide a means of monitoring response to treatment. Direct measurement of palpable tumour masses may be possible in some cases, e.g. lymphadenopathy. When describing lesions, the site, size and appearance should be noted as accurately as possible to reduce intra-observer variability. Clinical photography can also be a useful means of monitoring disease response where exact tumour dimensions are difficult to ascertain or multiple lesions are present, e.g. inflammatory breast cancer. It allows for accurate documentation of disease, and provides a useful tool for comparison of lesions before and after treatment.

### Biochemical tumour markers

Tumour markers are substances which are either released directly by a tumour or are released by normal tissue in response to the presence of a malignant tumour. These substances can be antigens, proteins, enzymes, hormones or other molecular substances. Their role in clinical practice varies. For example, prostate-specific antigen (PSA) is widely used to monitor disease and is under investigation as a screening marker, whereas other markers such as carcinoembryonic antigen (CEA) can be used to detect disease recurrence. Some of the most commonly used tumour markers are shown in Table 1.1, along with benign causes of elevation and their sensitivities.

| Table 1.1 | Commonly used tumour markers | | |
|---|---|---|---|
| Marker | Associated malignancy | Benign conditions | Sensitivity (%) |
| CA27.29 | Breast | Breast, liver and kidney disorders | 33 – early stage |
| | | | 67 – late stage |
| CEA | Colonic | In smokers, peptic ulcer disease, ulcerative colitis, Crohn's disease | 25 – early stage<br>75 – late stage |
| CA19.9 | Pancreatic and biliary tract | Pancreatitis, cirrhosis | 80–90 – in pancreatic |
| AFP | Hepatocellular and non-seminomatous germ cell tumours | Viral hepatitis, cirrhosis, pregnancy | 80 – in hepatocellular |
| βhCG | Non-seminomatous germ cell tumours | Hypogonadal states, marijuana use | 20 – early stage<br>85 – late stage |
| CA125 | Ovarian | Pregnancy, ascites, cirrhosis | 50 – early stage<br>85 – late stage |
| PSA | Prostate | Prostatitis, benign prostatic hypertrophy | 75 – in organ confined disease |

hCG, human chorionic gonadotrophin; AFP, α-fetoprotein; CEA, carcinoembryonic antigen; PSA, prostate-specific antigen.

Tumour markers can be used to assess response to chemotherapy. The rate of fall of the tumour markers can used to determine response to treatment, for example in the treatment of germ cell tumours. Studies have shown that normalization of α-fetoprotein (AFP) and β-human chorionic gonadotrophin (βhCG) in patients with germ cell tumours corresponds to complete remission with chemotherapy and survival.[3]

In ovarian cancer, studies have shown that defined responses of CA125 may be used as a means of assessing tumour response, and that this is as reliable as serial CT scanning of patients known to be CA125 responders.[4] The definition of what numerical change in the CA125 level is classed as a response is debatable, with several definitions having been proposed. One example, which has been validated, is that serial increases of 25% in four samples, 50% in three samples or levels persistently elevated at more than 100 μ/ml related to disease progression.[5] For this to be used in clinical practice to maintain accuracy it is necessary to use a computer program, which is not always feasible in routine clinical practice. Simpler definitions have been developed, for example a confirmed doubling of the CA125 from the nadir predicted progression with a sensitivity of 94% and specificity of almost 100% in patients on second-line chemotherapy.[6]

As there is ongoing debate with regard to the defined role of tumour markers, in practice tumour markers are often used in adjunct to clinical and radiological indices of tumour response. Inter-centre variation in the measurement of tumour markers can also cause difficulty in the interpretation of markers as these techniques are as yet not fully standardized.

## Radiological assessment

The most commonly used method of assessing tumour response in the clinical setting is radiological assessment. Comparison between pretreatment and mid or post-treatment scans can provide evidence of response to chemotherapy. The modality used depends on which marker lesion is being followed to monitor response to treatment. Where possible, plain radiographs or ultrasound is preferable as their use reduces the amount of ionizing radiation to which a patient is exposed; also in most centres they are more easily accessible.

Plain films are quick and simple to obtain and can be interpreted by non-radiologists. The information gained from them can be useful in determining response to treatment, for example in lung lesions in non-small cell lung cancer. However, the information is often limited. Ultrasound again is readily available but is operator dependent, which can introduce inaccuracy in the tumour measurement and make serial imaging difficult to interpret. The reproducibility of these methods is not as accurate as that of CT and magnetic resonance imaging (MRI). Therefore it may be necessary to perform assessment by CT or in some cases MRI to accurately assess disease response.

In an effort to standardize assessment of tumour response both in trial and non-trial settings, Response Evaluation Criteria in Solid Tumours (RECIST)[7] were developed in 2000, providing uni-dimensional criteria for tumour assessment. RECIST replaced the 1981 WHO criteria for tumour response[8] which had originally been developed mainly for use in relation to plain radiographs and early CT scanning, and used bi-dimensional criteria. RECIST criteria also define the use of tumour markers and clinical findings in the assessment of tumour response, although the main focus is on the radiological assessment of tumours. RECIST criteria categorizes lesions into:

● **Measurable lesions** – lesions that can be accurately measured in at least one dimension with the longest diameter ≥20 mm using conventional techniques or ≥10 mm with spiral CT scan.

● **Non-measurable lesions** – all other lesions, including small lesions (longest diameter <20 mm with conventional techniques or <10 mm with spiral CT scan), i.e. bone lesions, leptomeningeal disease, ascites, pleural/pericardial effusion, inflammatory breast disease, lymphangitis, cystic lesions, and also abdominal masses that are not confirmed.

Following identification of these baseline lesions a maximum of five lesions per organ or ten lesions in total are identified as target lesions. The sum of the longest diameters of the target lesions is then calculated. The response to treatment is determined by the serial assessment of these lesions. Table 1.2 shows the definitions of response according to RECIST criteria for target lesions and Table 1.3 shows definitions for non-target lesions.[9] RECIST is the most commonly used tool for assessing disease response. It provides standardized definitions of response in the setting of clinical trials, although its use in routine clinical practice is perhaps less structured.

| Table 1.2 Definitions of response of target lesions | |
| --- | --- |
| Complete response (CR) | Disappearance of all target lesions |
| Partial response (PR) | At least a 30% decrease in the sum of the longest diameter (LD) of target lesions, taking as reference the baseline sum LD |
| Progressive disease (PD) | At least a 20% increase in the sum of the LD of target lesions, taking as reference the smallest sum LD recorded since the treatment started or the appearance of one or more new lesions |
| Stable disease (SD) | Neither sufficient shrinkage to qualify for PR nor sufficient increase to qualify for PD, taking as reference the smallest sum LD since the treatment started |

| Table 1.3 Definitions for non–target lesions | |
| --- | --- |
| Complete response | Disappearance of all non-target lesions and normalization of tumor marker level |
| Incomplete response/ stable disease | Persistence of one or more non-target lesion(s) or/and maintenance of tumor marker level above the normal limits |
| Progressive disease | Appearance of one or more new lesions and/or unequivocal progression of existing non-target lesions |

# Discussion

### How do the methods apply to the patient?

The case history above is an example of where structured tools used routinely in trials are difficult to apply in routine clinical practice. There is one measurable lesion, the right mid-zone mass (the target lesion), and one non-measurable lesion, the left apical nodule (the non-target lesion), on the pre-treatment scan. By RECIST criteria the post-treatment scan shows stable disease of the target lesion as the maximum longitudinal diameter has reduced by 10%. The non-target lesion has resolved fully indicating complete response (although no tumour marker information is given). The presence of the new lesion in the liver in this case would not affect the best overall response, as the liver has not been imaged previously so there is the possibility that the lesion was present beforehand and it is unknown if it has altered with treatment. To determine best overall response both responses are taken into account (Table 1.4), and the patient would be said to have stable disease by RECIST.

If the WHO criteria are applied the outcome would differ from that of RECIST. WHO uses the sum of the products of the longitudinal and perpendicular measurements of the lesions, and does not specify a maximum number of lesions to be included in the assessment. In this example assessment of response by WHO would conclude that the patient had achieved a partial response. This highlights the need for standardization of response criteria, especially where comparison is being made between outcome measures, i.e. in multicentre clinical trials.

| Table 1.4 Assessing response with RECIST | | | |
| --- | --- | --- | --- |
| Target lesions | Non–target lesions | New lesions | Overall response |
| CR | CR | No | CR |
| CR | Incomplete response/SD | No | PR |
| PR | Non-PD | No | PR |
| SD | Non-PD | No | SD |
| PD | Any | Yes or No | PD |
| Any | PD | Yes or No | PD |
| Any | Any | Yes | PD |

CR, complete response; PR, partial response; PD, progressive disease; SD, stable disease.

The example also illustrates the need to take into account all indices of response. If the patient felt their symptoms had reduced in this case, one would be more inclined to think that the patient had a partial response to their treatment.

### What will you say to the patient?

The case demonstrates the difficulty in relaying information to patients. It is important to try to inform the patient fully and clearly about their condition from the outset. In this case the patient may see the new information with regard the liver metastases as being an indication of deterioration of their condition, when this may not necessarily be the case.

When discussing post-treatment results with patients, spend time going through results, explaining the implications of results and their impact on future management and addressing any questions that the patient may have.

## Conclusion

Assessment of tumour response is a complex process which involves the use of several modalities. The decisions made on the basis of these results have direct implications for patient care.

Tumour assessment is an area which will continue to become more complex. The development of new targeted agents has meant that present evaluation methods for tumour response are likely to be insensitive to these agents. This has led to the development of new molecular and radiological biomarkers which aim to determine more accurately the response of tumours to therapeutic intervention. These new methods will no doubt be translated into routine clinical practice in the future.

## Further Reading

1 Geels P, Eisenhauer E, Bezjak A, Zee B, Day A. Palliative effect of chemotherapy: objective tumour response is associated with symptom improvement in patients with metastatic breast cancer. *J Clin Oncol* 2000; **18**: 2395–405.

2 Velikova G, Booth L, Smith AB, Brown PM, Lynch P, Brown JM, Selby PJ. Measuring quality of life in routine oncology practice improves communication and patient well-being: a randomized controlled trial. *J Clin Oncol* 2004; **22**: 714–24.

3 Fizazi K, Culine S, Kramar A, Amato RJ, Bouzy J, Chen I, Droz JP, Logothetis CJ. Early predicted time to normalization of tumour markers predicts outcome in poor-prognosis non-seminomatous germ cell tumours. *J Clin Oncol* 2004; **22**: 3868–76.

4 Bridgewater JA, Nelstrop AE, Rustin GJ, Gore ME, McGuire WP, Hoskins WJ. Comparison of standard and CA125 response criteria in patients with epithelial ovarian cancer treated with platinium or paclitaxel. *J Clin Oncol* 1999; **17**: 501–8.

5 Rustin GJ, Nelstrop A, Stilwell J, Lambert HE. Savings obtained by CA-125 measurements during therapy for ovarian carcinoma: The North Thames Ovary Group. *Eur J Cancer* 1992; **28**: 79–82.

6 Rustin GJ, Marples M, Nelstrop AE, Mahmoudi M, Meyer T. Use of CA 125 to define progression of ovarian cancer in patients with persistently elevated levels. *J Clin Oncol* 2001; **19**: 4054–7.

7 Therasse P, Arbuck SG, Eisenhauer EA, Wanders J, Kaplan RS, Rubinstein L, Verweij J, Van Glabbeke M, van Oosterom AT, Christian MC, Gwyther SG. New guidelines to evaluate the response to treatment in solid tumours. *J Natl Cancer Inst* 2000; **92**: 205–16.

8 World Health Organization. *WHO Handbook for Reporting Results of Cancer Treatment.* Offset Publication, Geneva, Switzerland, 1979.

9 National Cancer Institute. Response Evaluation Criteria in Solid Tumors (RECIST) Quick Reference. Cancer Therapy Evaluation Guidelines, National Cancer Institute.

# Appendix 1.1

| Appendix Table 1.1 | Karnofsky performance score |
|---|---|
| 100 | Normal, no signs or symptoms |
| 90 | Minor signs or symptoms |
| 80 | Activity with effort, signs and symptoms present |
| 70 | Activity restricted, not working, self-caring, lives at home |
| 60 | Requires some help |
| 50 | Frequent medical care and help |
| 40 | Disabled |
| 30 | In hospital, death not near |
| 20 | Hospitalized and supported |
| 10 | Moribund |
| 0 | Dead |

| Appendix Table 1.2 | WHO/ECOG performance scores. KP, Karnofsky performance score | |
|---|---|---|
| 0 | Able to carry out all normal activity without restriction | KP: 100 |
| 1 | Restricted in physically strenuous activity but ambulatory and able to carry out light work | KP: 80, 90 |
| 2 | Ambulatory and capable of all self-care but unable to carry out any work; up and about more than 50% of waking hours | KP: 60, 70 |
| 3 | Capable only of limited self-care; confined to bed or chair more than 50% of waking hours | KP: 40, 50 |
| 4 | Completely disabled; cannot carry out any self-care; totally confined to bed or chair | KP: 20, 30 |

# 2 Chemotherapy Toxicity: Cisplatin Extravasation

## Case History

A woman who is receiving inpatient chemotherapy with cisplatin complains of pain at her cannula site. You examine the hand but apart from a little tenderness at the insertion site you cannot find any abnormality.

**What is chemotherapy extravasation?**

**What should be done?**

## Background

### What is chemotherapy extravasation?

Extravasation is the non-intentional leakage of an intravenous agent from a vessel into the surrounding subcutaneous tissues. Chemotherapeutic agents can be divided into vesicant, irritant and non-vesicant drugs (Table 2.1). Vesicant drugs have the potential to cause severe tissue necrosis and blistering and can be further divided into DNA-binding or non-DNA-binding subtypes. Irritant drugs cause local inflammatory reaction but without tissue necrosis. Cisplatin is classified as an irritant drug but at high doses it can have vesicant potential (if >20 ml of 0.5 mg/ml is extravasated).

The degree of soft tissue injury is related to the specific drug administered, the amount extravasated, duration of exposure and the site of extravasation. Prevention is of paramount importance and several factors need to be taken into account to reduce risk. These

**Table 2.1** Classification of chemotherapeutic agents according to vesicant potential

| Vesicant (DNA binding) | Vesicant (non–DNA binding) | Irritant | Non–vesicant |
|---|---|---|---|
| Anthracyclines | Vinca alkaloids | Alkylating agents | ● 5-Fluorouracil |
| ● Doxorubicin | ● Vincristine | ● Dacarbazine | ● Gemcitabine |
| ● Epirubicin | ● Vinblastine | ● Ifosfamide | ● Irinotecan |
| ● Daunorubicin | ● Vinorelbine | ● Melphalan | ● Methotrexate |
| | ● Vindesine | ● Carmustine | ● Cytarabine |
| Antitumour antibiotics | Taxane | Platinum analogues | |
| ● Mitomycin | ● Paclitaxel | ● Carboplatin | |
| ● Mitoxantrone | ● Cisplatin (<0.5mg/ml) | | |
| | ● Oxaliplatin | | |
| | Anthracycline | | |
| | ● Liposomal doxorubicin | | |

include: avoiding using veins in close proximity to important nerves and tendons, such as in the antecubital fossa, wrist and dorsum of hand; injection of vesicant drugs prior to any other agent and regular checks of vein patency with frequent saline flushes; and confirmation of venous return.[1] Patients should be asked to report any change in sensation, stinging or burning and it is important to check for swelling and inflammation regularly. Factors that can impair detection of extravasation injury include lymphoedema, peripheral neuropathy, obstruction of the superior vena cava and central line use. Only specially trained staff should administer cytotoxic agents.

## Discussion

 ### What should be done?

The management of chemotherapy extravasation is outlined in Figure 2.1. The first step for all suspected extravasation injuries is to stop and disconnect the infusion. Then

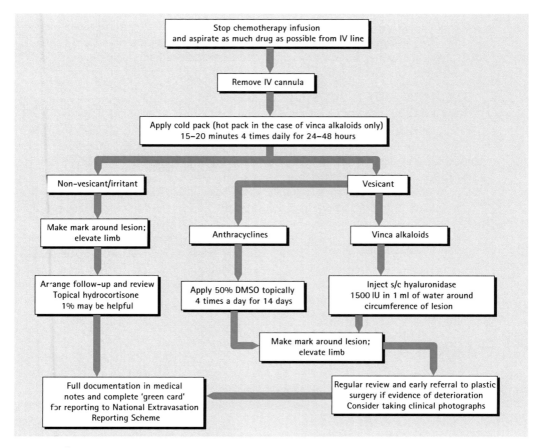

**Figure 2.1** Algorithm for management of chemotherapy extravasation. Refer to extravasation protocols that should be present on all chemotherapy units. DMSO, dimethylsulphoxide, s/c, subcutaneous.

aspirate as much drug as possible from the IV line followed by removal of the device. For irritant and non-vesicant drugs a cold pack should be applied immediately and then on/off for a 24-hour period to induce vasoconstriction and reduce local uptake of the drug by the tissues.[2] Elevation of the limb is also helpful. A mark should be made around the injury and arrangements made to follow up the patient within 24 hours.

Vesicant extravasation can cause severe soft tissue damage up to several days, weeks or even months following injury. Initial management should be as given in Figure 2.1, but specific antidotes are available for doxorubicin and vinca alkaloids.

- Doxorubicin and other anthracyclines (DNA-binding): Use cold pack to localize the injury. Apply 50% dimethylsulphoxide (DMSO) topically to the affected area four times a day for 14 days. DMSO is a potent free-radical scavenger that rapidly penetrates tissues.[2,3] The site should be observed closely with regular review and a plastic surgery opinion should be sought early if there is evidence of progression or inadequately healing ulceration.

- Vinca alkaloids (non-DNA-binding): Use hot pack (only indication) to disperse drug through tissues causing dilutional effect. Inject hyaluronidase 1500 IU in 1 ml of water at points of the compass around the circumference of the area of extravasation. This enzyme breaks down part of the interstitial fluid barrier and allows dispersion of the vesicant and increased absorption.[4] Again regular review is required and refer to plastic surgery if necessary.

Cisplatin is an irritant drug as indicated above but does have the potential for severe extravasation injury. As it is classed as irritant it does not warrant the same meticulous observation required for vesicant agents. In addition cisplatin is administered as an intravenous (IV) infusion usually over a period of 2–4 hours as opposed to vesicant agents administered as slow IV bolus. As cisplatin infusions are unlikely to be closely monitored there is potential for significant drug leakage into subcutaneous tissue prior to clinical detection. Patients also tend to be mobile, with greater risk of dislodgement or damage to the peripheral IV cannula. Serious attention should be given to these problems, and do not be complacent due to cisplatin's classification as an irritant.

The large, undetected, inadequately treated cisplatin extravasation can cause severe morbidity with soft tissue injury. Patients should observe their infusion and be encouraged to report any potential abnormalities. If >20 ml 0.5 mg/ml is considered to have leaked, a subcutaneous injection of sodium thiosulphate around the site has been shown to be of some benefit.[4] This is unnecessary for smaller cisplatin injuries. Regular review of the injury should be arranged.

## Conclusion

Any extravasation involving a central line, especially with vesicant agents should be referred to plastic surgery immediately. All injuries need to be fully documented in the medical notes and reported via the National Extravasation Reporting Scheme. Evidence for useful interventions is scarce due to inherent ethical issues in performing controlled clinical trials. Newer agents are, however, under investigation mainly in the context of animal models and include the use of dexrazoxane, granulocyte macrophage-colony stimulating factors (GM-CSFs) and hyperbaric oxygen.[1]

## Further Reading

1  Goolsby TV, Lombardo FA. Extravasation of chemotherapeutic agents: prevention and treatment. *Semin Oncol* 2006; **33**: 139–43.

2  Bertelli G. Prevention and management of extravasation of cytotoxic drugs. *Drug Saf* 1995; **12**: 245–55.

3  Olver IN, Aisner J, Hament A, Buchanan L, Bishop JF, Kaplan RS. A prospective study of topical dimethyl sulfoxide for treating anthracycline extravasation. *J Clin Oncol* 1988; **6**: 1732–5.

4  Dorr RT. Antidotes to vesicant chemotherapy extravasations. *Blood Rev* 1990; **4**: 41–60.

---

**PROBLEM**

# 3  Chemotherapy Toxicity: Delayed Nausea

---

## Case History

A patient's mother phones the ward to seek help for her daughter who has been having nausea and vomiting since discharge after having chemotherapy. She was well on the day of discharge but became unwell the next day.

**What is the differential diagnosis?**

**How can chemotherapy drugs and antiemetics be usefully classified? What are the general mechanisms involved in emesis?**

**How should the patient be assessed?**

**If you judge this patient sufficiently unwell to require admission what are the appropriate investigations and management?**

## Background

### What is the differential diagnosis?

There are many causes of nausea and vomiting in patients having treatment for cancer. The most likely cause in this case is the chemotherapy drugs, though other causes should also be considered. Other drugs, such as opioids may cause or exacerbate nausea and vomiting. Metabolic causes such as hypercalcaemia, gastrointestinal causes such as obstruction or gastric stasis, and raised intracranial pressure due to brain metastases are all possibilities in patients with cancer. Knowledge of the underlying malignancy along with results of recent relevant investigations will be helpful in excluding these non-chemotherapy causes of this patient's symptoms.

### How can chemotherapy drugs and antiemetics be usefully classified? What are the general mechanisms involved in emesis?

Nausea and vomiting remains a common side effect following the administration of chemotherapy in a significant number of patients despite concurrent therapy with antiemetics. Emesis following chemotherapy can be divided into acute emesis, i.e. occurring in the first 24 hours after the administration of cytotoxic drugs, and delayed emesis, which occurs after the first 24 hours. Chemotherapy drugs can themselves be divided into four according to the degree of emesis that they induce (Table 3.1), though this is limited by the fact that the potential of any drug to induce emesis has only been determined for a few agents. One of the most highly emetogenic drugs is cisplatin, which causes vomiting in more than 99% of treated patients unless an antiemetic is administered concurrently. Trials to date clearly show that if an antiemetic is effective against cisplatin-induced emesis it will be at least as effective with other chemotherapy drugs.

An understanding of the neurotransmitters and pathways involved in nausea and vomiting is helpful. Emesis is mediated centrally by two separate centres. The chemoreceptor trigger zone (CTZ) is located in the floor of the fourth ventricle. Neural pathways run from here to the vomiting centre in the medulla oblongata which in turn sends impulses via the efferent fibres of the vagal nerve to the stomach to induce vomiting. Afferent pathways carry impulses from different areas of the body to the vomiting centre. Various neurotransmitters and their receptors are thought to be involved in chemotherapy-induced nausea and vomiting. 5-Hydroxytryptamine (5-HT$_3$) receptors are important in acute nausea and vomiting, substance P and neurokinin-1 (NK-1) are important in both acute and delayed emesis, and other neurotransmitters are important in delayed symptoms.

**Table 3.1** The degrees of emesis induced by chemotherapy drugs

| Emetic risk (incidence of emesis without antiemetics) | Drug |
| --- | --- |
| High (>90%) | Cisplatin (>50 mg/m$^2$)<br>Cyclophosphamide (>1500 mg/m$^2$)<br>Dacarbazine |
| Moderate (30–90%) | Carboplatin<br>Doxorubicin<br>Oxaliplatin<br>Irinotecan |
| Low (10–30%) | Paclitaxel<br>Etoposide<br>Docetaxel<br>Fluorouracil<br>Gemcitabine |
| Minimal (<10%) | Vincristine<br>Vinorelbine |

Antiemetics can be classified according to the therapeutic index seen with each drug, with $5HT_3$ antagonists, corticosteroids (dexamethasone) and NK-1 receptor antagonists (aprepitant) having the highest therapeutic index. Many $5HT_3$ antagonists are available with studies to date demonstrating that these agents have equivalent efficacy and toxicity.[1] At biologically equivalent doses oral and intravenous preparations are felt to be equally effective. Corticosteroids are also effective antiemetics for preventing both acute and delayed emesis, with dexamethasone being the most widely used steroid. More recently NK-1 receptor agonists have been developed, with aprepitant being the first agent in this class of drugs. NK-1 receptors, the binding site of tachykinin substance P, are found in both the brainstem emetic centre and the gastrointestinal tract. Agents that block this receptor prevent emesis caused by almost all experimental emetic stimuli. An antiemetic protocol should be available in the cancer centre, outlining the most appropriate choice of antiemetics for each chemotherapy regimen. The American Society of Clinical Oncology (ASCO) also publishes guidelines, with the most recent update being in 2006.[2] For highly emetogenic regimens (including cisplatin-containing regimens) the three-drug combination of dexamethasone, a $5HT_3$ antagonist and aprepitant is recommended. Placebo-controlled trials have shown that with this regimen up to 86% of patients have no episodes of emesis.[3] Aprepitant is, however, less widely used in the UK, with dexamethasone, a $5HT_3$ antagonist and metoclopramide more routinely prescribed for highly emetogenic regimens. The ASCO recommended regimen for moderately emetogenic chemotherapy regimens is the two-drug combination of dexamethasone and a $5HT_3$ antagonist, with dexamethasone alone recommended for regimens of low emetic risk.

# Discussion

### How should the patient be assessed?

When assessing the severity of nausea and vomiting a detailed history of the current symptoms is important. Ask about the frequency of vomiting, how much oral intake is being achieved and associated symptoms that may increase the risk of dehydration, such as diarrhoea, along with comorbidities such as diabetes mellitus. Knowledge of the pre-scribed antiemetic regimen is important (and confirmation of compliance with the regimen). Oral antiemetics work best if taken regularly. Where vomiting persists despite regular oral antiemetics an alternative route of administration should be tried. The rectal route is a possibility, may be particularly helpful in the community and may allow a patient to remain at home. Simple measures such as regular sips of iced fluids can also be useful for some patients, however, with persistent symptoms admission to hospital may be warranted.

On admission to hospital a full history should be taken and the patient examined to assess the extent of dehydration and exclude other causes (Figure 3.1). Biochemical investigation will help to assess renal impairment and exclude other metabolic causes. Dehydrated patients should be appropriately resuscitated. Regular antiemetics should be prescribed and consideration given to the subcutaneous route, either as regular injections or via a syringe driver. Haloperidol blocks dopamine receptors in the CTZ and can be a useful first line antiemetic for drug-induced emesis (2.5–5 mg over 24 hours). The choice of drug should be reviewed after 24 hours, and further consideration given to the

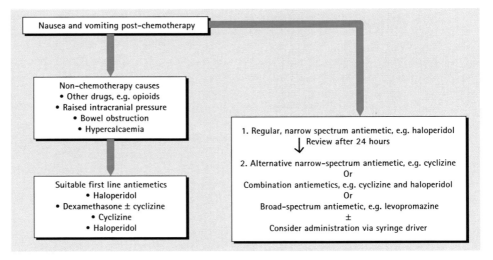

**Figure 3.1** Management of patients requiring admission for post-chemotherapy nausea and vomiting.

aetiology of ongoing symptoms. A second antiemetic could be tried as a single agent, but antiemetics have different modes of action and a combination of drugs can be helpful. Cyclizine, an antihistaminic antiemetic that acts on the vomiting centre can be useful in combination with haloperidol. Levopromazine, a sedating antihistaminic, which acts on various receptor sites may alone successfully replace an unsuccessful combination.

### If you judge this patient sufficiently unwell to require admission what are the appropriate investigations and management?

Once the symptoms are under control consideration needs to be given to reducing the risk of recurrence of severe emesis with the subsequent cycles of chemotherapy. Aprepitant can be substituted, or given in conjunction with a 5-HT$_3$ antagonist. Many patients are also helped by a continuous subcutaneous infusion of an antiemetic such as cyclizine, which can be administered in the community. Patients who have experienced significant chemotherapy-induced nausea and vomiting are at high risk of anticipatory nausea and vomiting. Lorazepam, which has amnesic and anti-anxiety effects, taken the night before and the day of chemotherapy can be useful for reducing such symptoms.

## Conclusion

 Once it has been confirmed that this patient's vomiting is due to the chemotherapy, antiemetic therapy should be instigated. Oral therapy is usually the first line approach. If the patient does not respond, a change in regimen will be needed, either by administering a different combination of drugs and/or considering alternative delivery routes. If emesis is severe and unresponsive to therapy, admission to hospital may be necessary.

## Further Reading

1   del Giglio A, Soares HP, Caparroz C, Castro PC. Granisetron is equivalent to ondansetron for prophylaxis of chemotherapy induced nausea and vomiting. *Cancer* 2000; **89**: 2301–8.

2   American Society of Clinical Oncology; Kris MG, Hesketh PJ, Somerfield MR, Feyer P, Clark-Snow R, Koeller JM, Morrow GR, Chinnery LW, Chesney MJ, Gralla RJ, Grunberg SM. American Society of Clinical Oncology Guideline for Antiemetics in Oncology: Update 2006. *J Clin Oncol* 2006; **24**: 2932–47.

3   Hesketh PJ, Grunberg SM, Gralla RJ, Warr DG, Roila F, de Wit R, Chawla SP, Carides AD, Ianus J, Elmer ME, Evans JK, Beck K, Reines S, Horgan KJ; Aprepitant Protocol 052 Study Group. The oral neurokinin-1 antagonist aprepitant for the prevention of chemotherapy-induced nausea and vomiting: a multinational randomised, double-blind, placebo-controlled trial in patients receiving high-dose cisplatin. *J Clin Oncol* 2003; **21**: 4112–19.

PROBLEM

# 4  Chemotherapy Toxicity: Febrile Neutropenia

## Case History

A 65-year-old patient is admitted unwell after the first cycle of cytotoxic chemotherapy. The full blood count reveals: Hb 78 g/l; WCC 0.2 × 10⁹/l; neutrophils 0.01 × 10⁹/l; platelets 48 × 10⁹/l. Vital signs: temperature 38.6 °C; pulse 120 bpm; blood pressure 150/84 mmHg. The central venous catheter (CVC) exit site is inflamed with a purulent discharge.

**What is febrile neutropenia?**

**How is it evaluated?**

**What is the treatment?**

## Background

### What is febrile neutropenia?

Febrile neutropenia is defined as single temperature reading above 38.5 °C while having an absolute neutrophil count (ANC) <0.5 × 10⁹/l. Bodey *et al.*'s seminal work first described the association between ANC and pyogenic infection and also identified that Gram-negative rod bacteraemia due to *Pseudomonas aeruginosa* is associated with a mortality rate of >50% within 48 hours.[1] Despite relatively high rates of neutropenia during standard dose chemotherapy regimens, rates of febrile neutropenia and mortality are now relatively low for most standard chemotherapy regimens (Table 4.1). The median time of onset for the first febrile neutropenic episode is day 12 of a cytotoxic cycle.[2] This correlates with the nadir of the neutrophil count and with the integumental damage to the intestinal mucosal epithelium. The most common sources of infection, in decreasing order are: gastrointestinal tract (especially the periodontium and oropharynx), bloodstream, skin (predominantly from indwelling CVCs), lower respiratory tract and the urinary tract.[3] There has been a shift in the causative organisms for bacteraemia over the past few decades from Gram-negative rods such as *Escherichia coli*, *Klebsiella pneumoniae* and *P. aeruginosa* to aerobic, Gram-positive cocci such as *Staphylococcus*, *Streptococcus* and *Enterococcus*.[4]

| Table 4.1 | Incidence of febrile neutropenia and other complications, and mortality[5] |
|---|---|
| Leukopenia WHO grade 4 | 2–28% |
| Febrile neutropenia | 10–57% |
| Infections WHO grade 3 or 4 | Up to 16% |
| Death in febrile neutropenia | 0–7% |
| WHO, World Health Organization. | |

# Discussion

### How is it evaluated?

The management of patients with febrile neutropenia includes a rapid and meticulous clinical evaluation to identify a clinical focus of infection and a causative pathogen, administration of broad-spectrum antibacterial therapy, and a strategy to monitor the patient for medical complications. Given that immunocompromised hosts rarely mount an adequate inflammatory response to infection, the classic signs and symptoms of infection may be minimal or absent. In particular, it is useful to enquire whether the patient has been administered any blood products in the past 24 hours and whether rigors are associated with the flushing of a central venous line. Physical examination should include oropharynx, sinuses, skin, fundi and perineum (defer rectal examination until antibiotics have been started). In addition, any indwelling lines or catheter should be inspected for signs of inflammation and exudates cultured.

The lack of adequate inflammatory response renders some laboratory tests unreliable. Initial investigations should include: full blood count, coagulation screen, urea and electrolytes, liver function tests, chest radiograph, and concomitant blood cultures from peripheral veins and/or central catheter. If clinically indicated, the following should be cultured: stool or urine samples, skin biopsies, respiratory secretions and cerebrospinal fluid. Viral and fungal serological tests should be done. In addition, high-resolution chest computed tomography may indicate early signs of invasive fungal infections in patients with a normal chest radiograph.[6]

Risk assessment is an important part of initial evaluation, allowing for the identification of those patients who are suitable for outpatient treatment and those patients at risk of complications. Two risk assessment systems have been developed by Talcott et al.[7] and the Multinational Association of Supportive Care in Cancer (MASCC).[8] Talcott et al. placed patients in one of three high-risk groups within 24 hours of diagnosis with neutropenic sepsis. The remaining patients, with no high-risk features were placed a separate control group. Serious medical complications occurred in 34% of patients with risk factors compared with 5% of the remaining patients. According to the MASCC system, factors associated with a better outcome are assigned a score (Table 4.2). A risk index score ≥21 identifies low-risk patients with a <5% risk of complications. However, the MASCC study included a relatively low percentage of patients with active acute leukaemia, who typically are high-risk patients and should not have outpatient therapy.

| Table 4.2 The Multinational Association of Supportive Care in Cancer Risk Scoring Index for identification of low–risk neutropenic patients at presentation | |
|---|---|
| Characteristic | Score* |
| Extent of illness[†] | |
| No symptoms | 5 |
| Mild symptoms | 5 |
| Moderate symptoms | 3 |
| No hypotension | 5 |
| No chronic obstructive pulmonary disease | 4 |
| Solid tumour or no fungal infection | 4 |
| No dehydration | 3 |
| Outpatient at onset of fever | 3 |
| Age <60 years[‡] | 2 |

*A risk index score of ≥21 indicates that the patient is likely to be at low risk for complications and morbidity.
†Choose one item only.
‡Does not apply to patients age ≤16 years.

## What is the treatment?

A landmark study from 1971 first identified that prompt initiation of broad-spectrum combination antibacterial therapy results in a dramatic reduction in mortality.[9] Empirical treatment should be started before the results of cultures are available, and antibiotics should be given in maximal therapeutic doses adjusted appropriately with respect to clinical condition, weight, and renal and hepatic function. If the cultures yield a specific pathogen, then the regimen should be modified accordingly. However, the infecting organism is confirmed microbiologically in only a third of neutropenic patients.

The issue of which antibiotics should be included in empirical therapy for febrile neutropenia remains controversial. The emergence of previously rare, resistant pathogens and the increasing resistance of common pathogens to antibiotics mean that there are no universal guidelines. Therefore, doctors should refer to their local guidelines.

Moderate-risk to high-risk patients should *always* be admitted to hospital and administered intravenous antibiotic therapy. In low-risk patients, oral antibiotics may be safely substituted for intravenous antibiotics, at the discretion of the responsible clinician. The best oral combination studied to date is that of quinolone with amoxicillin/clavulanate. However, the patient should be living with a responsible adult and be within close distance of the hospital with telephone and transport access. CVC removal should only be considered in patients when the tunnel or exit site is infected or when there is microbiologically confirmed CVC-related infection.

Febrile neutropenia can also have detrimental effects on clinical outcomes due to substantial delays in dose delivery or the discontinuation of chemotherapy. It is well documented that patients who are treated with suboptimal doses of the chemotherapy have lower survival and other options should be considered before reducing dose intensity. The use of haemopoietic colony-stimulating factors (hCSF) has been shown to allow the maintenance of dose intensity while reducing the duration of neutropenia and incidence of neutropenic sepsis.[10,11] The 2006 ASCO guidelines recommend the use of hCSF when the risk of febrile neutropenia is approximately 20% and no other equally effective regimen that does not require hCSFs is available.[12] Ideally, these drugs should be used for patients at greatest risk of neutropenic complications and thus the most likely to benefit.

## Conclusion

All patients who are treated with chemotherapy are at risk of developing neutropenic complications. Patients should be instructed on how to take their temperatures and given a list of symptoms to watch for. Clinic attendance and laboratory monitoring is essential during chemotherapy. Prompt initiation of empirical antibiotic therapy is vital and doctors are advised to follow local treatment algorithms.

## Further Reading

1 Bodey GP, Jadeja L, Eltin L. Pseudomonas bacteremia: retrospective analysis of 410 episodes. *Arch Intern Med* 1985; **145**: 1621–9.

2 Bow EJ. Management of the febrile neutropenic cancer patient: lessons from 40 years of study. *Clin Microbiol Infect* 2005; **11**(Suppl 5): 24–9.

3 Bow EJ. Infection risk and cancer chemotherapy: the impact of the chemotherapeutic regimen in patients with lymphoma and solid tissue malignancies. *J Antimicrob Chemother* 1998; **41**(Suppl D): 1–5.

4 Zinner SH. Changing epidemiology of infections in patients with neutropenia and cancer: emphasis on gram-positive and resistant bacteria. *Clin Infect Dis* 1999; **29**: 490–4.

5 Greil R, Jost LM. ESMO recommendations for the application of hematopoietic growth factors. *Ann Oncol* 2005; **16**(Suppl 1): i80–i82.

6 Heussel CP, Kauczor HU, Heussel GE, Fischer B, Begrich M, Mildenberger P, Thelen M. Pneumonia in febrile neutropenic patients and in bone marrow and blood stem cell transplant recipients: use of high resolution computed tomography. *J Clin Oncol* 1999; **17**: 796–805.

7  Talcott JA, Siegel RD, Finberg R, Goldman L. Risk assessment in cancer patients with fever and neutropenia: a prospective, two-center validation of a prediction rule. *J Clin Oncol* 1992; **10**: 316–21.

8  Klastersky J, Paesmans M, Rubenstein EB, Boyer M, Elting L, Feld R, Gallagher J, Herrstedt J, Rapoport B, Rolston K, Talcott J. The Multinational Association for Supportive Care in Cancer Risk Index: a multinational scoring system for identifying low-risk febrile neutropenic cancer patients. *J Clin Oncol* 2000; **18**: 3038–51.

9  Schimpff S, Satterlee W, Young VM, Serpick A. Empiric therapy with carbenicillin and gentamicin for febrile patients with cancer and granulocytopenia. *N Engl J Med* 1971; **284**: 1061–6.

10  Crawford J, Ozer H, Stoller R, Johnson D, Lyman G, Tabbara I, Kris M, Grous J, Picozzi V, Rausch G. Reduction by granulocyte colony stimulating factor of fever and neutropenia induced by chemotherapy in patients with small-cell lung cancer. *N Engl J Med* 1991; **325**: 164–70.

11  Trillet-Lenoir V, Green J, Manegold C, Von Pawel J, Gatzemeier U, Lebeau B, Depierre A, Johnson P, Decoster G, Tomita D, Ewen C. Recombinant granulocyte colony stimulating factor reduces the infectious complications of cytotoxic chemotherapy. *Eur J Cancer* 1993; **29A**: 319–24.

12  Smith TJ, Khatcheressian J, Lyman GH, Ozer H, Armitage JO, Balducci L, Bennett CL, Cantor SB, Crawford J, Cross SJ, Demetri G, Desch CE, Pizzo PA, Schiffer CA, Schwartzberg L, Somerfield MR, Somlo G, Wade JC, Wade JL, Winn RJ, Wozniak AJ, Wolff AC. Update of recommendations for the use of white blood cell growth factors: an evidence-clinical practice guideline. *J Clin Oncol* 2006; **24**: 3187–205.

## PROBLEM

# 5  Chemotherapy Toxicity: Drug Reaction

## Case History

You are called to the chemotherapy suite to see a patient who is receiving an infusion of carboplatin. The nurse is concerned that the patient is having a reaction to the drug.

**What is a carboplatin reaction?**

**How should a carboplatin reaction be managed, and how will you modify the patient's future treatment?**

## Background

### What is a carboplatin reaction?

About 2% of patients treated with carboplatin have a carboplatin hypersensitivity reaction (CHR), but this proportion is increasing as the therapeutic application of the agent expands. Typically hypersensitivity reactions occur after a median of eight cycles of carboplatin, suggesting sensitization to the agent is required. It is unusual to see these reactions during earlier cycles of treatment.[1] The symptoms of CHR can develop acutely (within 5–35 minutes of starting the infusion) or be delayed several hours or even days following administration. The former is thought to be mediated through type I IgE hypersensitivity and the latter through type IV delayed hypersensitivity reactions involving T-cell response.[2]

Symptoms of CHR include pruritus, urticaria, palmar erythema, anxiety, dyspnoea, facial or tongue oedema, erythematous rash to severe with rigors, tachycardia, hypotension, hypertension, bronchospasm, angina pectoris, diffuse erythroderma and potentially respiratory arrest, seizures or death.[2] Hypersensitivity grading systems vary greatly between studies, making comparisons difficult. A standardized grading system has recently been developed taking into account the correlation between clinical symptoms and pathophysiological response. It is based on the premise that unequivocal compromise of either the cardiovascular system or respiratory system defines a severe reaction. This grading system has been proposed as a new standard for both routine clinical practice and future clinical studies (Table 5.1).[3]

**Table 5.1** Grading system for generalized hypersensitivity reactions

| Grade | Defined by |
| --- | --- |
| 1 Mild (skin and subcutaneous tissues only) | Generalized erythema, urticaria, periorbital oedema, or angioedema |
| 2 Moderate (features suggesting respiratory, cardiovascular, or gastrointestinal involvement) | Dyspnoea, stridor, wheeze, nausea, vomiting, dizziness (presyncope), diaphoresis, chest or throat tightness, or abdominal pain |
| 3 Severe (hypoxia, hypotension, or neurologic compromise) | Cyanosis or $SpO_2$ ≥92% at any stage, hypotension (SBP <90 mmHg in adults), confusion, collapse, LOC or incontinence |

Reproduced from Brown.[3] SBP, systolic blood pressure; LOC, loss of consciousness.

# Discussion

### How should a carboplatin reaction be managed, and how will you modify the patient's future treatment?

The management of CHR is similar to that of other acute drug allergies and is outlined in Figure 5.1.

Once someone has developed hypersensitivity it is likely similar reactions will occur with subsequent administration. This risk needs to be balanced against the potential benefit of the agent, which will depend on the treatment scenario and specifically whether the intent is curative or palliative. Options include avoiding carboplatin in future treatment/converting to an alternative platinum analogue, reintroducing carboplatin with premedication or attempting a desensitization protocol.

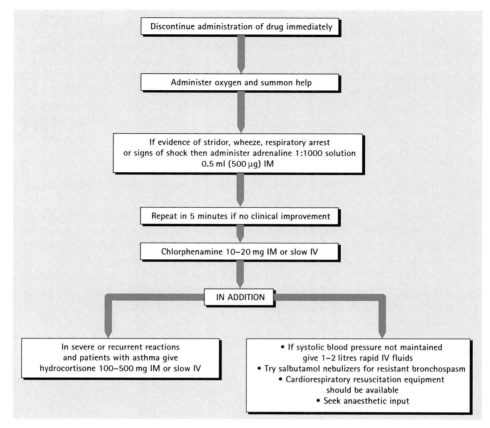

**Figure 5.1** Algorithm for management of anaphylactic reactions. (Adapted from Resuscitation Council (UK) guidelines.[4])

The use of premedication with dexamethasone and antihistamine has been investigated in several small studies but none have shown convincing evidence to support a significant reduction in re-challenge hypersensitivity.[1,5] If this method is used and ineffective, carboplatin must be discontinued. Desensitization involves re-introduction of carboplatin at an initial dilute strength with progressively increasing concentrations. Several groups have adapted protocols for this. Although the studies have been small there is evidence to support the effectiveness of this technique in reducing subsequent hypersensitivity and allowing successful continuation of treatment. In the largest patient cohort, Confino-Cohen et al.[6] used a 6-hour desensitization protocol. Initially 1/1000 of total dose was administered over 90 minutes, followed by 1/100 and 1/10 of total dose given over 90 minutes each, followed by the remainder of the dose over 90 minutes. Nineteen of 20 women (95%) were successfully desensitized with this technique thus representing a potentially acceptable protocol for those patients in whom it is beneficial to persevere with carboplatin.

In daily clinical practice it can be difficult to differentiate a true hypersensitivity reaction from an anxiety attack which may mimic some of the aforementioned symptoms.

Clinical judgement is paramount and if any doubt exists treatment should be administered accordingly. Reassurance has a pivotal role in the management of all cases of potential drug reaction and in certain circumstances this alone can be enough to settle supposed symptoms of hypersensitivity. Indeed it is often this patient group that we treat empirically with chlorphenamine and hydrocortisone to good effect. Whether this represents a true pharmacological response or placebo effect is debatable. Indeed the same argument may apply to the use of chlorphenamine and hydrocortisone as premedication for subsequent carboplatin administration and to the effectiveness of desensitization protocols in those patients who may not have true hypersensitivity. The new standardized grading system may aid in clarification of diagnosis for future studies.

Intradermal skin testing has been proposed as an effective means of predicting hypersensitivity to carboplatin. Markman et al.[7] studied 126 women with gynaecological cancers given a small dose of intradermal carboplatin 30 minutes prior to their treatment, in those who had previously received more than six cumulative cycles of carboplatin. They demonstrated a negative predictive value of 98.5%. The positive predictive value was difficult to assess as most patients with positive skin tests did not receive further carboplatin. However, six of seven patients with a positive test who did continue to receive treatment experienced signs and symptoms of hypersensitivity. Although not routine practice, with this sort of prediction judgements can be made about the benefits of continuing carboplatin or need for desensitization earlier in the course of treatment to prevent potentially serious reactions.

## Conclusion

A thorough clinical examination will confirm whether the symptoms are consistent with the diagnosis of hypersensitivity reaction to carboplatin. Treatment should be initiated even if there are some doubts. For future treatment, an alternative to carboplatin should be considered, or premedication with steroids and antihistamines if there are no suitable alternatives.

## Further Reading

1 Markman M, Kennedy A, Webster K, Elson P, Peterson G, Kulp B, Belinson J. Clinical features of hypersensitivity reactions to carboplatin. *J Clin Oncol* 1999; **17**: 1141.

2 Navo M, Kunthur A, Badell ML, Coffer LW 2nd, Markman M, Brown J, Smith JA. Evaluation of the incidence of carboplatin hypersensitivity reactions in cancer patients. *Gynecol Oncol* 2006; **103**: 608–13.

3 Brown SG. Clinical features and severity grading of anaphylaxis. *J Allergy Clin Immunol* 2004; **114**: 371–6.

4 Project Team of the Resuscitation Council (UK). *The Emergency Medical Treatment of Anaphylactic Reactions for First Medical Responders and for Community Nurses*. London: Resuscitation Council, 2002.

5 Polyzos A, Tsavaris N, Kosmas C, Arnaouti T, Kalahanis N, Tsigris C, Giannopoulos A, Karatzas G, Giannikos L, Sfikakis PP. Hypersensitivity reactions to carboplatin

administration are common but not always severe: a 10-year experience. *Oncology* 2001; **61**: 129–33.

6   Confino-Cohen R, Fishman A, Altaras M, Goldberg A. Successful carboplatin desensitization in patients with proven carboplatin allergy. *Cancer* 2005; **104**: 640–3.

7   Markman M, Zanotti K, Peterson G, Kulp B, Webster K, Belinson J. Expanded experience with an intradermal skin test to predict for the presence or absence of carboplatin hypersensitivity. *J Clin Oncol* 2003; **21**: 4611–14.

PROBLEM

# 6  Growth Factor Support in Chemotherapy

## Case History

A 65-year-old patient recovers from a neutropenic event without problems and is seen in clinic a week later. She has been receiving palliative chemotherapy for metastatic breast cancer. She asks why she was not given a granulocyte-colony stimulating factor (G-CSF) with her first cycle of chemotherapy and requests it with her next.

**How may neutropenia be avoided?**

**Can this be done for more intensive therapy?**

**Does this help older patients?**

**Is it useful for established neutropenia?**

## Background

**How may neutropenia be avoided?**

Neutropenia is a major dose-limiting toxicity in cancer patients treated with myelosuppressive chemotherapy. The incidence of chemotherapy dose reductions or treatment delays, which can impact on overall dose intensity and compromise treatment outcomes, may be reduced by the proactive use of drugs that stimulate the growth and development of neutrophils in the bone marrow such as granulocyte-colony stimulating factors (G-CSFs). To guide the targeted use of supportive care before complications occur, risk assessment should be conducted before the first cycle of chemotherapy treatment. For patients who do not receive G-CSF in the first cycle, risk should be re-evaluated before each subsequent cycle as a patient's risk categorization may change. If a patient experiences febrile neutropenia or a dose-limiting neutropenic event in any cycle, G-CSF use should be considered in the next cycle.

# Discussion

 Primary prophylactic use of G-CSF is its use to prevent febrile neutropenia in patients who are at a high risk based on age, medical history, disease characteristics, and myelotoxicity of the chemotherapy regimen. The American Society of Clinical Oncology (ASCO) guidelines, based on two large randomized clinical trials, support the use of G-CSF when the risk of febrile neutropenia is approximately 20% or higher and no other equally effective regimen that does not require G-CSF is available.[1] Vogel et al.[2] randomized 928 patients with breast cancer receiving 100 mg/m² docetaxel every 3 weeks for four cycles, to pegfilgrastim or no pegfilgrastim. The incidence of febrile neutropenia (1% versus 17%, respectively) and hospitalization (1% versus 14%, respectively) was reduced by more than 90% ($P < 0.001$). A trial in 171 patients with small cell lung cancer, with randomization to prophylactic G-CSF and/or antibiotics showed a reduction in the rate of overall febrile neutropenia from 32% to 18% ($P < 0.01$).[3]

Secondary prophylactic use of G-CSF is its use in patients who have experienced a neutropenic complication from a prior cycle of chemotherapy (for which primary prophylaxis was not received), in whom a reduced dose may compromise disease-free or overall survival or treatment outcome. Riveria et al.[4] conducted a prospective clinical trial in which women receiving adjuvant breast cancer chemotherapy who had experienced neutropenia <500/mm³ in cycle 1 were given G-CSF in subsequent cycles. The G-CSF recipients had lower rates of hospitalization for febrile neutropenia and greater dose intensity. Other significant outcomes (survival, quality of life, or cost) were not reported. There is no evidence that the use of G-CSF for dose maintenance or escalation in the palliative treatment of cancer improves clinically important outcomes, and in this setting dose reduction or delay is a reasonable alternative.

### Can this be done for more intensive therapy?

Although several trials have attempted to address the effects of dose-intense/dense chemotherapy by using G-CSF in a variety of tumour types, few trials have demonstrated a significant impact on the underlying disease itself. However, in breast cancer dose-dense chemotherapy with G-CSF versus standard chemotherapy has shown a disease-free and overall survival benefit.[5] In addition, patients aged 65 years and older, with diffuse aggressive lymphoma treated with curative dose-dense chemotherapy (CHOP or more aggressive regimens) should be given prophylactic G-CSF to reduce the incidence of febrile neutropenia, as one study has shown a statistically significant improvement in event-free survival and overall survival.[6] In the future it is possible that chemotherapy will be tailored so that patients receive equivalent doses based on tumour biology rather than the usual tissue side effects. Current ASCO recommendations are that dose-dense regimens, supported by the use of G-CSF, should only be used within the context of a clinical trial or if supported by convincing efficacy data.

### Does this help older patients?

Multiple studies have identified that the risk of febrile neutropenia following chemotherapy increases with age. The threshold for this effect varies among the studies, with ages ranging from ≥60 to 70 years. Mortality from febrile neutropenia is also increased in older patients, with most episodes of febrile neutropenia occurring in the first cycle of chemotherapy in treatment.[7] In addition, among patients aged ≥65 years, those with a performance status ≥2 are at increased risk of febrile neutropenia. However, due the subjective nature of assessment of performance status, it cannot be used reliably as a predictor for febrile neutropenia. Besides the data available for lymphoma, mentioned above, ASCO does *not* support the routine use of G-CSF in patients *solely* based on age, and additional risk factors for febrile neutropenia must be considered.

### Is it useful for established neutropenia?

G-CSF should not be routinely administered to patients who are afebrile and neutropenic following chemotherapy. In patients with febrile neutropenia, G-CSF is recommended for those who are at high risk for infection-associated complications or have poor prognostic factors. In a Cochrane meta-analysis of 1518 patients from 13 trials, patients who received G-CSF experienced less prolonged neutropenia, less prolonged hospitalization, marginally less infection-related mortality and there was significant difference in overall mortality.[8] However, the problem is identifying, prospectively, those patients with cancer who are at higher risk of complications as a result of fever and neutropenia. In a multivariate analysis of hospitalized patients with febrile neutropenia the independent risk factors associated with inpatient mortality were: age ≥65 years, cancer type (leukaemia, lung cancer), comorbidities (congestive heart failure, pulmonary embolism, and lung, renal, and cerebrovascular disease), and infectious complications (hypotension, pneumonia, bacteraemia, and fungal infection).[9]

No definitive conclusions can be reached from trials investigating different dosing schedules of G-CSF. Most doctors prescribe once daily G-CSF 24–72 hours after the administration of myelotoxic chemotherapy, continuing until the absolute neutrophil count is between $2 \times 10^9/l$ and $3 \times 10^9/l$. However, importantly, there is no evidence that G-CSF administered early after myelotoxic chemotherapy reduces the depth of the nadir although it can shorten its duration. The development of a longer-acting pegylated G-CSF injection (pegfilgrastim) has reduced the inconvenience associated with daily injections, with a once-per-cycle subcutaneous injection. Randomized trials have shown a significantly lower risk of febrile neutropenia in breast cancer patients and equal efficacy in reducing the severity of febrile neutropenia with the once-per-cycle injection compared with daily injections.

## Conclusion

Neutropenia is a major dose-limiting toxicity in patients with cancer who are treated with myelosuppressive chemotherapy. To guide the targeted use of supportive care before complications occur, risk assessment should be conducted before the first cycle of chemotherapy treatment. Use of G-CSF is recommended when the risk of febrile neutropenia is approximately 20% and no other equally effective regimen that does not require G-CSF is available.

# Further Reading

1   Smith TJ, Khatcheressian J, Lyman GH, Ozer H, Armitage JO, Balducci L, Bennett CL, Cantor SB, Crawford J, Cross SJ, Demetri G, Desch CE, Pizzo PA, Schiffer CA, Schwartzberg L, Somerfield MR, Somlo G, Wade JC, Wade JL, Winn RJ, Wozniak AJ, Wolff AC. 2006 Update of recommendations for the use of white blood cell growth factors: an evidence-based clinical practice guideline. *J Clin Oncol* 2006; **24**: 3187–205.

2   Vogel CL, Wojtukiewicz MZ, Carroll RR, Tjulandin SA, Barajas-Figueroa LJ, Wiens BL, Neumann TA, Schwartzberg LS. First and subsequent cycle use of pegfilgrastim prevents febrile neutropenia in patients with breast cancer: a multicenter, double-blind, placebo-controlled phase III study. *J Clin Oncol* 2005; **23**: 1178–84.

3   Timmer-Bonte JN, Adang EM, Smit H, Biesma B, Wilschut FA, Bootsma GP, de Boo TM, Tjan-Heijnen VC. Cost-effectiveness of adding granulocyte colony-stimulating factor to primary prophylaxis with antibodies in small-cell lung cancer. *J Clin Oncol* 2006; **24**: 2991–7.

4   Rivera E, Erder MH, Moore TD, Shiftan TL, Knight CA, Fridman M, Brannan C, Danel-Moore L, Hortobagyi GN; Risk Model Study Group. Targeted filgrastim support in patients with early-stage breast carcinoma: toward the implementation of a risk model. *Cancer* 2003; **98**: 222–8.

5   Citron ML, Berry DA, Cirrincione C, Hudis C, Winer EP, Gradishar WJ, Davidson NE, Martino S, Livingston R, Ingle JN, Perez EA, Carpenter J, Hurd D, Holland JF, Smith BL, Sartor CI, Leung EH, Abrams J, Schilsky RL, Muss HB, Norton L. Randomized trial of dose-dense versus conventionally scheduled and sequential versus concurrent combination chemotherapy as postoperative adjuvant treatment of node-positive primary breast cancer. First report of Intergroup Trial C9741/Cancer and Leukemia Group B Trial 9741. *J Clin Oncol* 2003; **21**: 1431–9.

6   Pfreundschuh M, Truemper L, Kloess M, Schmits R, Feller AC, Rube C, Rudolph C, Reiser M, Hossfield DK, Eimermacher H, Hasenclever D, Schmitz N, Loeffler M; German High-Grade Non-Hodgkin's Lymphoma Study Group. 2-weekly or 3-weekly CHOP chemotherapy with or without etoposide for the treatment of elderly patients with aggressive lymphomas: Results of the NHL-B2 trial of the DSHNHL. *Blood* 2004; **104**: 634–41.

7   Lyman GH, Lyman CH, Agboola O, for the Anc Study Group. Risk models for predicting chemotherapy-induced neutropenia. *Oncologist* 2005; **10**: 427–37.

8   Clark OA, Lyman GH, Castro AA, Clark LG, Djulbegovic B. Colony-stimulating factors for chemotherapy-induced febrile neutropenia: a meta-analysis of randomized controlled trials. *J Clin Oncol* 2005; **23**: 4198–214.

9   Kuderer NM, Crawford J, Dale DC, Lyman GH. Meta-analysis of prophylactic granulocyte colony-stimulating factor (G-CSF) in cancer patients receiving chemotherapy. 41st Annual Meeting of the American Society of Clinical Onocology, 14–17 May, 2005, Orlando, FL (abstract 8117).

# General Issues in Oncology

# 7  Unknown Primary: Work-up and Treatment

## Case History

A 65-year-old smoker presents with pain in the right hip and a plain radiograph shows a lytic lesion with a pathological fracture in the neck of the right femur. He has been reasonably well prior to this and a good-quality chest radiograph is reported as showing normal findings.

**What investigations are indicated? How extensive should be the search for the primary?**

**What is the value of serum tumour markers in the diagnosis of an unknown primary?**

**What about emerging technologies such as gene profiling?**

**What are the basic principles to guide management – looking for the treatable?**

**Assuming the final diagnosis is carcinoma of unknown primary, what are the results from treatment with chemotherapy?**

**What are the options and the optimal local treatment for the fracture?**

# Background

 **What investigations are indicated? How extensive should be the search for the primary?**

A cancer of unknown primary origin is defined as a biopsy-proved cancer that could not have arisen at the site of biopsy, with no primary tumour found after a careful history, physical examination and diagnostic work-up. The physical examination of a man with an unknown primary should include a testicle and prostate examination. A computed tomography (CT) scan of the thorax, abdomen and pelvis is the most appropriate radiological investigation to assess the extent of disease and to identify any potential primary sites of disease. Conventional radiography is, however, unable to determine the primary site of disease in most cases of UKP. Recently, positron emission tomography (PET) scans have been evaluated in the diagnostic work-up of unknown primary. The strongest evidence to support the use of PET is in patients with head and neck cancer. PET will identify primary sites of disease in up to a third of such patients in whom the sites have not been found on conventional radiography.[1] In patients with extracervical metastatic disease, primary sites of disease may be identified but the clinical benefit and cost-effectiveness is uncertain and needs to be confirmed by larger studies.

In this patient with pathological fracture a bone scan may also be useful to assess the extent of the bony disease. He requires a bone biopsy with routine light microscopy and immunohistochemistry carried out by an experienced histopathologist who may be able to define potential organs of origin. Assuming the pathologist excludes a primary bone tumour, the working diagnosis is that of unknown primary cancer.

## What is the value of serum tumour markers in the diagnosis of an unknown primary?

In men presenting with adenocarcinoma and bone metastases, a serum prostate-specific antigen (PSA) level can be useful to identify those with possible prostate cancer. In men in whom the histological examination shows poorly differentiated carcinomas, serum levels of human chorionic gonadotrophin (hCG) and α-fetoprotein (AFP) should be measured as significantly raised levels raise the possibility of a germ cell tumour which may respond well to chemotherapy. Other serum markers, including carcinoembryonic antigen (CEA), CA125, CA15–3 and CA19–9 are not specific and are not usually recommended to aid the diagnosis of unknown primary, but they can be a useful in monitoring response to treatment.

## What about emerging technologies such as gene profiling?

Recent developments in molecular biology have allowed scientists to screen a large number of genomic changes (e.g. comparative genomic hybridization) or expressed genes (oligonucleotide or cDNA arrays, SAGE [serial analysis of gene expression]) simultaneously. This may allow refinement of tumour classifications currently based on clinical staging and histology alone. This technology is currently also under investigation in patients with unknown primaries. Tothill *et al.*[2] examined cDNA microarrays of 229 primary and metastatic tumours from 14 different tumour types; 10 500 genes were represented on the microarray, with 79 of these genes found to differentiate the tumour by its site of origin. These genes were subsequently examined in 13 cases of unknown primaries. On the basis of these investigations, putative sites of origin were suggested for eleven of these cases, supported by the clinical course in some of them. Prospective studies are required to validate these interesting approaches.

# Discussion

## What are the basic principles to guide management – looking for the treatable?

The diagnosis of unknown primary occurs in a heterogeneous group of patients and it is apparent that some subsets of patients have a more favourable prognosis and response to treatment. Figure 7.1 summarizes the management of patients with unknown primary cancer.

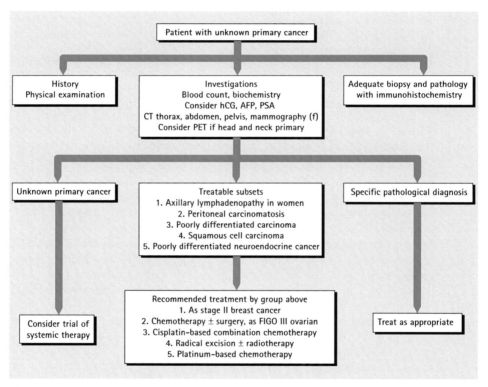

**Figure 7.1** Management of patients with unknown primary cancer. hCG, human chorionic gonadotrophin; AFP, α-fetoprotein; PSA, prostate-specific antigen; PET, positron emission tomography.

● Patients with poorly differentiated carcinomas may have atypical germ cell tumours. The extragonadal germ cell cancer syndrome was described in the 1970s and should be considered for patients with two or more of the following:[3]
  – men <50 years
  – midline tumour location

    – elevated serum β-hCG and/or AFP
    – short symptom interval with rapid tumour growth
    – a good response to chemotherapy or radiotherapy.

Recommended treatment is with cisplatin-based regimens as suitable for advanced germ cell tumours.

● Women with adenocarcinoma in axillary nodes should be considered to have breast cancer until proved otherwise, and should be treated as appropriate for the equivalently staged breast cancer.

● Women with peritoneal carcinomatosis may have primary peritoneal carcinoma and should be treated with platinum- and/or taxane-based chemotherapy as appropriate for the International Federation of Gynecology and Obstetrics (FIGO) stage III ovarian cancer.

● Patients with squamous cell carcinoma limited to cervical or inguinal lymph nodes should be considered for surgical dissection with or without radiotherapy.

● Poorly differentiated carcinomas staining positive for neurone-specific enolase (NSE), chromogranin and/or synaptophysin are consistent with a diagnosis of a neuroendocrine carcinoma. Such tumours may be highly sensitive to treatment with platinum- or doxorubicin-based regimens.

### Assuming the final diagnosis is carcinoma of unknown primary, what are the results from treatment with chemotherapy?

Most patients with unknown primaries do not fall into one of the subsets discussed above. Numerous chemotherapy regimens have been investigated in patients with metastatic cancer of unknown primary. Published trials have been generally small, non-randomised phase II trials. No randomised phase III trials have compared chemotherapy in unknown primary to best supportive care, but such trials are now unlikely to be done. Entry criteria in published trials have been variable in terms of pre-chemotherapy radio-logical and pathological work-up. It is difficult to determine how many patients who fall into a more treatable subset are included, particularly in the older trials. Documented response rates to the investigated chemotherapy regimens range from 0% to 50%.[3] From the available data it is difficult to recommend one regimen over another and treatment selection remains empirical. Many centres in the UK use a combination of epirubicin, cisplatin and 5-fluorouracil (ECF), with the rationale that these drugs have activity against common malignancies. However, the combination may be poorly tolerated. From the available evidence a platinum drug in combination with a taxane may also be one of the more effective regimens, with documented response rates of 20–40%. Furthermore, large-scale trials in patients with both lung and ovarian cancer have demonstrated the tolerability of the regimen.

### What are the options and the optimal local therapy for the fracture?

The pathological fracture of the femur should be discussed with a trauma surgeon for consideration of surgery with a construct that allows immediate weightbearing that will last the lifetime of the patient.[4] Postoperative radiotherapy (usually given as a single fraction) should be considered to encourage bone healing. Most pathological fractures rarely unite even if stabilized. In patients with pathological fractures that are not suitable for surgical intervention, palliative radiotherapy is also recommended.

## Conclusion

 Unless histopathology shows that the fracture is due to primary bone cancer, the most likely diagnosis is tumour of unknown origin. The site and type of the primary cancer should be sought, so as to optimize treatment and prognosis.

## Further Reading

1   Jungehulsing M, Scheidhauer K, Damm M, Pietrzyk U, Eckel H, Schicha H, Stennert E. 2[F]-fluoro-2-deoxy-D-glucose positron emission tomography is a sensitive tool for the detection of occult primary cancer (carcinoma of unknown primary syndrome) with head and neck lymph node manifestation. *Otolaryngol Head Neck Surg* 2000; **123**: 294–301.

2   Tothill RW, Kowalczyk A, Rischin D, Bousioutas A, Haviv I, van Laar RK, Waring PM, Zalcberg J, Ward R, Biankin AV, Sutherland RL, Henshall SM, Fong K, Pollack JR, Bowtell DD, Holloway AJ. An expression based site of origin diagnostic method designed for clinical application to cancer of unknown origin. *Cancer Res* 2005; **65**: 4031–40.

3   Greco FA, Hainsworth JD. Cancer of unknown primary site. In: DeVita Jr VT, Hellman S, Rosenberg SA, eds. Cancer Principles and Practice of Oncology. Lippincott Williams & Wilkins, Philadelphia, 2005: 2213–36.

4   www.library.nhs.uk/guidelinesfinder/ViewResource.aspx?resID=113614

**PROBLEM**

# 8  Large Abdominal Mass

## Case History

 A 45-year-old man presents with a vague history of feeling unwell, loss of appetite but no apparent loss of weight, and early satiety. Abdominal examination reveals an obviously distended abdomen with a large central non-tender mass.

**What is the differential diagnosis?**

**What investigations can help to determine the nature of the mass and what imaging techniques might be useful?**

**What is the choice of definitive diagnostic test?**

# Background

## What is the differential diagnosis?

Most abdominal masses are usually detected incidentally during routine physical examination. An abdominal mass may not be detected by the affected person because most abdominal masses develop slowly. If there are symptoms, abdominal masses are most often associated with pain or digestive problems. However, depending on the cause, masses may be associated with other signs and symptoms, such as jaundice or bowel obstruction.

An abdominal mass can be a sign of an abscess, an aneurysm, or an enlarged organ (such as the liver, spleen or kidney). Differential diagnosis includes all abdominal benign and malignant tumours and metastatic tumours, although in the present case, emphasis should be given to malignant tumours given the patient's symptoms (Table 8.1).

| Table 8.1 Most common causes of abdominal mass | | |
|---|---|---|
| | Tumours | |
| Benign | Malignant | Other |
| Adenomas | Stomach cancer | Abscess |
| Haemangiomas | Lower oesophageal carcinoma | Cyst |
| Leiomyomas | Abdominal lymphoma (Hodgkin's, non–Hodgkin's) | Crohn's disease |
| | NET – carcinoid tumours | Bowel obstruction |
| | Sarcomas (GIST) | Diverticulitis |
| | Colon cancer | Pancreatic abscess |
| | Metastatic carcinomas | Pancreatic pseudocyst |
| | Pancreatic cancer | Abdominal aortic aneurysm |
| | Hepatocellular carcinoma | Hepatomegaly |
| | Germ cell cancer | Splenomegaly |
| | Renal cancer | Hydronephrosis |
| | Bladder cancer | Bladder distension |

NET, neuroendocrine tumour; GIST, gastrointestinal stromal tumour.

The first steps in diagnosis are a medical history and physical examination. Important clues during history include weight loss and gastrointestinal symptoms. During physical examination, the clinician must identify and characterize the location of the mass, as well as assess whether it is rigid or mobile. Also characterize the mass for pulse or peristalsis, as these would help in further identification.

# Discussion

## What investigations can help to determine the nature of the mass and what imaging techniques might be useful?

Routine blood tests are usually the next step in diagnosis. They should include a full blood count and biochemistry (including serum amylase, total bilirubin and serum glucose). The tumour markers, βhuman chorionic gonadotrophin and α-fetoprotein, are useful to exclude treatable extragonadal germ cell tumours. Epithelial serum tumour markers (carcinoembryonic antigen (CEA), CA19–9), although not proved to have prognostic or diagnostic value, may be useful. Urine 5-hydroxyindoleacetic acid (5-HIAA) will help in the diagnosis of carcinoid tumours and serum hormone levels (insulin, gastrin, glucagons, vasoactive intestinal polypeptide [VIP], somatostatin) will help the differential diagnosis of neuroendocrine tumours.[1]

## What is the choice of definitive diagnostic test?

Several investigational tools are available to complete the assessment of an abdominal mass. Their use depends on availability and on the organ studied.

An abdominal radiograph may be useful. Generally, an ultrasound can identify the mass and provides information on its origin and nature. It is highly sensitive and specific for diagnosing a cystic abdominal lesion.[2] However, its efficacy in localizing the site of the lesion is not very good, especially in cases of a large mass. Ultrasound may also be used to direct a biopsy.

Computed tomography (CT) allows accurate detection, characterization and localization of abdominal masses, which helps the surgeon to plan the surgery. (Under CT guidance multiple fine needle aspiration and core biopsy specimens can also be obtained.)

Investigators have found both ultrasound and CT excellent for affirming or excluding a clinically suspected abdominal mass,[2-7] with sensitivity and specificity values in excess of 95%.[2,6] Both ultrasound and CT can visualize the organ from which a mass arises. The success of ultrasound in determining organ of origin has been 88–91%,[4,6] whereas that of CT has been slightly better at 93%.[2] Ultrasound studies have been shown to correctly predict the pathologic diagnosis in 77–81% of cases,[4,6,8] whereas CT suggested the diagnosis in 88% of cases.[2]

Some investigators have stressed the ability of CT and ultrasound to image masses no matter what their organ of origin and have touted them as first-line procedures for evaluating palpable masses.[3,8] Although certain combinations of clinical findings could lend themselves to a more targeted approach (for example, haematemesis plus a palpable gastric-region mass might merit endoscopy as the first study), cross-sectional imaging in general is well suited to initial evaluation of an abdominal mass. One study in 1981 showed that CT can result in savings with regard to time for diagnosis and overall cost of hospitalization compared with strategies not using CT.[3]

The non-organ-specific nature and multiplanar imaging capabilities of magnetic resonance imaging (MRI) seem quite suitable for evaluating an abdominal mass. However, the usefulness of MRI in evaluating palpable masses is not known. It is probably comparable with CT and ultrasound. MRI has been considered superior to CT in determining both the exact origin of a cyst and in assessing its exact extent because the lesion can be viewed in multiple planes. MRI helps characterize the cyst contents as well.[3]

Depending on presenting symptoms, barium enema, oesophagogastroduodenoscopy (OGD) or sigmoidoscopy might be useful to identify the mass or the primary tumour in case of metastatic disease. Exploratory laparotomy or laparoscopy will be necessary to make the diagnosis, or the patient might subsequently undergo laparotomy for removal of this mass. Definitive diagnosis is most reliably achieved by biopsy or surgical excision.

### Histopathological analysis

Cytokeratin (CK) monoclonal antibodies against various CK polypeptides are a useful tool in histopathological analysis of normal and cancerous epithelial cells. CK20 seems to be useful in diagnosing gastrointestinal adenocarcinomas, whereas CK7 is more common in lung cancer. In addition, determining the CK7/CK20 phenotype aids in the diagnosis of certain solid tumours. Overall, the CK7+/CK20– phenotype favours a lung origin, the CK7+/CK20+ phenotype favours urothelial-transitional cell carcinoma, the CK7–/CK20+ phenotype favours colorectal or gastric carcinoma, and the CK7–/CK20– phenotype favours prostatic, renal or liver adenocarcinoma[9] (Table 8.2).

| Table 8.2 Cytokeratin phenotypic expression in adenocarcinomas of different organs | |
| --- | --- |
| Organ | CK |
| Colon | CK7–/CK20+ |
| Stomach | CK7–/CK20+, CK7+/CK20+ |
| Biliary | CK7+/CK20–, CK7+/CK20+ |
| Pancreas | CK7+/CK20–, CK7+/CK20+ |
| Urothelial | CK7+/CK20+ |
| Prostate | CK7–/CK20– |
| Renal | CK7–/CK20– |
| Liver | CK7–/CK20– |
| Lung | CK7+/CK20– |

When gastrointestinal stromal tumour (GIST) is suspected – as opposed to other causes for similar tumours – the histopathologist can use immunohistochemistry (specific antibodies that stain the molecule CD117, also known as *c*-kit). Virtually all GISTs are CD117-positive.

The treatments depend on the cause, and may range from watchful waiting to radical surgery (Figure 8.1).

# Conclusion

The mass should be localized and characterized as far as possible on clinical examination, followed up by blood tests for tumour markers. Abdominal imaging, using ultrasound or CT, can further localize the tumour and help elucidate its origins. Histopathology following biopsy or surgical excision will provide a definitive diagnosis, to guide further treatment and diagnosis.

# Further Reading

1   Tomassetti P, Migliori M, Lalli S, Campana D, Tomassetti V, Corinaldesi R. Epidemiology, clinical features and diagnosis of gastroenteropancreatic endocrine tumours. *Ann Oncol* 2001; **12** Suppl 2: 95–9.

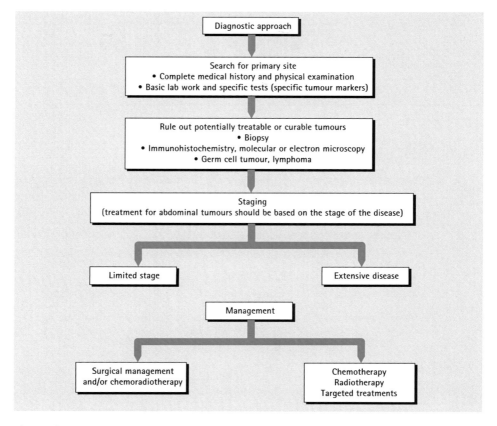

**Figure 8.1** Diagnostic approach and management of abdominal mass (tumour).

2   Williams MP, Scott IK, Dixon AK. Computed tomography in 101 patients with a palpable abdominal mass. *Clin Radiol* 1984; **35**: 293–6.

3   Dixon AK, Fry IK, Kingham JG, McLean AM, White FF. Computed tomography in patients with an abdominal mass: effective and efficient? A controlled trial. *Lancet* 1981; **1**: 1199–201.

4   Aspelin P, Hildell J, Karlsson S, Sigurjonson S. Ultrasonic evaluation of palpable abdominal masses. *Acta Chir Scand* 1980; **146**: 501–6.

5   Holm HH, Gammelgaard J, Jensen F, Smith EH, Hillman BJ. Ultrasound in the diagnosis of a palpable abdominal mass. A prospective study of 107 patients. *Gastrointest Radiol* 1982; **7**: 149–51.

6   Barker CS, Lindsell DR. Ultrasound of the palpable abdominal mass. *Clin Radiol* 1990; **41**: 98–9.

7   Colquhoun IR, Saywell WR, Dewbury KC. An analysis of referrals for primary diagnostic abdominal ultrasound to a general X-ray department. *Br J Radiol* 1988; **61**: 297–300.

8   Annuar Z, Sakijan AS, Annuar N, Kooi GH. Ultrasound in the diagnosis of palpable abdominal masses in children. *Med J Malaya* 1990; **45**: 281–7.

9   Pavlidis N, Briasoulis E, Hainsworth J, Greco FA. Diagnostic and therapeutic management of cancer of an unknown primary. *Eur J Cancer* 2003; **39**: 1990–2005.

# 9 Ascites in an Elderly Patient

## Case History

An 84-year-old woman with stable angina, a history of a previous transient ischaemic attack (TIA) and chronic obstructive pulmonary disease presents with abdominal distension, lower limb oedema and anorexia. Her Eastern Cooperative Oncology Group (ECOG) performance status is 2. Computed tomography (CT) of the abdomen shows the presence of marked ascites, diffuse omental thickening and a possible mass on the right ovary.

**What differential diagnoses would you consider?**

**How would you approach further diagnosis and management?**

## Background

**What differential diagnoses would you consider?**

Non-malignant causes account for about 80% of all cases of ascites. These include raised right atrial pressure secondary to cardiac disease or constrictive pericarditis, chronic pulmonary disease, and liver cirrhosis. The CT findings in the present case point to a malignant cause. The most likely diagnosis is epithelial carcinoma of the ovary or primary peritoneal carcinoma. This is compatible with the CT findings and a fairly common malignancy in this age group. It is also possible that the woman has an upper gastrointestinal malignancy such as gastric or pancreatic carcinoma, causing ascites and a secondary ovarian metastasis (Krukenberg's tumour). This is less likely, although not impossible, as the CT scan suggests no abnormality in the pancreas or stomach. Occasionally lobular breast cancer may present as pelvic disease with ascites and therefore a full clinical examination of the breast should be undertaken. However, it is more common in younger women than in this patient's age group. Finally, non-Hodgkin's lymphoma may occasionally present as ascites and peritoneal disease.

## Discussion

**How would you approach further diagnosis and management?**

The diagnosis and management should be approached with the twin goal of symptom control and pursuing a diagnosis insofar as further treatment would be feasible. The logical first step is therapeutic ascitic drainage, which may also yield a diagnosis on cytological examination. Guidelines have been developed on paracentesis for ascites related to malignancy. These emphasize carrying out ultrasound investigations only in cases of uncertainty, allowing up to 5 l of fluid to drain without clamping, leaving the drain in for no more that 6 hours and giving intravenous fluid only when specifically indicated.[1]

In the present case, particular attention should be paid to the patient's cardiovascular status during drainage because of her age and comorbidity. If adenocarcinoma cells are seen in the ascitic fluid, the morphology and/or immunohistochemical staining may support a diagnosis of ovarian or peritoneal carcinoma. This would also be supported by extremely elevated serum concentrations of CA125. However, serum CA125 is not specific for ovarian malignancy and may be moderately elevated in almost any cancer presenting with ascites and peritoneal disease. Gastrointestinal or lobular breast cancer may also be distinguishable on cytological examination, lobular breast cancer being characterized by hormone receptor positivity. A finding of peritoneal lymphocytosis may prove less definitive as reactive lymphocytosis can accompany ascites and a firm diagnosis of non-Hodgkin's lymphoma usually requires a tissue specimen.

If the diagnosis cannot be made based on the ascitic fluid, a CT-guided biopsy of the omentum may be possible. The patient's cardiovascular comorbidity means she may be on antithrombotic or anticoagulant agents, and treatment may need to be modified before any invasive procedure.

If a diagnosis of malignancy is made, the next step is to consider management. There is increasing evidence that a comprehensive geriatric assessment (CGA) can help to predict and guide toxicity of cancer therapy.[2–4] If this is ovarian carcinoma, in the normal course of events consideration would be given to debulking surgery. However, this patient's comorbidities make her a particularly high anaesthetic risk and, with CGA for guidance, primary chemotherapy may be a better approach.[5] Single-agent carboplatin at an area under the curve (AUC) of 4 or 5 is an effective and generally well-tolerated palliative treatment. It can prevent recurrence of ascites and improve quality of life and survival. In elderly patients, formal measurement of the glomerular filtration rate (GFR) before dose calculation should be considered as the Cockroft-Gault formula may not provide an accurate estimate of GFR in such patients.[6]

If this woman has radiological and histological evidence of hormone receptor-positive breast cancer, systemic hormonal treatment is relatively well tolerated and can produce meaningful responses and improvement in quality of life. Even in the elderly, non-Hodgkin's lymphoma may be successfully treated with judicious use of cytotoxics and steroids, so this diagnosis is also worth pursuing.[7]

If further investigations suggest an upper gastrointestinal primary the question of systemic therapy is more difficult. The prognosis is poor and the modest benefits of systemic chemotherapy have to be balanced against the risks of toxicity. In particular, 5-fluorouracil/capecitabine-based treatments are associated with an increased risk of endothelial damage and thrombotic events which may be significant given the patient's history of cardiovascular disease. Of course, if she developed local upper gastrointestinal symptoms it might still be worth investigation with a view to local palliative measures.

## Conclusion

In summary, the most likely diagnosis is an epithelial ovarian cancer, whose relative chemosensitivity to carboplatin warrants a definitive diagnosis. There is increasing evidence that CGA and multidisciplinary team involvement in patient care are beneficial in treating older patients with cancer.

## Further Reading

1   Stephenson J, Gilbert J. The development of clinical guidelines on paracentesis for ascites related to malignancy. *Palliat Med* 2002; **16**: 213–18.

2   Extermann M, Aapro M, Bernabei R, Cohen HJ, Droz JP, Lichtman S, Mor V, Monfardini S, Repetto L, Sorbye L, Topinkova E; Task Force on CGA of the International Society of Geriatric Oncology. Use of comprehensive geriatric assessment in older cancer patients: recommendations from the Task Force on CGA of the International Society of Geriatric Oncology (SIOG). *Crit Rev Oncol Hematol* 2005; **55**: 241–52.

3   Gosney M. Clinical assessment of elderly people with cancer. *Lancet Oncol* 2005; **6**: 790–7.

4   Lichtman SM. Therapy insight: therapeutic challenges in the treatment of elderly cancer patients. *Nat Clin Pract Oncol* 2006; **3**: 86–93.

5   Freyer G, Geay JF, Touzet S, Provencal J, Weber B, Jacquin JP, Ganem G, Tubiana-Mathieu N, Gisserot O, Pujade-Lauraine E. Comprehensive geriatric assessment predicts tolerance to chemotherapy and survival in elderly patients with advanced ovarian carcinoma: a GINECO study. *Ann Oncol* 2005; **15**: 291–5.

6   Marx GM, Blake GM, Galani E, Steer CB, Harper SE, Adamson KL, Bailey DL, Harper PG. Evaluation of the Cockroft-Gault, Jelliffe and Wright formulae in estimating renal function in elderly cancer patients. *Ann Oncol* 2004; **15**: 291–5.

7   Bairey O, Benjamini O, Blickstein D, Elis A, Ruchlemer R. Non-Hodgkin's lymphoma in patients 80 years of age or older. *Ann Oncol* 2006; **17**: 928–34.

# 10 Cancer in Teenagers and Young Adults: Special Issues

## Case History

A 19-year-old man presents with a high-grade synovial sarcoma in his left ankle. By the time a diagnosis is made the tumour is too advanced to allow resection without amputation. Staging investigations reveal no evidence of metastatic disease. The patient is studying music at university, his parents are separated but both attended with their son for the initial consultation. He has a younger brother aged 16 who is at school. During the consultation he is withdrawn and leaves the talking to his mother. She is confused and seems angry. They have been told he will probably need an amputation and chemotherapy lasting a year.

**Where should 19-year-old patients be treated?**

**What are the special issues in the management of teenagers and young adults that are different from managing cancer in an older patient?**

**Is there any alternative to amputation in this case?**

**What is the evidence for giving adjuvant chemotherapy to this patient postoperatively?**

## Background

### Where should 19-year-old patients be treated?

Patients in this age group have been described in different ways. They are much younger than the average referral to an adult oncology service and yet would on the whole no longer consider themselves to be children. Young adults, older teenagers, adolescents and 'thresholders' are just some the terms that attempt to describe the transitional state between dependent childhood and independent adulthood. The relatively small number of patients in this group who are diagnosed with cancer each year might be better managed in an 'age appropriate' environment. Some cancer centres have dedicated beds for these patients to allow the focusing of support services. Some have 'virtual' teams that try to coordinate the support while the patients stay either on paediatric or adult oncology wards. The Teenage Cancer Trust (www.teenagecancertrust.org) has been instrumental in raising funds for and awareness of this group of cancer patients. In some cases it has provided funding to allow dedicated units to develop.

The medical expertise required to manage a patient's specific illness is critical regardless of where the patient is actually admitted for treatment. The consultant in charge of this case should work as part of a multidisciplinary team looking after sarcomas. This will mean coming to the local cancer network 'centre' for most of the care. It may also involve the supra-regional sarcoma surgical services. The additional appropriate support services should then be built up around the specific needs of the individual once the medical plan is in place. The extent and style of this will vary depending on the local factors.

### What are the special issues in the management of teenagers and young adults that are different from managing cancer in an older patient?

#### Family dynamics

As a child develops into an adult the relationship between the child and the parents is re-negotiated. The stock of the family tends to drop while the stock of friends increases in value. Mental and emotional independence generally precede becoming financially and socially independent (i.e. moving out of home and supporting themselves). This process happens at different rates and at different ages, depending on the family style and individual's circumstances and personality.

If a young person is diagnosed with cancer at some point on this continuum towards full adult independence, it will inevitably alter the balance of the relationships between the patient and their family. The most common change is that the young person becomes more dependent on their parents again, reverting to a more child-like state. This is not something that either the parents or the patient were expecting and can be quite difficult. The young person may move back into the family home and require financial support as before. This re-adjustment of family roles after a cancer diagnosis is not unique to young adults, but the loss of such newly gained independence can lead to conflict. The incidence of intra-family conflict is high and often needs active management as part of the overall treatment plan. Dedicated community support nurses, social workers and/or clinical psychologists experienced in this field are therefore an indispensable part of the multidisciplinary team managing these patients.

#### Siblings

When treating young adults it is worth making an effort to remember the siblings of the patient. As parental energies and attention inevitably become focused on the patient, the lives of the siblings are also affected. They may not be involved in the discussions about the illness and feel uninformed or guilty about what is happening. They will often lose out on time with the parents because of hospital appointments and admissions. They may also end up with a lot more work to do around the house and even have to give up activities they enjoy because of time or financial constraints. Most teams that look after young adults and teenagers make an effort to get to know and include the siblings as much as possible.

#### Control

Acquisition of independence allows a person to gain control over what they do, how they look and how they behave. The changes in family dynamics, physical appearance, care needs and mobility that can come with a cancer diagnosis rob the young adult patient of this control. It is not uncommon for a patient who feels they have lost control over one element of their life to try to compensate by insisting on control over another. This might be how and when they take their medication, how they communicate (or don't!) or how and what they choose to eat. On the surface this can appear as if they are being 'difficult' and can lead to accusations of non-compliance. It adds to stress on the relationship with the parents as they also seek control over the elements that they can influence to help their child get better or tolerate treatment (diet, oral medicines at home, etc.). Be prepared to negotiate plans of treatment rather than dictate them if there are problems. Giving the patients the opportunity to be involved in decision making, and involving them as much as their capacity/wishes allow in the consenting process, will help in building rapport and improving adherence to the management plan.

### Life plans

Young adults have rarely developed a sense of their own mortality and are busy making plans – plans for the weekend, plans for the summer or plans for a career and family. A cancer diagnosis and treatment inevitably impacts on those plans and may change them forever. Education, work or training is commonly interrupted and patients need support to liaise with employers, universities or colleges, so that they do not fall too far behind their peers and are able to restart the course/job and catch up with their peers at the appropriate time.

The impact of treatment on relationships and fertility is a major consideration and needs to be discussed early on. Dealing with cancer around the time of a pregnancy or birth of a child is not that rare and brings another set of challenges to all involved. Mutilating or disabling surgery is not uncommon in the solid malignancies that effect young adults (sarcomas, germ cell tumours), and this has psychological and physical implications. A footballer or pianist may be more devastated by the loss of a leg than another patient.[1]

## Discussion

### Is there any alternative to amputation in this case?

Current evidence identifies a clear margin as one of the most important prognostic factors for long-term survival. Therefore, any treatment that is unlikely to achieve this may seem to be inadvisable. On closer scrutiny, the published data are based on relatively small numbers and are obviously biased because the studies compared patients with resectable and unresectable tumours. The significant reduction in amputation in favour of limb salvage surgery by most large sarcoma teams over the past 30 years has been associated with an increase in the rates of local recurrence. Despite this, recent series have shown no apparent difference in outcome from planned marginal excision compared with wide excision[2] and the impact of local recurrence on survival is somewhat controversial.

When primary radiotherapy is given as the definitive local treatment in synovial sarcomas that are considered to be unresectable, local control and survival is poor.[3] Primary radiotherapy should not be considered as a suitable alternative for a resectable tumour. However, when conservative surgery has been carried out, particularly if there are positive margins, then adjuvant radiotherapy has been shown to reduce the risk of local recurrence.[4,5]

Preoperative (neoadjuvant) intravenous chemotherapy with the intention of limb salvage surgery has been explored with modest success,[6] but no comparative trial data are available to guide the advice to patients. If considering chemotherapy in a fit patient, combination treatment with doxorubicin and ifosfamide (at doses higher than 9 g/m²) is advised in view of the higher response rates compared with single-agent treatment.[3]

Isolated limb perfusion is a novel technique in which the circulation of a limb is transferred to an isolated circuit (using cardiac bypass equipment). This allows infusing the limb with agents at higher concentrations than would be tolerable in systemic circulation via intravenous administration.[7] Particular success has been achieved with the combination of tumour necrosis factor (TNF) α and melphalan.[8]

Preoperative radiotherapy may also be a treatment option for this patient. It has many advantages over postoperative radiotherapy. A lower dose and a smaller target volume can be used, reducing the risk of local late effects, particularly arthropathy. A recent randomized controlled trial of pre- and postoperative radiotherapy showed an increase risk of wound complication in the preoperative arm (35% versus 17% in the postoperative arm; $P = 0.01$).[9] However, this may be manageable with modern techniques such as intensity-modulated radiation therapy (IMRT).

The wide variety of treatment options illustrates the complexity of treatment of soft tissue sarcomas generally and underlines the need for expert input from a specialist multidisciplinary team. The final decision needs to be sensitively discussed with the patient and his family to arrive at a management plan that incorporates the best possible medical care and is acceptable to the patient.

### What is the evidence for giving adjuvant chemotherapy to this patient postoperatively?

Synovial sarcomas are high-grade tumours with a high risk (~50%) of metastasis. Therefore, there is a clear rationale for considering systemic therapy as an adjunct to surgery. However, results from the meta-analysis of a number of rather small randomized controlled trials of doxorubicin-based chemotherapy do not suggest an improvement in overall survival.[10,11] This may be because these trials included a wide variety of subtypes of soft tissue sarcoma including leiomyosarcoma, liposarcoma, angiosarcoma and even gastrointestinal stromal tumour. There is some suggestion that synovial sarcoma is a more chemosensitive tumour than other types of adult soft tissue sarcoma. For example, one non-randomized series reported a response rate of 58% for patients with metastatic synovial sarcoma[12] in comparison with 28–47% reported in other series of mixed sub-types of soft issue sarcomas. In adult sarcoma practice, therefore, adjuvant chemotherapy is recommended only in the context of clinical trials. This may conflict with standard paediatric oncology practice where adjuvant treatment may be advised as standard care.[13] Harmonious resolution of interdisciplinary differences in the patient's best interest is another frequently encountered challenge in the management of patients in this age group.[14,15]

# Conclusion

It is important to engage this young patient and make sure he understands the diagnosis and treatment, and discuss the possibility of adjuvant chemotherapy. Such situations are never easy but may be further complicated by psychosocial issues related to his age and family relationships.

# Further Reading

1 Grinyer A. *Cancer in Young Adults: Through Parents' Eyes*. Milton Keynes: Open University Press, 2002.

2 Brennan MF, Casper ES, Harrison LB. The role of multimodality therapy in soft tissue sarcoma. *Surgery* 1991; **214**: 328–36.

3 Patel SR, Vadhan-Raj S, Burgess MA, Plager C, Papadopolous N, Jenkins J, Benjamin RS. Results of two consecutive trials of dose intensive chemotherapy with doxorubicin and ifosfamide in patients with sarcomas. *Am J Clin Oncol* 1998; **21**: 317–21.

4 Fein DA, Lee WR, Lanciano RM, Corn BW, Herbert SH, Hanlon AL, Hoffman JP, Eisenberg BL, Coia LR. Management of extremity soft tissue sarcomas with limb-sparing surgery and postoperative irradiation: do total dose, overall treatment time, and the surgery-radiotherapy interval impact on local control? *Int J Radiat Oncol Biol Phys* 1995; **32**: 969–77.

5 Yang JC, Chang AE, Baker AR, Sindelar WF, Danforth DN, Topalian SL, DeLaney T, Glatstein E, Steinberg SM, Merino MJ, Rosenberg SA. Randomized prospective study of the benefit of adjuvant radiation therapy in the treatment of soft tissue sarcomas of the extremity. *J Clin Oncol* 1998; **16**: 197–203.

6 Grobmyer SR, Maki RG, Demetri GD, Mazumdar M, Riedel E, Brennan MF, Singer S. Neo-adjuvant chemotherapy for primary high-grade extremity soft tissue sarcoma. *Ann Oncol* 2004; **15**: 1667–72.

7 Eggermont AM, de Wilt JH, ten Hagen TL. Current uses of isolated limb perfusion in the clinic and a model system for new strategies. *Lancet Oncol* 2003; **4**: 429–37.

8 Eggermont AM, Schraffordt Koops H, Klausner JM, Kroon BB, Schlag PM, Lienard D, van Geel AN, Hoekstra HJ, Meller I, Nieweg OE, Kettelhack C, Ben-Ari G, Pector JC, Lejeune FJ. Isolated limb perfusion with tumour necrosis factor and melphalan for limb salvage in 186 patients with locally advanced soft tissue extremity sarcomas. The multicenter European experience. *Ann Surg* 1996; **224**: 756–64.

9 O'Sullivan B, Davis AM, Turcotte R, Bell R, Catton C, Chabot P, Wunder J, Kandel R, Goddard K, Sadura A, Pater J, Zee B. Preoperative vs postoperative radiotherapy in soft-tissue sarcoma of the limbs: a randomised trial. *Lancet* 2002; **359**: 2235–41.

10 Adjuvant chemotherapy for localised resectable soft tissue sarcoma of adults: meta-analysis of individual data. Sarcoma meta-analysis collaboration. *Lancet* 1997; **350**: 1647–54.

11 Bramwell VH. Adjuvant chemotherapy for adult soft tissue sarcoma: is there a standard of care? *J Clin Oncol* 2001; **19**: 1235–7.

12 Spurrell EL, Fisher C, Thomas JM, Judson IR. Prognostic factors in advanced synovial sarcoma: an analysis of 104 patients treated at the Royal Marsden Hospital. *Ann Oncol* 2005; **16**: 437–44.

13 Ferrari A, Brecht IB, Koscielniak E, Casanova M, Scagnellato A, Bisogno G, Alaggio R, Cecchetto G, Catania S, Meazza C, Int-Veen C, Kirsch S, Dantonello T, Carli M, Treuner J. The role of adjuvant chemotherapy in children and adolescents with surgically resected, high-risk adult-type soft tissue sarcomas. *Pediatr Blood Cancer*. 2005; **45**: 128–34.

14 Okcu MF, Despa S, Choroszy M, Berrak SG, Cangir A, Jaffe N, Raney RB. Synovial sarcoma in children and adolescents: thirty-three years of experience with multimodal therapy. *Med Pediatr Oncol* 2001; **37**: 90–6.

15 Ferrari A, Gronchi A, Casanova M, Meazza C, Gandola L, Collini P, Lozza L, Bertulli R, Olmi P, Casali PG. Synovial sarcoma: a retrospective analysis of 271 patients of all ages treated at a single institution. *Cancer* 2004; **101**: 627–34.

PROBLEM

# 11 Spinal Cord Compression

## Case History

A 56-year-old previously fit woman presents with paraparesis of 24 hours duration on a background of 4 weeks of mild malaise and progressive back pain. An urgent magnetic resonance scan of the spine reveals destructive vertebral lesions at T8–T9 causing spinal cord compression (Figure 11.1). A chest radiograph shows a right lower lobe infiltrate.

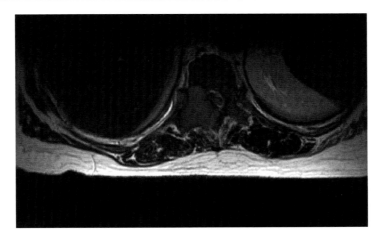

**Figure 11.1** Detail from magnetic resonance scan showing an epidural soft tissue metastasis encroaching on the spinal canal and cord at the level of a thoracic vertebra.

**What underlying malignancies would you consider in the differential diagnosis?**

**What is the immediate management?**

**What are the treatment options and how should the decision be based?**

# Background

## What underlying malignancies would you consider in the differential diagnosis?

Breast cancer is common in women of this patient's age and may present like this. The chest radiograph appearances may be due to an obstructing bronchial lesion, so primary lung carcinoma metastatic to the spine should be considered. The picture of localized destructive bony lesions also fits with multiple myeloma, which may present with concurrent respiratory tract infection due to associated immune suppression.

Other less common malignancies that have an affinity for bone and may present as spinal cord compression include renal and thyroid cancers. Of course lymphoma may present with almost any clinical picture and should always be considered in the differential diagnosis of metastatic spinal cord compression.

# Discussion

## What is the immediate management?

Metastatic spinal cord compression (MSCC) is an oncological emergency as the process and consequent neurological deficits are remediable if treated early enough. Extrinsic compression of the cord, either by bony fragments or metastatic tumour, leads to vasogenic oedema. At this stage the process is potentially reversible but if the oedema progresses to ischaemia, neuronal death and permanent neurological deficit will occur.

High-dose dexamethasone should be initiated immediately as steroids can play a vital role in reducing oedema, inhibiting prostaglandin synthesis and possibly downregulating vascular endothelial growth factor. Some evidence suggests that patients treated with very high-dose corticosteroids (i.e. dexamethasone 100 mg) have improved motor function and longer maintenance of ambulation compared to those receiving moderate doses (e.g. dexamethasone 10–30 mg) (reviewed in Loblaw et al.[1]). This is at the expense of more frequent serious adverse events related to steroid use. One phase II study suggested that in patients with good motor function at the time of diagnosis of MSCC, corticosteroids might not be necessary prior to radiotherapy treatment,[2] but their omission is not standard practice.

## What are the treatment options and how should the decision be based?

The choice of definitive initial emergency treatment for MSCC lies between surgery and radiotherapy. Selected patients should be considered for surgery. These include patients with spinal instability, bony fragments as a cause for cord compression and patients with rapid deterioration and no tissue diagnosis.

The role of surgery in MSCC was addressed by a randomized controlled trial.[3] The study population consisted of relatively fit patients with magnetic resonance imaging (MRI)-proved spinal cord compression at a single site, at least one neurological symptom and/or paraparesis of onset within 48 hours of study entry. They were randomized to receive either decompressive surgery followed by radiotherapy (30 Gy in 10 fractions) or radiotherapy alone. Interim analysis showed a clear difference in the proportion of patients able to walk after surgery (84%) compared with those who only received radiotherapy (57%) ($P = 0.001$). In addition, patients who underwent surgery remained ambulatory for longer and had higher rates of maintaining continence, muscle strength and functional ability than those who did not. There was also a greatly reduced need for opioid analgesics and corticosteroids in the surgical group. In that study, 30-day mortality rates did not differ significantly between the two groups, but figures of 0–13% for postoperative mortality and 0–54% for postoperative complication rates have been reported elsewhere. In general, complication rates for vertebral body resection are higher than for laminectomy. Therefore the benefits of surgery need to be weighed against the potential morbidity and mortality; careful selection of patients is mandatory.

For most patients with MSCC, immediate radiotherapy is the definitive treatment. The aim of radiotherapy is to decompress the spinal cord and nerve roots by targeted induction of cell death thereby preventing progression of neurological deficits and providing pain relief, as well as improvement of motor function. A prospective study assessing radiotherapy response rates in MSCC (total dose 30 Gy) reported recovery of ambulation in 11% of patients with paraplegia, 60% of patients with paraparesis and 94% of patients with assisted ambulation;[4] 44% of patients with sphincter dysfunction experienced an improvement in function and 54% of patients with back pain noted complete resolution. The evidence suggests that patients with MSCC due to a soft tissue tumour do better with radiotherapy than those with bony collapse or bony fragments as a cause.[4-7] Other important prognostic factors predicting for response following radiotherapy treatment include:

- favourable histology (breast cancer, multiple myeloma, prostate cancer, lymphoma, renal cancer)

- absence of visceral metastases

- slower development of motor dysfunction

- long interval from cancer diagnosis to MSCC

- good pretreatment ambulatory function.

Most patients with spinal cord compression have a limited life expectancy in the order of months. However patients with favourable histology may live for much longer. Survival is adversely affected by[6-8] poor performance status, rapid progression of motor dysfunction, presence of visceral and other bone metastases and deterioration of symptoms following radiotherapy.

Radiotherapy schedules for MSCC need to be individualized to take into account life expectancy, among other factors. Rades *et al.*[9] retrospectively looked at the outcomes of five radiotherapy schedules given over an 11-year period (1992–2003) to 1304 patients. Schedules of 1 × 8 Gy, 5 × 4 Gy, 10 × 3 Gy, 15 × 2.5 Gy and 20 × 2 Gy were assessed for impact on motor function, ambulatory status and recurrences within the radiotherapy field. No single regimen conferred any marked advantage over the others when immediate functional outcomes were assessed. However, at 2 years, recurrences in the radiotherapy field were greatly reduced with the more protracted regimens.

A recently published randomized controlled trial in almost 300 patients addressed the issue of the optimum schedule in patients with poor prognosis. The eligibility criteria included patients with progressive disease and MSCC diagnosed by MRI and/or computed tomography (CT), no indication for initial surgery, short life expectancy (<6 months for poor risk histology or favourable risk histology but a low performance status and motor and/or sphincter dysfunction). These criteria were designed to exclude those patients in whom surgery or protracted course radiotherapy would be appropriate as initial management. Patients were randomized to receive either short-course schedule of 8 Gy × 2 given a week apart or a split-course schedule of 5 Gy × 3, 4 days rest then 3 Gy × 5. There were no notable differences in toxicity, response rate, response duration or survival. The authors concluded that for patients with a prognosis of months, short-course schedules are effective and may be appropriate to limit potential toxicities of treatment and to minimize the number of visits to hospital.[10] However, for patients with a favourable prognosis, protracted course radiotherapy should be considered to reduce the risk of in-field recurrences.

If there is disease recurrence within a previous radiotherapy field, the options for further management include surgery, systemic chemotherapy (depending on tumour type), further radiotherapy and best supportive care. The role of surgery where compression has occurred in a previous radiotherapy field is difficult. On the one hand, there are likely to be major limitations in the capacity to deliver a second effective dose of radiotherapy because of tissue tolerance. On the other hand, appreciably higher surgical morbidity is reported in patients who have received prior radiotherapy.[11]

## Conclusion

The options for the definitive management of the index patient therefore are radiotherapy, surgery or chemotherapy if the tumour is highly chemosensitive, e.g. multiple myeloma, lymphoma, etc. This patient is young and fit with limited spinal disease. Also, there is no tissue diagnosis and her neurological symptoms are of short duration and potentially reversible. In view of the evidence, she would be a candidate for surgery, possibly followed by radiotherapy, depending on the tissue diagnosis. If she turns out to have a chemosensitive cancer, then early chemotherapy could be considered after surgery.

## Further Reading

1 Loblaw DA, Perry J, Chambers A, Laperriere NJ. Systematic review of the diagnosis and management of malignant extradural spinal cord compression: the Cancer Care Ontario Practice Guidelines Initiative's Neuro-Oncology Disease Site Group. *J Clin Oncol* 2005; **23**: 2028–37.

2 Maranzano E, Latini P, Beneventi S, Perruci E, Panizza BM, Aristei C, Lupattelli M, Tonato M. Radiotherapy without steroids in selected metastatic spinal cord compression patients: a phase II trial. *Am J Clin Oncol* 1996; **19**: 179–83.

3 Patchell RA, Tibbs PA, Regine WF, Payne R, Saris S, Kryscio RJ, Mohiuddin M, Young B. Direct decompression surgical resection in the treatment of spinal cord compression caused by metastatic cancer: a randomised trial. *Lancet* 2005; **366**: 643–8.

4 Maranzano E, Latini P. Effectiveness of radiation therapy without surgery in metastatic spinal cord compression: final results from a prospective trial. *Int J Radiat Oncol Biol Phys* 1995; **32**: 959–67.

5　Pigott K, Baddeley H, Maher EJ. Pattern of disease in spinal cord compression on MRI scan and implications for treatment. *Clin Oncol (R Coll Radiol)* 1994; **6**: 7–10.

6　Helweg-Larsen S, Sorensen PS, Kreiner S. Prognostic factors in metastatic spinal cord compression: a prospective study using multivariate analysis of variables influencing survival and gait function in 153 patients. *Int J Radiat Oncol Biol Phys* 2000; **46**: 1163–9.

7　Rades D, Veninga T, Stalpers LJ, Schulte R, Hoskin PJ, Poortmans P, Schild SE, Rudat V. Prognostic factors predicting functional outcomes, recurrence-free survival, and overall survival after radiotherapy for metastatic spinal cord compression in breast cancer patients. *Int J Radiat Oncol Biol Phys* 2006; **64**: 182–8.

8　Rades D, Fehlauer F, Schulte R, Veninga T, Stalpers LJ, Basic H, Bajrovic A, Hoskin PJ, Tribius S, Wildfang I, Rudat V, Engenhart-Cabilic R, Karstens JH, Alberti W, Dunst J, Schild SE. Prognostic factors for local control and survival after radiotherapy of metastatic spinal cord compression. *J Clin Oncol* 2006; **24**: 3388–93.

9　Rades D, Stalpers LJ, Veninga T, Schulte R, Hoskin PJ, Obralic N, Bajrovic A, Rudat V, Schwarz R, Hulshof MC, Poortmans P, Schild SE. Evaluation of five radiation schedules and prognostic factors for metastatic spinal cord compression. *J Clin Oncol* 2005; **23**: 3366–75.

10　Maranzano E, Bellavita R, Rossi R, De Angelis V, Frattegiani A, Bagnoli R, Mignogna M, Beneventi S, Lupattelli M, Ponticelli P, Biti GP, Latini P. Short-course versus split-course radiotherapy in metastatic spinal cord compression: results of a phase III, randomized, multicenter trial. *J Clin Oncol* 2005; **23**: 3358–65.

11　Ghogawala Z, Mansfield F, Borges L. Spinal radiation before surgical decompression adversely affects outcomes of surgery for symptomatic metastatic spinal cord compression. *Spine* 2001; **26**: 818–24.

# Urological Cancers

## PROBLEM

# 12  Primary Germ Cell Tumours

## Case History

 A 26-year-old man with no significant past medical or sexual history presents to his general practitioner with a 1-week history of a painful swollen left testicle. He is initially treated for epididymo-orchitis with a course of antibiotics, but his symptoms do not resolve. He is referred urgently to a urologist. Clinical assessment and a scrotal ultrasound scan reveal a highly suspicious lesion in the left testicle, and he proceeds to a radical inguinal orchidectomy. This confirms a germ cell tumour invading the rete testis but not the spermatic cord. Lymphovascular invasion is also seen. Postoperative staging is negative.

**What is the initial differential diagnosis?**

**What pre- and postoperative tests are essential to fully stage this patient and what is his stage?**

**What adjuvant treatment should be considered if the histological examination revealed a non-seminomatous germ cell tumour (NSGCT)?**

**What adjuvant treatment should be considered if the histological examination revealed a seminoma?**

# Background

### What is the initial differential diagnosis?

Testicular tumours usually present as a painless testicular nodule or swelling of the whole testicle, with acute pain being a feature in only 10%. The differential diagnosis of a testicular mass include epididymitis/epididymo-orchitis, testicular torsion, varicocele, hydrocoele and haematoma. Up to 40% of patients may present with a sensation of heaviness or a dull ache in the scrotum or perianal region.

### What pre- and postoperative tests are essential to fully stage this patient and what is his stage?

The baseline tumour markers (β-human chorionic gonadotrophin [hCG], α-fetoprotein [AFP] and lactate dehydrogenase [LDH]) are vital prognostic indicators, used to stratify patients into prognostic groups according to the International Germ Cell Cancer Collaborative Group (IGCCCG) guidelines,[1] if they have metastatic disease. These markers are not specific for germ cell tumours and may occasionally be falsely raised (e.g. marijuana use and liver damage may raise β-hCG and AFP levels, respectively). In 25% of patients with NSGCTs they are not raised; only up to 35% of seminomas produce β-hCG, with pure seminomas not producing AFP at all. Postoperatively the tumour markers should be repeated if they were raised preoperatively. Serial weekly measurements are required until normal values are reached to ensure the levels are falling according to the serum half life of the markers (18–36 hours for β-hCG, and 4–5 days for AFP). Failure to do so implies metastatic disease.

Postoperative imaging consists of a computed tomography (CT) scan of the chest, abdomen and pelvis to fully stage the patient. Positron emission tomography (PET) has not been shown to be useful in confirming stage 1 disease.

The stage of this patient is stage 1B,[2] which equates to pT2 N0 M0 S0. Invasion of the rete testis, although prognostic for seminomas, is not part of the staging system; tunica vaginalis invasion, however, will upstage it to pT2, as does the presence of lymphovascular invasion.

# Discussion

### What adjuvant treatment should be considered if the histological examination revealed NSGCT?

The cure rate of patients with stage 1 NSGCT is in the region of 99%. Because of this there has been a shift in the focus of patient management towards reducing treatment-related morbidity. There are three main options for the management of stage 1 NSGCTs (see also Figure 12.1).[3,4]

#### Surveillance

Surveillance involves strong commitment by both the patient and oncologist, with careful adherence to follow-up protocols. It is generally only appropriate for highly motivated patients with a low risk of relapse. Careful patient selection, using histopathological findings to stratify patients into high or low risk groups, as well as sound patient education about the importance of complying with the follow-up regimen make surveillance a good option for the management of stage 1 NSGCT.

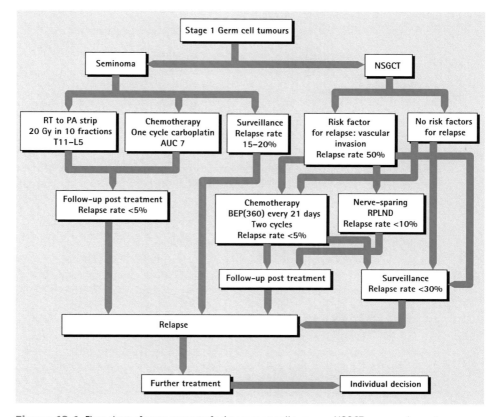

**Figure 12.1** Flow chart of management of primary germ cell tumours. NSGCT, non-seminomatous germ cell tumour; RPLND, retroperitoneal lymph node dissection; AUC, area under the curve; RT, radiotherapy; PA, para-aortic nodes.

Stage 1 NSGCT has a recurrence rate of 25–30%, and 95% of these occur in the first 2 years after orchidectomy – 55–80% occur in the retroperitoneum, 15–30% in the lungs, and 10–20% are marker only relapse. Patients rarely relapse in more than one visceral organ. The relative risk (RR) of relapse has been found to correlate with four key histological features:[5]

- invasion of blood vessels:          3–4 features – 58% RR
- invasion of lymphatic vessels:      2 features – 24% RR
- absence of yolk sac elements:       1 feature – 10% RR
- presence of embryonal cell carcinoma elements:   0 features – 0% RR.

The single most important factor for predicting relapse is lymphovascular invasion, which is associated with a 40–50% risk of relapse.

Low-risk patients are defined as those without lymphovascular invasion. These patients have a 75–85% chance of not requiring further treatment, but if they relapse, still have a cure rate of close to 100% with salvage chemotherapy. High-risk patients are defined as those with lymphovascular invasion, and they have a significant risk of relapse. With close surveillance, more than 98% will have favourable stage disease on relapse and will be cured with salvage chemotherapy. However, many clinicians favour adjuvant chemotherapy in this setting.

### Adjuvant chemotherapy

The rationale for adjuvant chemotherapy is to treat occult systemic disease with fewer cycles of chemotherapy than would be required for more disseminated disease, hence less toxicity. In patients with high-risk disease (as described above), two courses of adjuvant BEP (bleomycin [30 000 IU], etoposide [360 mg/m$^2$] and cisplatin [100 mg/m$^2$]) every 21 days has been shown in a non-randomized study to reduce the risk of relapse from 40% to 1–2%.[6] The overall cure rate is >99%. The side effects include the short-term toxicities and the long-term risks to fertility (ensure sperm storage prior to the therapy), hearing and pulmonary function.

### Retroperitoneal lymph node dissection (RPLND)

RPLND is more popular in the USA than Europe and developed because NSGCT generally has an orderly pattern of spread, with regional nodal metastasis generally appearing in the retroperitoneal nodes first. RPLND allows accurate identification of micrometastasis and thereby accurate pathological staging. A proportion of patients are upstaged by RPLND and may require postoperative chemotherapy. Relapse occurs in ~10% of patients who have a negative RPLND, and this is almost exclusively in the lungs. RPLND can be associated with significant morbidity, including ejaculatory dysfunction.

In view of the presence of lymphovascular invasion, this patient, in many institutions would be offered adjuvant chemotherapy, using two cycles of BEP.

## What adjuvant treatment should be considered if the histological examination revealed a seminoma?

Approximately 80% of all patients with seminomas present with stage 1 disease for which there are three options (see also Figure 12.1).

### Surveillance

Surveillance is potentially less reliable in seminomas than NSGCT. There are no good tumour markers, and seminomas have a potential for late relapse, up to 10 years after orchidectomy. In view of the risk of late relapse patients have to be especially motivated. Approximately 20% of patients on surveillance will have recurrence, 80% of which will be in the retroperitoneal lymph nodes. This will require higher doses of radiotherapy or more intense chemotherapy than in the adjuvant setting. The risk of relapse is higher if the tumour is ≥4 cm (20–35% compared with 5% if less than 4 cm) or the tumour invades the rete testis. Protocols for surveillance are similar to those used for NSGCT follow-up.

### Adjuvant radiotherapy

Adjuvant radiotherapy traditionally had been the treatment of choice as seminomas are very radiosensitive and characteristically relapse in the retroperitoneum. Relapse rates have been reduced to 3–4%, the majority of which are outside the treatment field using this approach. To minimize toxicity, both the volume treated and the dose delivered have been reduced. Standard therapy now is to deliver treatment to the para-aortic (upper border of T11 to lower border of L5) and ipsilateral renal hilar nodes only. The iliac and inguinal nodes are only covered by the addition of an ipsilateral 'dog leg' when there has been prior inguino-scrotal surgery.[7] This modification of the radiotherapy field results in less azoospermia (11% versus 35% before), and no change in the total number of relapses. As seminomas are so radiosensitive the dose used in the adjuvant setting has been reduced to 20 Gy in ten fractions.[8] This regimen results in the same disease-free survival rate (97% 4-year disease-free survival) and less acute toxicity than 30 Gy in 15 fractions. The side effects of radiotherapy include acute gastrointestinal toxicity (nausea, vomiting, and diarrhoea) and the potential risk of a second malignancy.

### Adjuvant chemotherapy

Seminomas are very sensitive to platinum-based chemotherapy. Adjuvant chemotherapy with carboplatin has been investigated as its acute toxicity profile is quite similar to that of radiotherapy, with the potential advantage of fewer late effects (particularly infertility and secondary malignancies). The TE19 trial compared radiotherapy with carboplatin (area under the curve 7).[9] After 4 years of follow-up, there was no difference in relapse rate, although the pattern of relapse was different, with more pelvic relapses with adjuvant radiotherapy and more retroperitoneal relapses with the carboplatin. There was also a suggestion of more second malignancies in the radiotherapy group.

## Conclusion

For stage 1 disease consideration of the risk of relapse versus the toxicity of treatment needs to be addressed. Options should be discussed with the patient.

## Further Reading

1   International Germ Cell Consensus classification: a prognostic factor-based staging system for metastatic germ cell cancers. *J Clin Oncol* 1997; **15**: 594.

2   American Joint Committee on Cancer. *Cancer Staging Manual*, 6th edition. AJCC, 2002

3   Royal College of Radiologists' COIN Guidelines on the management of adult testicular germ cell tumours. *Clin Oncol* 2000; **12**: S173.

4   European consensus on the diagnosis and treatment of germ cell cancer: a report of the European Germ Cell Cancer Consensus Group. *Ann Oncol* 2004; **15**: 1377.

5   Freedman LS, Parkinson MC, Jones WG, Oliver RT, Peckham MJ, Reed G, Newlands ES, Williams CJ. Histopathology in the prediction of relapse of patients with stage I testicular teratoma treated by orchidectomy alone. *Lancet* 1987; **2**: 294.

6   Cullen MH, Stenning SP, Parkinson MC, Fossa SD, Kaye SB, Horwich AH, Harland SJ, Williams MV, Jakes R. Short-course adjuvant chemotherapy in high-risk stage I nonseminomatous germ cell tumours of the testis: a Medical Research Council report. *J Clin Oncol* 1996; **14**: 1106–13.

7   Fossa SD, Horwich A, Russell JM, Roberts JT, Cullen MH, Hodson NJ, Jones WG, Yosef H, Duchesne GM, Owen JR, Grosch EJ, Chetiyawardana AD, Reed NS, Widmer B, Stenning SP. Optimal planning target volume for stage I testicular seminoma: a Medical Research Council

randomized trial. Medical Research Council Testicular Tumor Working Group. *J Clin Oncol* 1999; **17**: 1146.

8   Jones WG, Fossa SD, Mead GM, Roberts JT, Sokal M, Horwich A, Stenning SP. Randomised trial of 30 Gy vs 20 Gy in the adjuvant treatment of stage I testicular seminoma. A report on the Medical Research Council trial TE18, European organization for the research and treatment of cancer trial. *J Clin Oncol* 2005; **23**: 1200–8.

9   Oliver RT, Mason M, Von der Masse H, *et al.* on behalf of the MRC Testis Tumour Group and the EORTC GU Group. A randomised trial of single agent carboplatin with radiotherapy in the adjuvant treatment of stage I seminoma of the testis, following orchidectomy (MRC TE19). *Lancet* 2005; **366**: 293.

## PROBLEM

# 13   Advanced Testicular Cancer

## Case History

A previously healthy 29-year-old man was admitted through the accident and emergency department with a history of a swollen left testis, weight loss and more recently breathing difficulties. A chest radiograph reveals multiple pulmonary metastases with an α-fetoprotein (AFP) of 65 000 ng/ml and β human chorionic gonadotrophin (hCG) 205 000 IU/l.

**What further investigations should he have?**

**What is the prognosis and treatment?**

**If he relapses what chemotherapy options are there?**

## Background

### What further investigations should he have?

The immediate concern is to stabilize the patient. A computed tomography (CT) scan (head, chest, abdomen and pelvis) should be done to determine the extent of the disease. Tissue diagnosis is not mandatory in this case as it would delay the time to treatment, and the diagnosis of a non-seminomatous germ cell tumour is clear from the raised tumour markers (both AFP and β-hCG). However, if possible, tissue diagnosis is valuable, particularly if the patient is stable.

### What is the prognosis and treatment?

The prognosis of patients with germ cell cancer is derived from the International Germ Cell Consensus Classification (IGCCC) published in 1997[1] (Table 13.1). It relies on the extent of disease and tumour markers and the primary site. The IGCCC was developed because of the variations in the classifications and staging systems used worldwide, making it difficult to compare trial data. Approximately 60% of all patients with metastatic non-seminomas come under the good prognosis category, 25% in the intermediate and 15% in the poor category; 90% of patients with metastatic seminoma come under the good prognosis category and 10% in the intermediate. Treatment is based on the IGCCC prognostic classification. BEP (bleomycin, etoposide and cisplatin) is the universal chemotherapy regimen and no other regimen to date has been shown to be superior. Scheduling of treatment and number of cycles depend on the prognosis. In 2001, the European Organisation for Research and Treatment of Cancer (EORTC) published data confirming that for good prognostic disease three cycles of 3-day BEP (500 mg/m$^2$ etoposide) was sufficient with a progression-free survival (PFS) at 2 years of 90.4%.[2] For patients with intermediate and poor prognosis four cycles of 5-day BEP is the standard. Bleomycin is an important component of the regimen, but in disease with good prognosis four cycles of EP (500 mg/m$^2$ etoposide + cisplatin) have been shown to be equivalent to three cycles of BEP.

## Discussion

There is significant interest in improving the outcome using different regimens of chemotherapy. The Medical Research Council is currently investigating the CBOP/BEP (carboplatin, bleomycin, vincristine and cisplatin followed by BEP) regimen. A phase II

| Prognosis | Non–seminomatous germ cell tumour | Seminoma |
|---|---|---|
| Good | ALL of:<br>Testis or retroperitoneal primary<br><br>No non-pulmonary visceral metastases (i.e. lung metastasis only)<br>AFP <1000 ng/ml<br>β-hCG <5000 IU/l<br>LDH <1.5 × ULN | Any primary site<br>No non-pulmonary visceral metastases (i.e. lung metastasis only)<br>Normal AFP<br><br>Any β-hCG, any LDH |
| Intermediate | Testis or retroperitoneal primary<br>No non-pulmonary visceral metastases and ANY of:<br>AFP >1000 – <10 000 ng/m<br>β-hCG >5000 – <50 000 IU/l | Any primary site<br>Non-pulmonary visceral metastases<br>Normal AFP<br>Any β-hCG, any LDH<br>LDH >1.5 × <10 × ULN |
| Poor | ANY of:<br>Mediastinal primary; non-pulmonary visceral metastases<br>AFP >10 000 ng/ml<br>β-hCG >50 000 IU/l<br>LDH >10 × ULN | No patients in this group |

**Table 13.1  International Germ Cell Consensus Classification (IGCCC)**

ULN, upper limit of normal; AFP, α-fetoprotein; hCG, human chorionic gonadotrophin; LDH, lactate dehydrogenase.

study showed 87.6% 5-year survival,[3] and has led to a phase III study comparing this regimen with BEP, which is currently recruiting. The present patient has an approximately 50% chance of long-term survival according to the prognostic classification, given that he is in the poor prognostic group. So he will receive four cycles of standard dose BEP unless he opts to participate in a clinical study; in some centres he would be given a colony-stimulating factor as well.

Following chemotherapy those patients with residual disease in the retroperitoneum, and also the mediastinum and neck, should be considered for surgery to render them disease free. If the pathological review of the resected specimen confirmed viable tumour it would suggest a significant risk of relapse. Long-term side effects of the treatment also have to be considered as a significant proportion of men with germ cell tumours are cured. Issues include fertility, psychological problems, cardiovascular disease, neuropathy, hearing problems and second tumours.

### If he relapses what chemotherapy options are there?

Relapsed germ cell cancer is still a chemosensitive disease and potentially curable in approximately 30% of cases. Several relapse regimens using cytotoxics, which have shown activity in the relapse setting, have been investigated. The optimum salvage regimen still needs to be defined, but most patients retain platinum sensitivity at relapse. Vinblastine, etoposide and cisplatin (VIP) as a salvage regimen is associated with a complete response rate of 50% and long-term survival of 30%.[4] More recently paclitaxel has been added to other active drugs, notably ifosfamide and cisplatin (TIP) with a 19–77% complete response rate[5,6] and 85% 2-year survival.[6] Suggested prognostic factors at relapse are poor response to initial therapy, progression-free interval less than 2 years and non-testicular primary.

High-dose chemotherapy has been investigated as a second- or third-line treatment. Several phase II studies and retrospective analyses have demonstrated efficacy with acceptable toxicity. Long-standing complete remission has been reported in 15–25% of patients. In a retrospective series, Einhorn's group (see Bhatia *et al.*[7]) reported a disease-free rate of 57% at a median follow-up of 39 months.[7] However, a recent study suggested no difference in outcome between conventional standard treatment (cisplatin, ifosfamide and etoposide or vinblastine) and high-dose therapy (carboplatin, etoposide and cyclophosphamide).[8] Complete and partial response rates were similar in both arms and there were no significant differences in overall survival.

## Conclusion

This patient is in the poor prognostic group for this category of cancer and has approximately a 50% chance of long-term survival. Treatment would usually involve four cycles of standard dose BEP; if the cancer relapses it may still be treatable.

## Further Reading

1  International Germ Cell Cancer Collaborative Group. International germ cell consensus classification: A prognostic factor based staging system for metastatic germ cell cancers. *J Clin Oncol* 1997; **15**: 594–603.

2   de Wit R, Roberts JT, Wilkinson PM, de Mulder PH, Mead GM, Fossa SD, Cook P, de Prijck L, Stenning S, Collette L. Equivalence of three or four cycles of bleomycin, etoposide, and cisplatin chemotherapy and of a 3- or 5-day schedule in good-prognosis germ cell cancer: a randomized study of the European Organisation for Research and Treatment of Cancer Genitourinary Tract Cancer Cooperative Group and the Medical Research Council. *J Clin Oncol* 2001; **19**: 1629–40.

3   Christian J, Huddart, R, Norman A, Mason M, Fossa S, Aass N, Nicholl EJ, Dearnaley DP, Horwich A. Intensive induction chemotherapy with CBOP/BEP in patients with poor prognosis germ cell tumours. *J Clin Oncol* 2003; **21**: 871–7.

4   Loehrer PJ Sr, Gonin R, Nichols CR, Weathers T, Einhorn LH. Vinblastine plus ifosfamide plus cisplatin as initial salvage therapy in recurrent germ cell tumour. *J Clin Oncol* 1998; **16**: 2500–4.

5   Mead GM, Cullen MH, Huddart R, Harper P, Rustin GJ, Cook PA, Stenning SP, Mason M; MRC Testicular Tumour Working Party. A phase II trial of TIP (paclitaxel, ifosfamide and cisplatin) given as second-line (post BEP) salvage chemotherapy for patients with metastatic germ cell cancer: a Medical Research Council trial. 2005. *Br J Cancer* 2005; **93**: 178–84.

6   Motzer RJ, Sheinfeld J, Mazumdar M, Bajorin DF, Bosl GJ, Herr H, Lyn P, Vlamis V. Paclitaxel, ifosfamide, and cisplatin second-line therapy for patients with relapsed testicular germ cell cancer. *J Clin Oncol* 2000; **18**: 2413–18.

7   Bhatia S, Abonour R, Porcu P, Seshadri R, Nichols CR, Cornetta K, Einhorn LH. High dose chemotherapy as initial salvage chemotherapy in patients with relapsed testicular cancer. *J Clin Oncol* 2000; **18**: 3346–51.

8   Pico JL, Rosti G, Kramar A, Wandt H, Koza V, Salvioni R, Theodore C, Lelli G, Siegert W, Horwich A, Marangolo M, Linkesch W, Pizzocaro G, Schmoll HJ, Bouzy J, Droz JP, Biron P; Genito-Urinary Group of the French Federation of Cancer Centers (GETUG-FNCLCC), France; European Group for Blood and Marrow Transplantation (EBMT). A randomised trial of high dose chemotherapy in the salvage treatment of patients failing first line platinum chemotherapy for advanced germ cell tumours. *Ann Oncol* 2005; **16**: 1152–9.

PROBLEM

# 14 Bladder Cancer

## Case History

An otherwise healthy 65-year-old female smoker is admitted as an emergency with acute bilateral loin pain and anuria. There is history of recurrent haematuria and dysuria over the last few months. An ultrasound reveals that she has bilateral hydronephrosis secondary to a lesion in the trigone of the bladder. Her renal function is partly restored with bilateral ureteric stents.

**What are the next steps in the diagnostic work-up of this patient?**

Biopsies confirm the presence of a transitional cell carcinoma (TCC) of the bladder that is invading the muscle but not beyond.

**What treatment options are available?**

**Is there any evidence for the use of neoadjuvant chemotherapy in this setting?**

**What factors may influence the decision to use neoadjuvant chemotherapy in this particular patient?**

**Is adjuvant chemotherapy a reasonable/valid option?**

## Background

### What are the next steps in the diagnostic work-up of this patient?

Cytological examination alone may be sufficient to confirm the presence of a neoplastic lesion, although it has low sensitivity for low-grade lesions. Nevertheless, cystoscopy with examination under anaesthesia is essential, to allow for accurate clinical and pathological staging. Biopsies taken from macroscopically normal parts of the bladder surface allow detection of field change, which would influence management. Radiological imaging will demonstrate nodal and/or visceral involvement and allows estimation of the local extent of disease. Computed tomography (CT) is usually adequate, however, small lesions (<1 cm) especially in the trigone and dome of the bladder may be missed, and sensitivity for low-volume nodal disease is quite low; magnetic resonance imaging (MRI) may be preferable in those circumstances. Finally, full staging should be done, including chest and abdominal CT and, if bone pain is present, a nuclear medicine bone scan.

### What treatment options are available?

For patients with localized muscle-invasive disease, the choice of treatment is between radical surgery, with cystectomy and subsequent reconstructive procedures, and a bladder-sparing multimodality approach with salvage cystectomy on recurrence. Neoadjuvant chemotherapy may be given with either of these options. Preoperative radiotherapy has fallen out of favour despite improved local control, as it has not been shown to improve overall survival and makes urological reconstructive procedures more difficult.[1]

## Discussion

Unfortunately, no large randomized clinical trials have directly compared the two treatment options (radical surgery versus multimodality treatment). Relatively small (n <1000) population-based retrospective studies (e.g. see Chahal *et al.*[2]) have suggested equivalence in terms of overall survival, but the issue has not been addressed prospectively. A meta-analysis of older trials comparing preoperative radiotherapy followed by radical surgery with upfront radical radiotherapy found a benefit for surgery in terms of overall survival.[3] However, it included only three small trials and some radiotherapy was given to both arms thus making extrapolation of the results difficult.

More recent studies have shown that, in carefully selected patient groups, multimodality approaches including radical radiotherapy and (neo-) adjuvant chemotherapy may offer results comparable with definitive surgery.[4] Pertinent selection criteria include: T2 disease; adequate renal function to allow administration of chemotherapy; no associated ureteric obstruction or hydronephrosis; and a visibly complete transurethral resection of bladder tumour and CR following combined radio-chemotherapy. This approach is ideal for patients who are medically unfit for a major surgical procedure but able to tolerate combination treatment. Other benefits include preservation of the bladder and usually its continence mechanism, and thus potentially improved quality of life.

A phase II/III study is currently underway in the UK, aiming to determine how effective conservative treatment (neoadjuvant chemotherapy followed by radiotherapy) is compared with radical treatment (neoadjuvant chemotherapy followed by radical cystectomy).

Currently a wide range of techniques are available for cystoscopy, ranging from ileal conduits to continent reservoirs to orthotopic neobladders, which allow different levels of functional and subsequent quality-of-life outcomes. The choice will depend partly on the patient's preference and also on medical considerations (such as tumour location, previous surgery/radiotherapy and preoperative renal function) and factors such as the patient's physiological age, manual dexterity, and level of social support.

In this patient's case, multimodality treatment is inadvisable in view of disease location, ureteric obstruction and renal dysfunction. The preferred option would be radical cystectomy.

### Is there any evidence for the use of neoadjuvant chemotherapy in this setting?

Numerous trials have attempted to show a survival benefit in favour of preoperative chemotherapy for patients with muscle-invasive bladder cancer. Most produced, at best, results of borderline statistical significance owing to small sample sizes and/or suboptimal treatment regimens. However, two recent meta-analyses[5,6] have shown that there is a definite 5–6.5% absolute survival benefit favouring the use of neoadjuvant treatment over localized treatment. Treatment-related morbidity was an issue, with 1.1% mortality attributable to chemotherapy, but overall was thought to be acceptable.

The meta-analyses show that cisplatin regimens confer a clear benefit compared with the alternatives, and MVAC (methotrexate, vincristine, doxorubicin and cisplatin) seems superior (at least in the metastatic setting) to single-agent cisplatin and CISCA (cisplatin, cyclophosphamide and doxorubicin). The use of CM (methotrexate and cisplatin) is controversial, with one study showing non-inferiority[7] in an adjuvant setting. The gemcitabine/cisplatin combination has not been adequately tested in this setting to date.

In summary, the current evidence favours MVAC as the preferred regimen, given in three preoperative cycles. It is the only regimen with level I evidence (large prospective randomized controlled trials and meta-analyses thereof) in its favour. The use of high-dose intensity MVAC (2-week cycles with granulocyte-colony stimulating factor support) has been also advocated. It potentially minimizes delay to surgical treatment, has a better toxicity profile and at least similar if not better outcomes as shown in a recent European Organisation for Research and Treatment of Cancer (EORTC) trial in the palliative setting.[8] However, it has not been formally assessed in the neoadjuvant setting.

### What factors may influence the decision to use neoadjuvant chemotherapy in this particular patient?

In this relatively young and otherwise fit patient the main factor determining whether she should be offered neoadjuvant treatment will be the degree of recovery of her renal function. This should be established in an accurate fashion, e.g. nuclear medicine EDTA creatinine clearance estimation, and followed closely throughout the course of treatment.

### Is adjuvant chemotherapy a reasonable/valid option?

Concerns with regard to treatment delay adversely affecting outcomes[9] have prompted investigation into the use of postoperative adjuvant chemotherapy. Unfortunately most studies done to date were small and/or prematurely terminated, e.g. see references 10 and 11. A recent meta-analysis of individual patient data in patients receiving cisplatin-based chemotherapy has shown an absolute survival benefit of up to 9% at 3 years,[12] although it was commented that 'the current evidence is clearly limited with too few trials and too few patients on which to base reliable treatment decisions'. A large-scale randomized controlled trial comparing immediate and deferred chemotherapy (EORTC 30994) at time of relapse is ongoing to attempt to clarify the situation.

Of note, to date, no direct comparisons have been made comparing pure adjuvant with neoadjuvant regimens. Treatment decisions should be tailored to the individual patient, taking into account their overall performance score, comorbidities (especially renal impairment), personal preference and extent of the disease. In this patient's case, given the lack of definite evidence, adjuvant treatment is not advised as a treatment option. Participation in a clinical trial would be appropriate.

Figure 14.1 summarizes the steps in the management of bladder cancer.

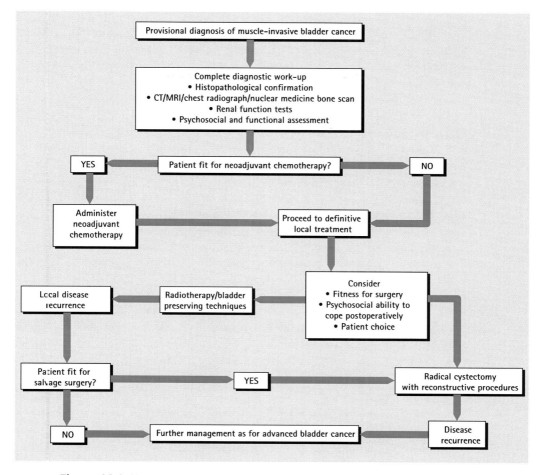

**Figure 14.1** Algorithm for management of localized muscle-invasive bladder cancer.

## Conclusion

The extent of this patient's cancer should be explored by cystoscopy and imaging. Once the cancer has been diagnosed and staged, appropriate treatment can be instigated, of which surgery will be a major component.

## Further Reading

1 Bondavalli C, Dall'Oglio B, Schiavon L, Luciano M, Guatelli S, Parma P, Galletta V. Complications of urinary diversion after radiotherapy. *Arch Ital Urol Androl* 2003; **75**: 10–13.

2 Chahal R, Sundaram SK, Iddenden R, Forman DF, Weston PM, Harrison SC. A study of the morbidity, mortality and long-term survival following radical cystectomy and radical radiotherapy in the treatment of invasive bladder cancer in Yorkshire. *Eur Urol* 2003; **43**: 246–57.

3 Shelley MD, Barber J, Wilt T, Mason MD. Surgery versus radiotherapy for muscle invasive bladder cancer. *Cochrane Database Syst Rev* 2002; **1**: CD002079.

4 Rodel C, Grabenbauer GG, Kuhn R, Papadopoulos T, Dunst J, Meyer M, Schrott KM, Sauer R. Combined-modality treatment and selective organ preservation in invasive bladder cancer: long-term results. *J Clin Oncol* 2002; **20**: 3061–71.

5 Advanced Bladder Cancer Overview Collaboration. Neoadjuvant chemotherapy for invasive bladder cancer. *Cochrane Database Syst Rev* 2005; **2**: CD005246.

6 Winquist E, Kirchner TS, Segal R, Chin J, Lukka H; Genitourinary Cancer Disease Site Group, Cancer Care Ontario Program in Evidence-based Care Practice Guidelines Initiative. Neoadjuvant chemotherapy for transitional cell carcinoma of the bladder: a systematic review and meta-analysis. *J Urol* 2004; **171**: 561–9.

7 Lehmann J, Retz M, Wiemers C, Beck J, Thuroff J, Weining C, Albers P, Frohneberg D, Becker T, Funke PJ, Walz P, Langbein S, Reiher F, Schiller M, Miller K, Roth S, Kalble T, Sternberg D, Wellek S, Stockle M; AUO-AB 05/95. Adjuvant cisplatin plus methotrexate versus methotrexate, vinblastine, epirubicin, and cisplatin in locally advanced bladder cancer: results of a randomized, multicenter, phase III trial (AUO-AB 05/95). *J Clin Oncol* 2005; **23**: 4963–74.

8 Sternberg CN, de Mulder P, Schornagel JH, Theodore C, Fossa SD, van Oosterom AT, Witjes JA, Spina M, van Groeningen CJ, Duclos B, Roberts JT, de Balincourt C, Collette L; EORTC Genito-Urinary Cancer Group. Seven year update of an EORTC phase III trial of high-dose intensity M-VAC chemotherapy and G-CSF versus classic M-VAC in advanced urothelial tract tumours. *Eur J Cancer* 2006; **42**: 50–4.

9 Fahmy NM, Mahmud S, Aprikian AG. Delay in the surgical treatment of bladder cancer and survival: systematic review of the literature. *Eur Urol* 2006; **50**: 1176–82.

10 Studer UE, Bacchi M, Biedermann C, Jaeger P, Kraft R, Mazzucchelli L, Markwalder R, Senn E, Sonntag RW. Adjuvant cisplatin chemotherapy following cystectomy for bladder cancer: results of a prospective randomized trial. *J Urol* 1994; **152**: 81–4.

11 Lehmann J, Franzaring L, Thuroff J, Wellek S, Stockle M. Complete long-term survival data from a trial of adjuvant chemotherapy vs control after radical cystectomy for locally advanced bladder cancer. *BJU Int* 2006; **97**: 42–7.

12 Advanced Bladder Cancer (ABC) Meta-analysis Collaboration. Adjuvant chemotherapy for invasive bladder cancer (individual patient data). *Cochrane Database Syst Rev* 2006; Issue 3.

# 15 Advanced Bladder Cancer

## Case History

A 70-year-old retired textile factory worker presents with recurrent haematuria and groin pain. Investigations confirmed the presence of a bladder tumour that is locally advanced and invading the lateral pelvic wall. Biopsies confirm multiple-site nodal involvement, including the retroperitoneum, but no visceral metastases. He has a good performance status.

**What are the risk factors for bladder cancer?**

**Describe the clinical staging system used in bladder cancer. What are its prognostic implications?**

**Does palliative chemotherapy have a role in this setting?**

**What is the likely prognosis in this patient?**

**If the patient showed a good response to first-line chemotherapy would there be a role for second-line treatment on disease recurrence?**

## Background

### What are the risk factors for bladder cancer?

Environmental factors are thought to account for most bladder neoplasms. Exposure to potentially toxic compounds, such as aromatic amines, accounts for up to 20% of all bladder cancer cases. The risk has been well documented. For employees in the aluminium, petrochemical and textile industries; more recent studies have suggested increased risk also for people constantly exposed to diesel fumes, such as professional drivers.

Smoking confers up to three times increased risk of developing a transitional cell carcinoma (TCC); this appears to increase approximately linearly with duration of exposure. Smoking cessation reduces it by about 40% within four years, but it never returns to baseline. Up to two-thirds of all bladder cancers could be directly attributable to smoking, due to its high prevalence.[1]

Chronic bladder inflammation, e.g. secondary to urinary stones or schistosomiasis, is also known to predispose to neoplasia, although in this setting squamous cell carcinomas are more common.

Radiotherapy to the pelvis and previous chemotherapy with cyclophosphamide-containing regimens have also been shown to be associated with secondary bladder malignancies with relatively short (<10 years) latency periods. The risk has been variously reported to range from 1.5 to 9 times the baseline risk.

### Describe the clinical staging system used in bladder cancer. What are its prognostic implications?

The currently used staging system is based on the 2002 TNM classification,[2] in which the clinical/pathological T stage has the most important role (Tables 15.1 and 15.2). This classification is still somewhat debated, with considerable inter- and intra-observer variability, especially for pT1 tumours. Substaging of the T2 and T3 categories also remains controversial, with several studies failing to find remarkable differences in survival or recurrence rates in subdivisions of the current stages.

Up to 30% of T1 lesions are multifocal at diagnosis or will go on to develop metachronous lesions. Up to 80% will recur after 12 months of complete transurethral resection of bladder tumour (TURBT), and overall up to 30% will go on to develop muscle-invasive

**Table 15.1  TNM classification of bladder cancer**

| T value | Maximum tumour depth invasion |
| --- | --- |
| 1 | Subepithelial connective tissue (lamina propria) |
| 2 | Bladder muscle (muscularis propria) |
| 3 | Perivesical tissue |
| 4a | Prostate/bladder/uterus |
| 4b | Pelvic wall or other adjacent viscera |

**Table 15.2  Staging bladder cancer**

| Stage | TNM |
| --- | --- |
| I | T1 N0 M0 |
| II | T2 N0 M0 |
| III | T3/4a N0 M0 |
| IV | T4b N>0 M1 |

**Table 15.3  Five- and 10-year survival rates and 10-year recurrence-free rates**

| Stage | 5-year overall survival (%) | 10-year overall survival (%) | 10-year recurrence-free rate (%) |
| --- | --- | --- | --- |
| pT2 N0 | 77 | 57 | 87 |
| pT3a N0 | 64 | 44 | 76 |
| pT3b N0 | 49 | 29 | 61 |
| pT4a N0 | 44 | 23 | 45 |
| LN positive | 31 | 23 | 34 |

disease even with optimal local treatment.[3] Once the disease spreads into the muscularis propria (T2 and higher) then the survival rates start dropping sharply. Even with radical cystectomy, patients with bladder-confined disease have an up to 50% 5-year recurrence rate (Table 15.3) – although this is less in lower-stage disease.[4]

# Discussion

### Does palliative chemotherapy have a role in this setting?

Once the disease has spread beyond the confines of the bladder (T4b N≥2 M1), the outlook is bleak; even with the best supportive treatment the median survival is in the region of 5 months. As TCC of the bladder is relatively chemosensitive, different regimens have been devised to take advantage of this and have pushed overall survival to 12–14 months in this category of patients. More importantly, patients who show a complete response (up to 20% using modern regimens such as MVAC [methotrexate, vincristine, doxorubicin and cisplatin] + granulocyte-colony stimulating factor [G-CSF] and gemcitabine + cisplatin[5]) can remain disease free for considerable lengths of time.

In terms of available regimens, the evidence currently favours the use of cisplatin-containing ones. For a long time MVAC remained the standard of care, as it was shown to be superior to single-agent cisplatin,[6] and various other cisplatin-containing regimens (e.g. CMV, CIMV, CM, CISCA [cisplatin, cyclophosphamide and doxorubicin]) had comparable results in phase II trials. Though overall response rates are >50%, toxicity remained high (neutropenic sepsis occurs in about 10%, treatment-related death in up to 4% of patients[7]) and 5-year survival rates are low at around 10%.

More recently a large phase III European Organisation for Research and Treatment of Cancer (EORTC) trial has shown high dose intensity (HD) MVAC with G-CSF support to be superior to the standard regimen (in terms of response, 62% versus 50% and PFS 9.1 months versus 8.2 months for HD-MVAC and classic MVAC, respectively) with appreciably less toxicity.[5] However, there was no statistical difference in overall survival.

The combination of gemcitabine with cisplatin has also been recently compared in a randomized trial. It was shown to be equivalent in terms of survival and response rates, but again with a much better toxicity profile.[8] Platinum-taxane combinations, although promising in phase II clinical trials, have considerable side effects and have not been shown to be superior to MVAC or gemcitabine + cisplatin. Carboplatin has been substituted for cisplatin in patients with poor performance status and/or inadequate renal function, and although it does show activity, response rates tend to be lower and it is considered to be inferior.[9]

### What is the likely prognosis in this patient?

Certain prognostic indicators in bladder cancer have been well documented.[10] Visceral metastases and poor performance status appear to be the most crucial, with considerable differences between the median survival times for patients who had zero, one, or two of these factors (33, 13.4 and 9.3 months, respectively). Thus this patient appears to be in a favourable prognostic group. Moreover, if he shows a complete response to chemotherapy with no evidence of residual disease, he will be eligible for consolidation treatment with surgery or radiotherapy. This has been found to enhance outcomes further,[11] although it should be noted that there is still a high possibility of relapse.

### If the patient showed a good response to first-line chemotherapy would there be a role for second-line treatment on disease recurrence?

Second-line chemotherapy in TCC is a difficult proposition, as by the time of relapse the patient's performance status and renal function will probably make eligibility for further aggressive treatment a remote possibility. Moreover, the likely previous use of a cisplatin-containing regimen also limits the choice of available agents. Regimens containing ifosfamide, taxane and oxaliplatin have been tried with response rates of up to 20% but their use is often limited by the associated toxicities and/or the patient's performance status. There are few data on the use of gemcitabine/cisplatin in patients previously treated with MVAC and vice versa. However, it remains a possibility if the renal function is good and there is a prolonged disease-free interval.

Research on monoclonal antibody and molecular-targeted small molecule therapy and also newer agents such as vinflunine and pemetrexed is currently under way. Patients in this situation should be considered for clinical trials.

## Conclusion

Although metastatic bladder cancer is generally associated with poor long-term survival, this patient has good performance status and no visceral metastases, so may have an improved prognosis if the tumour responds significantly to the chemotherapy regimen selected.

## Further Reading

1 Brennan P, Bogillot O, Cordier S, Greiser E, Schill W, Vineis P, Lopez-Abente G, Tzonou A, Chang-Claude J, Bolm-Audorff U, Jockel KH, Donato F, Serra C, Wahrendorf J, Hours M, T'Mannetje A, Kogevinas M, Boffetta P. Cigarette smoking and bladder cancer in men: a pooled analysis of 11 case-control studies. *Int J Cancer* 2000; **86**: 289–94.

2 American Joint Committee on Cancer. *AJCC Cancer Staging Manual*. Springer, New York, 2002.

3 Lamm DL, Riggs DR, Bugaj M. Proceedings of the first Lübeck symposium on superficial bladder cancer. D Juchan, A Böhle, eds. Oxford, Toronto, Philadelphia: The Medicine Publishing Foundation; 1997. 63–74.

4 Stein JP, Lieskovsky G, Cote R, Groshen S, Feng AC, Boyd S, Skinner E, Bochner B, Thangathurai D, Mikhail M, Raghavan D, Skinner DG. Radical cystectomy in the treatment of invasive bladder cancer: long-term results in 1,054 patients. *J Clin Oncol* 2001; **19**: 666–75.

5 Sternberg CN, de Mulder P, Schornagel JH, Theodore C, Fossa SD, van Oosterom AT, Witjes JA, Spina M, van Groeningen CJ, Duclos B, Roberts JT, de Balincourt C, Collette L; EORTC Genito-Urinary Cancer Group. Seven year update of an EORTC phase III trial of high-dose intensity M-VAC chemotherapy and G-CSF versus classic M-VAC in advanced urothelial tract tumours. *Eur J Cancer* 2006; **42**: 50–4.

6 Loehler PJ, Einhorn LH, Elson PJ, *et al.* A randomized comparison of cisplatin alone or in combination with methotrexate, vinblastine, and doxorubicin in patients with metastatic urothelial carcinoma. *J Clin Oncol* 1992; **10**: 1066–73.

7 Bamias A, Tiliakos I, Karali MD, Dimopoulos MA. Systemic chemotherapy in inoperable or metastatic bladder cancer. *Ann Oncol* 2006; **17**: 553–61.

8   von der Maase H, Sengelov L, Roberts JT, Ricci S, Dogliotti L, Oliver T, Moore MJ, Zimmermann A, Arning M. Long-term survival results of a randomized trial comparing gemcitabine plus cisplatin, with methotrexate, vinblastine, doxorubicin, plus cisplatin in patients with bladder cancer. *J Clin Oncol* 2005; **23**: 4602–8.

9   Chester JD, Hall GD, Forster M, Protheroe AS. Systemic chemotherapy for patients with bladder cancer – current controversies and future directions. *Cancer Treat Rev* 2004; **30**: 343–58.

10  Bajorin DF, Dodd PM, Mazumdar M, *et al.* Long-term survival in metastatic transitional-cell carcinoma and prognostic factors predicting outcome of therapy. *J Clin Oncol* 1999; **17**: 3173–81.

11  Herr HW, Donat SM, Bajorin DF. Post-chemotherapy surgery in patients with unresectable or regionally metastatic bladder cancer. *J Urol* 2001; **165**: 811–14.

**PROBLEM**

# 16  Treatment Options in Early Prostate Cancer

## Case History

A 68-year-old man with newly diagnosed prostate cancer has a prostate-specific antigen (PSA) of 11 ng/ml, Gleason score of 7 (4 + 3), and asymmetrically enlarged nodular prostate on digital rectal examination. The clinical stage of the tumour is cT2b (TNM classification). He has no medical problems and leads an active life.

**What are the treatment options?**

**What is watchful waiting?**

**What are the options for radical treatment?**

**What is the prognosis?**

## Background

### What are the treatment options?

Which is most effective therapy for clinically localized prostate cancer is not clear. The three standard treatment options for men with early stage (organ-confined) prostate cancer are: radical prostatectomy; radiotherapy (external beam radiotherapy (EBRT) or brachytherapy or both); and watchful waiting.

### What is watchful waiting?

The term watchful waiting is used when men choose to forego or defer active treatment for observation. Therapy is typically started if one of the following occurs: a marked increase in serum PSA[1] or a decrease in PSA doubling time to 3 years or less, a change on digital rectal examination, or detection of disease progression on surveillance biopsies.

The rationale for watchful waiting is that not all prostate cancers are clinically important, and that radical therapy constitutes over-treatment. This approach is based on data from Sweden.[2] However, longer follow-up in that study (21 years) showed that only 36% remained progression-free at 15 years, and 50% had developed metastases.[3] Randomized controlled trials are lacking in men with early stage prostate cancer, and only one trial has directly compared watchful waiting and radical prostatectomy in men with clinically localized disease, demonstrating a marked improvement in disease-specific survival as well as overall survival in men undergoing surgery.[4] In 1994, Epstein *et al.*[5] developed a set of criteria that could be used at the time of biopsy to predict the presence of clinically unimportant disease, which then could be used to decide if watchful waiting was an option. Men aged 70–75 years and older, and those with substantial comorbidity that may severely limit their life expectancy (e.g. to less than 10 years) may be considered for watchful waiting. Although younger men with favourable tumour characteristics may also do well with watchful waiting, published data show a considerably higher death rate with watchful waiting than with radical prostatectomy, particularly in those aged 65 and younger.[4] Men who are considering watchful waiting should be aware that the risk of cancer progression and death is increased if treatment is deferred.

## Discussion

### What are the options for radical treatment?

Radical treatment is given with curative intent and consists of radical prostatectomy or radiotherapy. No published trials have directly compared radical prostatectomy with either EBRT or brachytherapy. Observational series provide the only available data comparing outcomes following radical prostatectomy and radiotherapy, but they are fraught with bias. One important reason is that young, healthy men are typically encouraged to undergo radical prostatectomy and older men tend to be steered toward radiotherapy or observation. Radical prostatectomy can be carried out by a retropubic or perineal approach, or laparoscopically. For men who undergo radical prostatectomy, outcome prediction can be refined based on pathological characteristics such as seminal vesicle involvement, extraprostatic extension, surgical margin status, and whether nodal metastases are present.[6] Severe or life-threatening complications are rare. The adverse effects of greatest concern are damage to the urinary sphincter and penile nerves, resulting in urinary incontinence and impotence, respectively.[7]

Radical prostate radiotherapy is of two types: EBRT and interstitial implantation (brachytherapy). Complications after EBRT include bladder irritation (urgency, pain, frequency) in up to 5% of men, and impotence in 40–50%.[8] In contrast with surgery, these complications tend to increase over time. However, non-randomized data have shown that important differences in urinary, bowel, and sexual function continue to be evident at 2 years following treatment with either EBRT or radical prostatectomy, but are less marked at 5 years.[9] Newer three-dimensional conformal radiotherapy (3D-CRT) with sophisticated computer modelling minimizing damage to surrounding normal tissues, may help reduce the complications of radiotherapy. Brachytherapy usually involves placing radioactive, rice-sized pellets directly into the prostate gland; radiation is emitted from within the gland for a specified period of time and then dissipates.

The advantage of brachytherapy over EBRT is primarily convenience; interstitial implantation requires only a one-time insertion in an outpatient setting. Prostate inflammation and swelling can occur acutely following brachytherapy, suggesting that men with major urinary symptoms or a large prostate are not good candidates. Later complications include irritative voiding symptoms, urinary retention, rectal urgency, bowel frequency, rectal bleeding or ulceration, and prostatorectal fistula.[10] The incidence of erectile dysfunction varies.

Brachytherapy can be considered a reasonable option for men with low-risk disease. It is not recommended as monotherapy for higher-risk disease. Hormone therapy in men with early-stage disease can be used as definitive treatment or as an adjunct to local treatment (neoadjuvant hormone treatment), or, less commonly, in the adjuvant setting. Practice patterns in the USA suggest that the use of primary hormone treatment is increasing over time.[11] A randomized phase III study from France has shown evidence that immediate androgen suppression with an luteinizing hormone releasing hormone (LHRH) analogue given during and for 3 years after EBRT improves disease-free and overall survival of patients with locally advanced prostate cancer.[12]

### What is the prognosis?

In the USA, the 5-year survival for patients with early stage prostate cancer is 100% and in Europe it is around 50–60%. This difference is thought to be due to non-standardized screening in Europe.

The prognosis can be divided into clinical, pathological and molecular prognosis. The most important clinical prognostic indicators of disease outcome in prostate cancer are the pretreatment PSA level and Gleason score. Partin *et al.*'s normogram is widely used to predict pathological stage for men with clinically localized prostate cancer based on pretreatment PSA level, Gleason score and clinical stage.[13] Tumour stage and Gleason score are the most important pathological prognostic markers following surgery, with the pathological stage of the tumour being a strong predictor of outcome. Molecular and cellular prognostic markers are helpful in patients whose PSA levels and Gleason scores are intermediate so that accurate prognostication may be difficult. Most of these potential markers are still under investigation. Markers of potential value are: p53 tumour suppressor gene, bcl-2 proto-oncogene, proliferation marker (Ki-67), the apoptotic index, and angiogenesis.

## Conclusion

This patient has an intermediate prognosis. The three treatment options should be discussed with him.

# Further Reading

1   Carter CA, Donahue T, Sun L, Wu H, McLeod DG, Amling C, Lance R, Foley J, Sexton W, Kusuda L, Chung A, Soderdahl D, Jackmaan S, Moul JW. Temporarily deferred therapy (watchful waiting) for men younger than 70 years and with low-risk localized prostate cancer in the prostate-specific antigen era. *J Clin Oncol* 2003; **21**: 4001.

2   Johansson JE, Adami HO, Andersson SO, Bergstrom R, Holmberg L, Krusemo UB. High 10-year survival rate in patients with early, untreated prostatic cancer. *JAMA* 1992; **267**: 2191.

3   Johansson JE, Andren O, Andersson SO, Dickman PW, Holmberg L, Magnuson A, Adami HO. Natural history of early, localized prostate cancer. *JAMA* 2004; **291**: 2713.

4   Holmberg L, Bill-Axelson A, Helgesen F, Salo JO, Folmerz P, Haggman M, Andersson SO, Spangberg A, Busch C, Nordling S, Palmgren J, Adami HO, Johansson JE, Norlen BJ; Scandinavian Prostatic Cancer Group Study Number 4. A randomized trial comparing radical prostatectomy with watchful waiting in early prostate cancer. *N Engl J Med* 2002; **347**: 781–9.

5   Epstein JI, Walsh PC, Carmichael M, Brendler CB. Pathologic and clinical findings to predict tumor extent of nonpalpable (stage T1c) prostate cancer. *JAMA* 1994; **271**: 368–74.

6   Gerber GS, Thisted RA, Scardino PT, Frohmuller HG, Schroeder FH, Paulson DF, Middleton AW Jr, Rukstalis DB, Smith JA Jr, Schellhammer PF, Ohori M, Chodak GW. Results of radical prostatectomy in men with clinically localized prostate cancer. *JAMA* 1996; **276**: 615–19.

7   Naitoh J, Zeiner RL, Dekernion JB. Diagnosis and treatment of prostate cancer [see comments]. *Am Fam Physician* 1998; **57**: 1531.

8   Hamilton AS, Stanford JL, Gilliland FD, Albertsen PC, Stephenson RA, Hoffman RM, Eley JW, Harlan LC, Potosky AL. Health outcomes after external-beam radiation therapy for clinically localized prostate cancer: results from the prostate cancer outcomes study. *J Clin Oncol* 2001; **19**: 2517–26.

9   Potosky AL, Legler J, Albertsen PC, Stanford JL, Gilliland FD, Hamilton AS, Eley JW, Stephenson RA, Harlan LC. Health outcomes after prostatectomy or radiotherapy for prostate cancer: results from the prostate cancer outcomes study. *J Natl Cancer Inst* 2000; **92**: 1582–92.

10   Gelblum DY, Potters L. Rectal complications associated with transperineal interstitial brachytherapy for prostate cancer. *Int J Radiat Oncol Biol Phys* 2000; **48**: 119.

11   Cooperberg MR, Grossfeld GD, Lubeck DP, Carroll PR. National practice patterns and time trends in androgen ablation for localized prostate cancer. *J Natl Cancer Inst* 2003; **95**: 981–9.

12   Bolla M, Collette L, Blank L, Warde P, Dubois JB, Mirimanoff RO, Storme G, Bernier J, Kuten A, Sternberg C, Mattelaer J, Lopez Torecilla J, Pfeffer JR, Lino Cutajar C, Zurlo A, Pierart M. Long term results with immediate androgen suppression and external irradiation in patients with locally advanced prostate cancer (an EORTC study): a phase III randomised trial. *Lancet* 2002; **13**: 103–6.

13   Partin AW, Kattan MW, Subong EN, Walsh PC, Wojno KJ, Oesterling JE, Scardino PT, Pearson JD. Combination of prostate specific antigen, clinical stage and Gleason score to predict pathologic stage of localised prostate cancer. A multi-institutional update. *JAMA* 1997; **277**: 1445–51.

# 17 Treatment Options in Locally Advanced Prostate Cancer

## Case History

A 77-year-old man is diagnosed as having prostate cancer. His prostate-specific antigen (PSA) level is 15 ng/ml, there is a nodular, asymmetrical prostate on digital rectal examination, his Gleason score is 8 (4 + 4) and his staging is pT3a N0 M0 on imaging. He lives alone, has no relatives close by, and he walks 4.5–6.5 km every day. He is referred to the oncology clinic from the urology department.

**What are the treatment options for pT3 disease?**

**What drugs are available for hormone treatment?**

**What are the side effects of hormone treatment?**

## Background

The patterns of diagnosis and treatment of prostate cancer have changed in the past 15 years coinciding with the introduction of prostate-specific antigen (PSA) screening in the late 1980s. Between 1984 and 1991, 30–40% of men presented with advanced disease, whereas currently only 5% have distant metastases at the time of diagnosis.[1] In contemporary series, approximately 10–12% of men with newly diagnosed disease have locally advanced (clinical stage T3–T4) or metastatic disease at diagnosis.[2] Hormone treatment or androgen deprivation treatment (ADT) is the primary therapeutic approach for advanced prostate cancer because the suppression of androgens decreases tumour progression. As the testes are the major source of androgenic steroids, ADT can be accomplished with bilateral orchidectomy or with medical treatments.

## Discussion

### What are the treatment options for pT3 disease?

Locally advanced prostate cancer (cT3) can be treated with radiotherapy and hormone treatment is usually started 2 months before and continued during radiotherapy. Radiotherapy should be delivered in a way that ensures a curative dose to the prostate and minimizes rectal and bladder toxicity. A standard dose is 55 Gy over 20 fractions.

The outcome for radiotherapy is as good as for radical prostatectomy, and use of Partin *et al.*'s tables can help to define the likelihood of organ-confined disease.[3]

Radical prostatectomy has not been widely accepted but may be appropriate in younger men.[4] Pretreatment prognostic variables, using Epstein's criteria,[5] may help the selection of a subgroup of men with cT3 disease with the most favourable long-term outcomes following radical prostatectomy. Most men with locally advanced prostate cancer are advised to undergo some form of definitive local treatment (such as radiotherapy) but hormone treatment alone may represent a reasonable option for men who are medically unfit or who have a limited life expectancy.

### What drugs are available for hormone treatment?

Hormone treatment or ADT is the primary therapeutic approach for men with T4 and metastatic prostate cancer, alleviating metastatic bone pain in 80–90% and leading to objective responses in serum PSA level, and soft tissue and bone disease. Although ADT may modestly prolong survival,[6] it is palliative and not curative. Most of the men who initially respond to ADT progress to a 'hormone-refractory' state within 18–24 months, and the median survival is 24–30 months.

The following drugs for ADT are available:

- Continuous treatment with luteinizing hormone releasing hormone (LHRH) agonists, such as leuprolide and goserelin, reduces LH production, and, therefore, production of testicular androgens. These drugs cause a flare phenomenon, which can be avoided by concomitant use of anti-androgens such as bicalutamide.

- Oestrogen reduces LH production by its inhibitory effect on the hypothalamic/pituitary axis and diethylstilbestrol (DES) is most often used in metastatic prostate cancers.

- Non-steroidal anti-androgens, such as flutamide, bicalutamide, and nilutamide block the androgen receptors.

The optimal method of initial ADT has not been established. Much of the debate centres on the utility of complete androgen blockade (CAB), which can be achieved by using anti-androgens and LHRH agonists rather than monotherapy.[7] Published guidelines from the American Society of Clinical Oncology (ASCO) do not recommend CAB in preference to monotherapy as first-line ADT for men with metastatic prostate cancer. Instead orchidectomy or an LHRH agonist, such as goserelin, is recommended.[8] Most men prefer an LHRH agonist to bilateral orchidectomy for psychosocial reasons.

The timing of initiating treatment is also controversial. Many clinicians advocate starting treatment at the time of diagnosis in the hope of delaying disease progression and extending survival. Others argue that there is no evidence for a marked survival benefit with any form of ADT, and that treatment is best deferred until symptoms develop. However, early treatment seems to have more benefits.[9] In an attempt to minimize treatment-related adverse effects, potency-preserving strategies are under study and intermittent androgen deprivation has been used. Anti-androgen monotherapy with bicalutamide is a possibility, but concerns about inferior survival and the cost of higher-dose therapy have limited its use. Furthermore, bicalutamide (at any dose) is not approved as monotherapy for treatment of prostate cancer.

### What are the side effects of hormone treatment?

Management of side effects and quality of life issues are important when considering treatment in men who have advanced prostate cancer. Many adverse effects are common to ADT in general and include: sexual dysfunction; osteoporosis and bone fractures; vasomotor symptoms; and gynaecomastia.

## Conclusion

The case study patient has locally advanced prostate cancer and should be started on first-line hormone treatment such as goserelin. Radiotherapy should also be considered.

## Further Reading

1  Jemal A, Siegel R, Ward E, Murray T, Xu J, Smigal C, Thun MJ. Cancer statistics, 2006. *CA Cancer J Clin* 2006; **56**: 106–30.

2  Cooperberg MR, Moul JW, Carroll PR. The changing face of prostate cancer. *J Clin Oncol* 2005; **23**: 8146.

3  Partin AW, Kattan MW, Subong EN, Walsh PC, Wojno KJ, Oesterling JE, Scardio PT, Pearson JD. Combination of prostate specific antigen, clinical stage and Gleason score to predict pathologic stage of localised prostate cancer. A multi-institutional update. *JAMA* 1997; **277**: 1445–51.

4  Ward JF, Slezak JM, Blute ML, Bergstralh EJ, Zincke H. Radical prostatectomy for clinically advanced (cT3) prostate cancer since the advent of prostate-specific antigen testing: 15-year outcome. *BJU Int* 2005; **95**: 751–6.

5  Epstein JI, Walsh PC, Carmichael M, Brendler CB. Pathologic and clinical findings to predict tumor extent of nonpalpable (stage T1c) prostate cancer. *JAMA* 1994; **271**: 368–74.

6  Robson M, Dawson N. How is androgen-dependent metastatic prostate cancer best treated? *Hematol Oncol Clin North Am* 1996; **10**: 727.

7  Eisenberger MA, Blumenstein BA, Crawford ED, Miller G, McLeod DG, Loehrer PJ, Wilding G, Sears K, Culkin DJ, Thompson IM Jr, Bueschen AJ, Lowe BA. Bilateral orchiectomy with or without flutamide for metastatic prostate cancer. *N Engl J Med* 1998; **339**: 1036–42.

8  Loblaw DA, Mendelson DS, Talcott JA, Virgo KS, Somerfield MR, Ben-Josef E, Middleton R, Porterfield H, Sharp SA, Smith TJ, Taplin ME, Vogelzang NJ, Wade JL Jr, Bennett CL, Scher HI; American Society of Clinical Oncology. American Society of Clinical Oncology recommendations for the initial hormonal management of androgen-sensitive metastatic, recurrent, or progressive prostate cancer. *J Clin Oncol* 2004; **22**: 2927–41.

9  Nair B, Wilt T, MacDonald R, Rutks I. Early versus deferred androgen suppression in the treatment of advanced prostatic cancer (Cochrane Review). *Cochrane Database Syst Rev* 2002; **1**: CD003506.

**PROBLEM**

# 18 Treatment Options in Relapsing Prostate Cancer

## Case History

A 65-year-old man attends the outpatient department 1 year after undergoing radical radiotherapy. He feels well and leads an active life. Biochemistry reveals increased levels of prostate-specific antigen (PSA). He is not on any medication and examination is unremarkable.

**What are the treatment options for PSA-only progression?**

**What are the treatment options for patients in whom prostatectomy has been unsuccessful?**

**What are the treatment options for patients in whom radiotherapy has been unsuccessful?**

**What are the hormonal treatment options?**

**What other treatments are available?**

## Background

Because of the changing demographic patterns of prostate cancer[1] and changing clinical practice, clinicians see a growing population of men who have received primary treatment for localized prostate cancer and who require follow-up for disease progression and monitoring for the complications of radical therapy. Regular history taking, physical examination and PSA testing every 6–12 months are thought to be sufficient.[2] Follow-up strategies for these men should focus on identifying relapse and the potential complications of progression (e.g. bone pain, spinal cord compression). Disease recurrence may manifest by biochemical (PSA-only) relapse, local recurrence or metastatic (systemic) disease.

## Discussion

### What are the treatment options for PSA-only progression?

PSA-only early progression (biochemical failure) after radical prostatectomy or radiotherapy for early-stage disease is a common scenario. In 1997, a consensus panel convened by the American Society for Therapeutic Radiology and Oncology (ASTRO) agreed guidelines to define PSA recurrence after radiotherapy,[3] but these are neither widely used nor binding.

For men with a rising serum PSA level following definitive local treatment for early-stage disease, a thorough diagnostic evaluation including history, examination, haematology and biochemistry testing including PSA, and computed tomography (CT) and bone scans are indicated. Consideration can be given to repeating the biopsy. The main goal is to assess the likelihood of recurrence of localized rather than systemic disease to select those men who are candidates for potentially curative local salvage therapy. The curative options for men with a PSA-only recurrence include prostate bed irradiation in the situation of failed prior prostatectomy, and salvage prostatectomy and possibly cryotherapy in the situation of failed primary radiotherapy. Factors that help to identify patients at risk of not responding to primary treatment are: short time to biochemical recurrence, rapid PSA doubling time and high Gleason score.[4]

### What are the treatment options for patients in whom prostatectomy has been unsuccessful?

For men with failed prostatectomy, who are thought to have a localized recurrence, irradiation provides durable benefit if there is no adverse pathology (i.e. Gleason score <8, negative seminal vesicles or nodes), a low serum PSA (<1.5 ng/ml) at recurrence, and at least a 1-year recurrence-free interval. Although a persistently detectable serum PSA level following prostatectomy most often indicates occult metastatic disease, emerging data suggest that radiotherapy can cure a small but consistent proportion of these patients. Men who have a rapidly rising PSA (particularly a PSA doubling time of 3 months or less) early after radical prostatectomy are least likely to be cured. A consensus panel convened by ASTRO recommended that when salvage radiotherapy to the prostate bed is considered, it should be administered before the serum PSA rises above 1.5 ng/ml, and with radiotherapy doses ≥64 Gy.[5]

### What are the treatment options for patients in whom radiotherapy has been unsuccessful?

For patients with radiation failure and apparently locally recurrent disease prostatectomy should be considered only in those who had organ-confined disease prior to the original radiotherapy and probably still have clinically organ-confined disease. Preoperative evaluation should be directed towards minimizing the possibility of extraprostatic extension and occult micrometastatic disease (using bone scans). In general, appropriate candidates should have a Gleason score <6, pretreatment serum PSA <10 ng/ml, and T1c or T2a tumor stage at initial presentation. At the time of recurrence, the same conditions should be met (ideally, Gleason score <6, tumor stage <T2b, and serum PSA <4.0 ng/ml). The best outcomes are seen in men with a post-radiotherapy PSA doubling time longer than 12 months; a PSA doubling time less than 3 months is a relative contraindication to salvage radical prostatectomy. Before embarking on salvage prostatectomy, men should be counselled about the potential for morbidity, particularly incontinence, and documented informed consent must be obtained.

### What are the hormonal treatment options?

Hormone treatment is the best treatment for men with systemic recurrence, although the optimal timing of therapy is controversial. It is effective in over 90% of men with advanced disease, however, it is not curative. Response to treatment is temporary, with most patients showing disease progression within 2 years. Furthermore, treatment-related side effects can adversely affect the quality of life.

Clinical trials support the view that early hormone treatment may provide a survival advantage in men with positive lymph nodes or asymptomatic systemic disease.[6] Hormone treatment is also commonly used in men with PSA-only recurrence; choices include traditional hormone monotherapy (a luteinizing hormone releasing hormone [LHRH] agonist, orchidectomy), complete androgen block (CAB), or non-traditional (potency-sparing) treatments, such as intermittent androgen deprivation or anti-androgen monotherapy. Although early hormonal treatment may provide a survival benefit for men with node-positive or locally advanced non-metastatic prostate cancer, this has not been proved for PSA-only recurrence. A large multicentre study from the UK provides preliminary evidence that life expectancy may be increased by early detection and immediate treatment of men with localized and PSA-only recurrence.[6] Potency-sparing treatments are appealing, but long-term efficacy is unknown.

### What other treatments are available?

Other treatment options include cryotherapy, participation in clinical trials, second-line hormone treatment and, in some patients, chemotherapy or biological treatments. (However, there is limited long-term experience with salvage cryotherapy for irradiated patients and treatment-related morbidity may be substantial and long-term outcomes are poorly defined.) Chemotherapy is generally reserved for men with hormone-refractory disease, however, in one report, 10 of 23 such men who received docetaxel 70 mg/m² every 21 days had a ≥50% decline in their serum PSA level for at least 4 weeks, and mean testosterone levels were not reduced in the 17 patients who were assessed before and after therapy.[7] Further trial experience of this approach is needed. High frequency ultrasound (HIFU) is a possible alternative to surgery for localized prostate cancers. In March 2005, the National Institute for Health and Clinical Excellence (NICE) issued guidance for the usage of HIFU in prostate cancer.[8]

For men who present with nodal involvement or distant metastatic disease, or who develop a systemic recurrence after initial local treatment, androgen ablation by medical means (e.g. LHRH agonist with or without an anti-androgen) or orchidectomy is the primary mode of treatment.

## Conclusion

This patient should be offered radical prostatectomy if he has no evidence of metastases and if his restaging shows a Gleason score <6, tumor stage <T2b, and serum PSA <4.0 ng/ml, ideally. If he does not meet these criteria he should be given hormone treatment.

## Further Reading

1   Cooperberg MR, Moul JW, Carroll PR. The changing face of prostate cancer. *J Clin Oncol* 2005; **23**: 8146.

2   Prostate-specific antigen (PSA) best practice policy. American Urological Association (AUA). *Oncology (Huntingt)* 2000; **14**: 267.

3   Consensus statement: guidelines for PSA following radiation therapy. American Society for Therapeutic Radiology and Oncology Consensus Panel. *Int J Radiat Oncol Biol Phys* 1997; **37**: 1035.

4   Freedland SJ, Humphreys EB, Mangold LA, Eisenberger M, Dorey FJ, Walsh PC, Partin AW. Risk of prostate cancer-specific mortality following biochemical recurrence after radical prostatectomy. *JAMA* 2005; **294**: 433–9.

5   Cox JD, Gallagher MJ, Hammond EH, Kaplan RS, Schellhammer PF. Consensus statements on radiation therapy of prostate cancer: guidelines for prostate re-biopsy after radiation and for radiation therapy with rising prostate-specific antigen levels after radical prostatectomy. American Society for Therapeutic Radiology and Oncology Consensus Panel. *J Clin Oncol* 1999; **17**: 1155.

6   Immediate versus deferred treatment for advanced prostatic cancer: initial results of the Medical Research Council Trial. The Medical Research Council Prostate Cancer Working Party Investigators Group. *Br J Urol* 1997; **79**: 235.

7   Goodin S, Medina P, Capanna T, Shih WJ, Abraham S, Winnie J, Doyle-Lindrud S, Todd M, DiPaola RS. Effect of docetaxel in patients with hormone-dependent prostate-specific antigen progression after local therapy for prostate cancer. *J Clin Oncol* 2005; **23**: 3352.

8   High intensity focused ultrasound for prostate cancer. London: National Institute for Health and Clinical Excellence. c.2005. Available from: http://guidance.nice.org.uk/IPG118

PROBLEM

# 19  Treatment Options in Hormone-refractory Prostate Cancer

## Case History

A 72-year-old man with known prostate cancer is followed up regularly in clinic. He was diagnosed as having locally advanced cancer and was started on goserelin 23 months ago. His prostate-specific antigen (PSA) level has continued to rise over the past 6 months despite the addition of bicalutamide. He feels very well and has no comorbidities.

**What other hormone treatments can be used?**

**Is chemotherapy an option?**

**What other options are available for him?**

## Background

Hormone ablation treatment with luteinizing hormone releasing hormone (LHRH) agonists alone or in combination with complete androgen blockade (CAB) has become the mainstay of treatment for patients with advanced/metastatic prostate cancer. The definition of hormone-refractory prostate cancer (androgen-independent, androgen-refractory, or hormone-independent) in a man who has undergone androgen deprivation treatment (ADT) requires the demonstration of functionally castrate levels of serum testosterone (<1.7 nmol/l [50 ng/dl]) with biochemical and/or clinical evidence of disease progression. The options for systemic treatment in such men include second-line hormone treatment, systemic chemotherapy and adjunctive treatment including experimental therapies. However, there is no standard approach.

## Discussion

### What other hormone treatments can be used?

● Second-line hormone treatment options are withdrawal of anti-androgens

● administration of other anti-androgens (non-steroidal anti-androgens such as flutamide, bicalutamide and nilutamide; steroidal antiandrogens such as cyproterone acetate and megestrol)

● other hormones including oestrogen (diethylstilbestrol and glucocorticoids, e.g. dexamethasone or prednisone).

The overall response rates vary from 20% to 60% depending on when used but tend to be short lived.
Current guidelines recommend that the first approach should be:[1]

● discontinuation of anti-androgens if the patient is receiving CAB

or

● addition of an anti-androgen if LHRH agonist monotherapy is being administered.

The 'anti-androgen withdrawal syndrome' occurs in approximately 20% of men in whom CAB is unsuccessful and some experience symptomatic or objective improvement. Diethylstilbestrol is a non-steroidal oestrogen and clinical trials showed that it is as effective as orchidectomy in treating metastatic prostate cancer. However, there are more cardiovascular and thromboembolic complications.[2] A dose of 1 mg/day appears to be as effective as 5 mg/day, but it does not lower serum testosterone to castrate levels in all men. The testosterone level frequently begins to rise after 6 to 12 months of treatment.[3] Continuation of primary testicular androgen deprivation is recommended. The median survival of men with hormone-refractory prostate cancer is approximately 12 months.[4]

### Is chemotherapy an option?

Chemotherapy was previously considered to be relatively ineffective in hormone-refractory prostate cancer.[5] In early trials, objective response rates were 8.7%,[6] and median survival did not exceed 12 months. Estramustine phosphate (EMP) alone or in combination with taxanes or vinca alkaloids showed PSA response rates in 25–86% of patients.

Regimens containing taxanes, particularly those that include docetaxel, are associated with higher rates of both objective and biochemical response, and, importantly, a marked prolongation in median survival, approaching 20 months when compared with mitoxantrone.[7] Two landmark trials, TAX 327[7] and SWOG 9916,[8] involved nearly 1800 patients and have shown that docetaxel-based regimens markedly improved survival and reduced the risk of death by 24% and 20%, respectively. Investigators in the TAX 327 trial also reported that docetaxel significantly improved PSA levels by 43% ($P = 0.0005$) and reduced pain by 59% ($P = 0.0107$), relative to the response rates to mitoxantrone.[7] Docetaxel was well tolerated and had a generally predictable and manageable safety profile in both studies. These data have established 3-weekly docetaxel plus daily prednisone as a new standard of care for men with hormone-refractory prostate cancer, and further support the use of 3-weekly rather than the weekly schedule.[7,8] Based on the available evidence the National Institute for Health and Clinical Excellence (NICE) has issued guidance for the use of docetaxel as a treatment option for men with metastatic prostate cancer that is no longer responding to hormone treatment.[9]

### What other options are available for him?

In addition to systemic anti-tumour treatment, adjunctive treatments are often considered for men with progressive hormone-refractory prostate cancer, particularly if they have symptomatic bone metastases. Bone is the most common metastatic site (over 97%[10]), and these lesions are frequently symptomatic – causing pain and functional impairment. Treatment of bone pain is primarily palliative and aims to relieve discomfort, improve mobility, and prevent complications such as pathological fractures or cord compression. In general, treatment does not alter the natural history of the disease, although bisphosphonates may slow the progression of symptomatic bone metastases. Analgesics, local field radiotherapy, radiopharmaceuticals and radiofrequency ablation can be used as well. Whenever possible, patients should be entered into trials and referral to tertiary centres should be considered early in the course.

## Conclusion

This patient has a performance status of 1. The bicalutamide should be withdrawn, followed by treatment with steroids or diethylstilbestrol and then by docetaxel. He should also be offered a place in a clinical trial. If he has evidence of bony metastases on imaging he should be given bisphosphonates, particularly if he is symptomatic.

## Further Reading

1 Chang SS, Benson MC, Campbell SC, Crook J, Dreicer R, Evans CP, Hall MC, Higano C, Kelly WK, Sartor O, Smith JA Jr; Society of Urologic Oncology, Shaumberg, Illinois. Society of Urologic Oncology position statement: redefining the management of hormone-refractory prostate carcinoma. *Cancer* 2005; **103**: 11–21.

2   Byar DP. Proceedings: The Veterans Administration Cooperative Urological Research Group's studies of cancer of the prostate. *Cancer* 1973; **32**: 1126.

3   Byar DP, Corle DK. Hormone therapy for prostate cancer: results of the Veterans Administration Cooperative Urological Research Group studies. *Natl Cancer Inst Monogr* 1988; 165.

4   Smaletz O, Scher HI, Small EJ, Verbel DA, McMillan A, Regan K, Kelly WK, Kattan MW. Nomogram for overall survival of patients with progressive metastatic prostate cancer after castration. *J Clin Oncol* 2002; **20**: 3972–82.

5   Eisenberger MA, Simon R, O'Dwyer PJ, Wittes RE, Friedman MA. A re-evaluation of nonhormonal cytotoxic chemotherapy in the treatment of prostatic carcinoma. *J Clin Oncol* 1985; **3**: 827–41.

6   Yagoda A, Petrylak D. Cytotoxic chemotherapy for advanced hormone-resistant prostate cancer. *Cancer* 1993; **71**: 1098–1109.

7   Tannock IF, de Wit R, Berry WR, Horti J, Pluzanska A, Chi KN, Oudard S, Theodore C, James ND, Turesson I, Rosenthal MA, Eisenberger MA; TAX 327 Investigators. Docetaxel plus prednisone or mitoxantrone plus prednisone for advanced prostate cancer. *N Engl J Med* 2004; **351**: 1502–12.

8   Petrylak DP, Tangen CM, Hussain MH, Lara PN Jr, Jones JA, Taplin ME, Burch PA, Berry D, Moinpour C, Kohli M, Benson MC, Small EJ, Raghavan D, Crawford ED. Docetaxel and estramustine compared with mitoxantrone and prednisone for advanced refractory prostate cancer. *N Engl J Med* 2004; **351**: 1513–20.

9   NICE approves docetaxel as a treatment option for men with advanced prostate cancer. Press release, NICE 2006/031 (www.nice.org.uk/page.aspx?o=335999, accessed 5 May 2007).

10  Small EJ, Halabi S, Dawson NA, Stadler WM, Rini BI, Picus J, Gable P, Torti FM, Kaplan E, Vogelzang NJ. Antiandrogen withdrawal alone or in combination with ketoconazole in androgen-independent prostate cancer patients: a phase III trial (CALGB 9583). *J Clin Oncol* 2004; **22**: 1025–33.

# 20 Screening in Prostate Cancer

## Case History

A 73-year-old white man sees his general practitioner (GP) as he thinks he might have prostate cancer. His medical history is unremarkable other than osteoarthritis. He has prostatism but has no history of urinary tract infection. On digital rectal examination (DRE) his prostate is found to be symmetrically enlarged. His prostate-specific antigen (PSA) level is 5.5 ng/ml and was checked 1 week after the rectal examination.

**What are the causes of raised PSA?**

**What is the importance of the PSA level?**

**What is the likely diagnosis in this patient?**

## Background

Prostate cancer is being detected with increasing frequency, due in part to the widespread availability of serum PSA testing, although the incidence was increasing even before its introduction.

A 'prostate cancer risk management programme' was published in 2002 by Watson *et al.* on behalf of Cancer Research UK.[1] The programme aims to help the primary care team in giving clear and balanced information to men who ask about testing for prostate cancer.

### What are the causes of raised PSA?

The PSA may be raised for many reasons (Box 20.1) and these should be considered prior to a PSA test. In primary care, DRE is usually not recommended as a screening test in asymptomatic men. In men with symptoms, the PSA should be tested before a DRE. If the DRE is done before, the PSA test should be delayed for a week. This issue, however, is controversial and some feel that a PSA can be done immediately after a DRE.[2]

## Discussion

### What is the importance of the PSA level?

Key issues to be discussed with the patient are as follows.

PSA testing aims to detect localized prostate cancer when potentially curative treatment can be offered. It should be made clear that PSA testing is controversial and that profes-

---

**Box 20.1 Benign causes of raised PSA**

- Benign prostatic hypertrophy
- Acute prostatitis
- Subclinical inflammation
- Prostate biopsy in previous 6 weeks
- Cystoscopy
- Trans-urethral resection of the prostrate
- Urinary retention
- Ejaculation
- DRE
- Perineal trauma
- Prostatic infarction

---

sionals disagree on the usefulness of the test for population screening.[3] To date there is no good evidence that screening for prostate cancer using PSA testing reduces mortality.[4]

The traditional cut-off level for the PSA is 4.0 ng/ml,[5] however, some men (up to 20%) with clinically important prostate cancer will not have a raised PSA; and in about two-thirds of men with a raised PSA, prostate cancer is not diagnosed. Many modifications of the PSA test have been attempted, including lowering of cut-offs, serial PSA tests, usage of PSA velocity–PSA density–free PSA–complexed PSA, age-specific reference ranges, and race-specific reference ranges. However, no consensus has been reached and none of the approaches have resulted in a reduction in the number of unnecessary biopsies.[6]

An algorithm for management following PSA testing is given in Box 20.2.

The PSA test is not diagnostic and if raised, a prostate biopsy is required for diagnosis (Box 20.1). There may be complications following the biopsy, including bleeding (~1 in 3 men get haematuria/haematospermia after biopsy) and infection. Up to 20% of clinically important prostate cancers will be missed at biopsy, and if the biopsy is negative consider follow-up and possibly re-biopsy.[10] Biopsy is an uncomfortable experience, and both the PSA test and prostate biopsy may cause much anxiety in men undergoing such a procedure.[11]

---

**Box 20.2 PSA test results and management options**

- If the PSA is >10 ng/ml a prostate biopsy is recommended because the chance of finding prostate cancer is greater than 50%. However, in many men the disease is no longer organ confined and is not amenable to cure[7]

- If the PSA is between 4 ng/ml and 10 ng/ml, a prostate biopsy is usually advised regardless of the DRE findings. However, for every prostate cancer that is detected, four additional men will undergo an unnecessary biopsy

- If the PSA is <4 ng/ml the management is less clear because the majority will have negative biopsy. However, a substantial number of men with prostate cancer have PSA values below 4.0 ng/ml.[8] Men with PSA less than 4.0 ng/ml have a higher likelihood of organ-confined disease[9]

Another difficulty is that treatment may be of benefit only for some men with potentially aggressive tumours detected following PSA testing. Others may have slow-growing cancers that neither cause any symptoms nor shorten life expectancy. For this reason, some men who are tested face unnecessary anxiety, medical tests and treatments with side effects, and it has cost implications for the National Health Service (NHS) or any healthcare system. A Cochrane review by Ilic *et al.* concluded that 'no robust evidence from randomised controlled trials is available regarding the impact of screening on quality of life, harms of screening, or its economic value'.[12] To date published economic analyses (i.e. cost-identification, cost-benefit, cost-effectiveness or cost-utility analysis) for prostate cancer are inconclusive, and on the basis of available data routine screening is still questionable.[13]

PSA testing is not usually recommended for an asymptomatic man with less than 10 years life expectancy,[14] and therefore men most likely to benefit from screening are those who are 50–70 years of age or those who are older than 45 years of age and at higher risk for prostate cancer, such as African American men or those with a family history of prostate cancer.

It is emphasised that informed decision making is very important and that the patient should be involved in the decision.

## Conclusion

### What is the likely diagnosis in this patient?

The case study probably has benign prostatic hyperplasia. However, a history of urinary tract infection or rigorous exercise 48 hours prior to testing the PSA should be sought.

## Further Reading

1 Watson *et al.* Prostate cancer risk management programme; an information pack for primary care. www.primarycare.ox.ac.uk/research/crukpcerg/publications/prostate/PCRMP

2 Chybowski FM, Bergstralh EJ, Oesterling JE. The effect of digital rectal examination on the serum prostate specific antigen concentration: results of a randomized study. *J Urol* 1992; **148**: 83.

3 Whitmore WF Jr. Natural history of low-stage prostatic cancer and the impact of early detection. *Urol Clin North Am* 1990; **17**: 689.

4 Barry MJ. Health decision aids to facilitate shared decision making in office practice. *Ann Intern Med* 2002; **136**: 127.

5 Mettlin C, Lee F, Drago J, Murphy GP. The American Cancer Society National Prostate Cancer Detection Project. Findings on the detection of early prostate cancer in 2425 men. *Cancer* 1991; **67**: 2949–58.

6 Carroll P, Coley C, McLeod D, Schellhammer P, Sweat G, Wasson J, Zietman A, Thompson I. Prostate-specific antigen best practice policy–part I: early detection and diagnosis of prostate cancer. *Urology* 2001; **57**: 217–24.

7 Catalona WJ, Smith DS, Ratliff TL, Dodds KM, Coplen DE, Yuan JJ, Petros JA, Andriole GL. Measurement of prostate-specific antigen in serum as a screening test for prostate cancer. *N Engl J Med* 1991; **324**: 1156–61.

8  Partin AW, Carter HB, Chan DW, Epstein JI, Oesterling JE, Rock RC, Weber JP, Walsh PC. Prostate specific antigen in the staging of localized prostate cancer: influence of tumor differentiation, tumor volume and benign hyperplasia. *J Urol* 1990; **143**: 747–52.

9  Catalona WJ, Smith DS, Ornstein DK. Prostate cancer detection in men with serum PSA concentrations of 2.6 to 4.0 ng/ml and benign prostate examination. *JAMA* 1997; **277**: 1452.

10  Ellis WJ, Brawer MK. Repeat prostate needle biopsy: who needs it? *J Urol* 1995; **153**: 1496.

11  National Cancer Institute. SEER mortality statistics, 1999 to 2001. Available at: http://srab.cancer.gov/devcan/canques.html

12  Ilic D, O'Connor D, Green S, Wilt T. Screening for prostate cancer. *Cochrane Database Syst Rev* 2006; 3. CD004720

13  Albertsen PC. Screening for prostate cancer is neither appropriate nor cost-effective. *Urol Clin North Am* 1996; **23**: 521–30.

14  Roobol MJ van der, Cruijsen IW, Schroder FH. No reason for immediate repeat sextant biopsy after negative initial sextant biopsy in men with PSA level of 4.0 ng/ml or greater (ERSPC, Rotterdam). *Urology* 2004; **63**: 892.

PROBLEM

# 21  Local Ablative Therapy in Renal Cancer

## Case History

A 65-year-old man is found to have microscopic haematuria during a routine follow-up examination for his hypertension. He has an extensive history of vascular disease and smokes 20 cigarettes a day. He is referred urgently to a urologist, and further investigations reveal a 3 cm malignant looking lesion in his right kidney. On review at the multidisciplinary team meeting, he is deemed not to be a suitable candidate for surgery in view of his comorbidities.

**How should this patient be initially investigated by the urologist?**

**What is the differential diagnosis?**

**What local treatments are available for this patient?**

# Background

### How should this patient be initially investigated by the urologist?

Patients with renal malignancies may be asymptomatic at presentation, developing symptoms once there is local extension (pain, macroscopic haematuria, varicocele) or metastatic disease, or with the development of paraneoplastic syndromes (anorexia, cachexia, erythrocytosis, thrombocytosis, hypercalcaemia and polymyalgia). The classic triad of flank pain, haematuria and a flank mass is only seen in about 10% of patients and suggests locally advanced disease.

Patients with microscopic haematuria need investigations that include assessment of the degree of anaemia, assessment of renal disease (e.g. glomerulonephritis, interstitial nephritis), urine cytological examination (which may demonstrate casts suggesting renal parenchymal disease or malignant cells shed into the urinary tract) and imaging (including a kidney–ureter–bladder [KUB] radiograph to look for calcification, e.g. calculi, calcified haematomas, calcified carcinomas).

Ultrasound is helpful in determining renal size and demonstrated the presence of renal masses. It is less sensitive than computed tomography (CT) in detecting small masses but is able to distinguish a simple cyst from a more complex one. CT urography (CTU) has largely replaced intravenous urethrography in the diagnostic pathway as it is more sensitive and provides other anatomical information. If a malignant lesion of the renal tract is seen, full staging is completed with a chest CT, which is more sensitive than a chest radiograph in detecting metastatic disease. A flexible cystoscopy is also needed to reveal any mucosal abnormality of the bladder, and it allows taking biopsy specimens for histopathological assessment. This can be done with minimal sedation, but if abnormal findings are present, examination under anaesthesia and further cystoscopy are warranted.

### What is the differential diagnosis?

The differential diagnosis of a solid mass in the kidney includes malignant causes such as renal cell carcinomas (RCCs) (clear cell 75–85%, papillary 15%, chromophobe 5%, collecting duct 1%), transitional cell carcinomas or less commonly lymphomas and sarcomas. Secondary deposits (e.g. lung, ovary, breast and colon) can also occur. Benign causes include angiomyolipomas/hamartomas, oncocytomas and benign adenomas.

Of all small solid CT-enhancing renal masses 83–90% prove to be RCC on histopathological analysis,[1,2] the remainder including renal adenomas and oncocytomas.

# Discussion

### What local treatments are available for this patient?

Radical nephrectomy is the gold standard in managing localized RCC. Resection of the primary tumour should be considered even in metastatic disease. Although spontaneous regression of the disease has been reported,[3] more certainly it will improve the response to systemic treatment[4] and reduce the risk of troublesome local symptoms. Partial nephrectomy can be considered in patients with small (<4 cm) polar tumours, compromised renal function, bilateral tumours, tumours in solitary kidneys, or in those at risk of second primaries (e.g. van Hippel–Lindau disease). This patient is, however, inoperable due to his comorbidities, so other options have to be considered.

Surveillance could be an option. Historically, tumour size had been used to differentiate between benign and malignant lesions with 3 cm being the cut-off. The rate of metastatic disease with tumours <3 cm in size has been reported as 1–3%. Studies have shown slow growth rates of renal neoplasms up to 1.1 cm/year.[5] This suggests that small lesions can be kept under observation with appropriate intervention if they show reasonable growth. The local treatments available to this patient are as follows.

### Local ablative treatments

These were pioneered in patients with multiple or bilateral lesions to try to minimise damage to the normal kidney and preserve renal function. They are now used as minimally invasive techniques to treat patients with localized but inoperable disease.

### Cryotherapy

Cryoprobes are inserted into the lesion under image guidance and light sedation. Argon is then circulated through the probes to generate very low temperatures (−100 °C to −40 °C). This causes disruption of cellular integrity, resulting in cell death. A study in 20 patients with RCC showed in the 10 patients with measurable disease 3 had no visible tumour at 12 months, and the rest all showed some degree of tumour shrinkage.[6] No survival data are available.

### Radiofrequency ablation

Radiofrequency ablation is the destruction of viable tumour using temperatures up to 60 °C. Under image guidance and light sedation electrodes are placed in the tissue and high-frequency alternating currents are passed down the electrodes, generating ionic agitation. This produces localized heat that results in coagulative necrosis of the tumour. The process may need to be repeated at several sittings.

The evidence for its use comes from case studies in relatively small numbers of patients with limited follow-up. The rate of ablation ranges from 79% to 100%, with modest durability at up to 12 months of follow-up. Complications include abdominal pain, haematomas, uteropelvic obstruction requiring surgical repair, and calyceal leaks which required stent placement.

### High intensity focused ultrasound

This procedure involves extra-corporeal high frequency ultrasound to the tumour to heat a defined volume thereby destroying the cells by coagulative necrosis. Histological examination of the region reveals a sharp demarcation between dead and unaffected cells. The process is non-invasive and the lesions are targeted with real-time ultrasound imaging. Data on its efficacy are limited to case studies with limited follow up, but the results are encouraging.[7,8] The side effects are minimal, including mild skin burns and mild discomfort in the region treated.

### Embolization

Embolization is occasionally used to reduce the vascularity of renal tumours prior to nephrectomy to reduce the risk of serious haemorrhage. Rarely, in patients with symptomatic (e.g. pain and haematuria), inoperable lesions, it can be used to try to shrink tumours and provide symptom relief.[9] The key side effects are pain, fever and nausea, which may persist for several days. Patients need to have a relatively good performance status to tolerate this procedure.

## Conclusion

As this patient is not a suitable candidate for surgery, options such as surveillance of the cancer growth or local ablation need to be considered. Chemotherapy is not currently associated with a high success rate.

## Further Reading

1 Silver DA, Morash C, Brenner P, Campbell S, Russo P. Pathologic findings at the time of nephrectomy for renal masses. *Ann Surg Oncol* 1997; **4**: 570–4.

2 Lich MR. Renal adenoma and oncocytoma. *Semin Urol Oncol* 1995; **13**: 254–61.

3 Montie JE, Stewart BH, Straffon RA, Banowsky LH, Hewitt CB, Montague DK. The role of adjunctive nephrectomy in patients with metastatic renal cell carcinoma. *J Urol* 1977; **117**: 272–5.

4 Flanigan RC, Salmon SE, Blumenstein BA, Bearman SI, Roy V, McGrath PC, Caton JR Jr, Munshi N, Crawford ED. Nephrectomy followed by interferon alfa-2b compared with interferon alfa-2b alone for metastatic renal-cell cancer. *N Engl J Med* 2001; **345**: 1655–9.

5 Bosniak MA, Birnbaum BA, Krinsky GA, Waisman J. Small renal parenchymal neoplasms: further observations of growth. *Radiology* 1995; **197**: 589–97.

6 Shingleton WB, Sewell PE Jr. Percutaneous renal tumor cryoablation with magnetic resonance imaging guidance. *J Urol* 2001; **165**: 773.

7 Wu F, Wang ZB, Chen WZ, Bai J, Zhu H, Qiao TY. Preliminary experience using high intensity focused ultrasound for the treatment of patients with advanced stage renal malignancy. *J Urol* 2003; **170**(6 Pt 1): 2237–40.

8 Illing RO, Kennedy JE, Wu F, *et al.* The safety and feasibility of extracorporeal high-intensity focused ultrasound (HIFU) for the treatment of liver and kidney tumours in a Western population. *Br J Cancer* 2005; **93**: 890.

9 Swanson DA, Wallace S, Johnson DE. The role of embolization and nephrectomy in the treatment of metastatic renal carcinoma. *Urol Clin North Am* 1980; **7**: 719.

# 22 Penile Cancer

## Case History

A 65-year-old South American man presents with an ulcerated lesion on the glans penis; the only relevant clinical findings are phimosis and bilateral low-volume inguinal lymphadenopathy. A biopsy confirms squamous cell carcinoma.

**Is this a typical presentation?**

**What is the next step in this patient's management?**

Imaging confirms localized, possibly T1/2 disease.

**What treatment options are available for this patient?**

**What is the importance of the inguinal lymphadenopathy? How does this influence the management options in this patient?**

The patient had a penile-sparing procedure and re-presents 2 years later with a local recurrence.

**What are the outlook and management options for this patient? Is there any role for chemotherapy?**

## Background

### Is this a typical presentation?

Penile cancer is a rare disease in developed countries. However, in certain parts of the developing world it can account for up to 10% of all male malignancies. Known predisposing factors include smoking and phimosis, which confer a threefold and 10-fold increased risk, respectively; neonatal circumcision appears to be protective. The commonest presentation is a solid lesion, however, ulcerated lesions are also common and occasionally inflammatory lesions are seen.

### What is the next step in this patient's management?

Pathological and radiological staging should be the first priority. This should be established with a biopsy sufficient to assess the depth of invasion and to obtain adequate histological information. Furthermore, radiological imaging – computed tomography (CT)/magnetic resonance imaging (MRI) and urethroscopy – should be done to

**Table 22.1 TNM classification of penile cancers**

| T level | Depth of invasion | N level | |
|---------|-------------------|---------|---|
| Ta | Non-invasive verrucous carcinoma | N1 | Single superficial inguinal node |
| Tis | Carcinoma *in situ* | N2 | Multiple superficial lymph nodes |
| T1 | Subepithelial connective tissue | N3 | Deep inguinal/pelvic nodes |
| T2 | Corpus spongiosum/cavernosum | M level | |
| T3 | Urethra/prostate | M0 | No known metastases |
| T4 | Adjacent structures | M1 | Distant metastases |

**Table 22.2 Staging of penile cancers**

| Stage | TNM | | |
|-------|-----|-----|-----|
| 0 | Ta/Tis | N0 | M0 |
| I | T1 | N0 | M0 |
| II | T≤2 | N≤1 | M0 |
| III | T≤3 | N≤2 | M0 |
| IV | Any T4 | Any N3 | Any M1 |

investigate any distant spread. The currently used staging system is the TNM classification, updated in 2002[1] (Tables 22.1 and 22.2).

# Discussion

## What treatment options are available for this patient?

The gold standard for management of invasive penile cancer remains surgical excision. The extent will depend primarily on the depth of invasion. For T1 lesions the surgical excision margin should be sufficient to obtain at least 10 mm for grade 2 and 15 mm for grade 3 clear histological margin.[2] Provided >2.5–3 cm penile length remains postoperatively, the possible benefits in urinary and psychosexual function justify a partial penectomy. Otherwise, and also for T2/3 disease, a radical procedure (penectomy) should be done.

The major functional and psychological morbidities associated with the above procedures have led to the development of organ-sparing treatment modalities for T1 and T2 disease, such as Mohs' micrographic surgery,[3] surgical laser techniques and radiotherapy-based approaches.[4] No large randomized studies have been done to compare these treatments with a radical surgical approach. However, from the results of published case series, it seems that they do offer a reasonable alternative if the patient is prepared to accept a markedly higher rate of local recurrence (up to 65%), especially for T≥2 disease. Provided there is close follow-up to detect loco-regional recurrence early, salvage surgery can be done.

### What is the importance of the inguinal lymphadenopathy? How does this influence the management options in this patient?

Nodal status is extremely important as it has grave prognostic and treatment implications. Node positivity reduces the 5-year overall survival appreciably, in some series down to 50%.[5] The prognosis is particularly poor with pelvic node disease.

A survival benefit, however, has been documented for bilateral inguinal lymphadenectomy, especially for T≥2 disease,[6] and this procedure is the gold standard for determining the N stage. Unfortunately it is associated with considerable complications and long-term morbidity. Therefore other approaches have been proposed to limit this procedure to patients who are truly node positive.

Clinical examination is insufficient as up to 50% of palpable lymph nodes turn out to be non-metastatic, whereas 10–20% of clinically impalpable groin regions harbour metastatic disease, with higher rates in high-grade (2–3) and T2–4 stage disease (up to 50% in one series[7]). Simple surveillance with late salvage procedures is also clearly inferior in terms of survival.[8]

More recently proposed approaches are modified or selective lymphadenectomy and sentinel node biopsy. These approaches suffer from false-negative rates of up to 20% and no large randomized studies have been conducted so far comparing them with each other or with the gold standard.

The final decision regarding the management plan will need to be made by the patient, who needs to be informed of the possible morbidities and risks of recurrence associated with each modality. As there is insufficient evidence available, patient preference, taking into account individual social and psychological circumstances, will be critical for the final treatment plan.

### What are the outlook and management options for this patient? Is there any role for chemotherapy?

Local recurrence needs to be managed promptly and aggressively with completion penectomies or even anterior exenterations in some cases with urethral spread in view of their aggressive potential.[9] Nodal status should also be reassessed with bilateral inguinal lymphadenectomy if not already done. Disease localized to the penis and unilateral superficial inguinal nodes carries a median 5-year survival rate of about 55%, but once it spreads beyond this the prognosis is bleak with overall 5-year survival less than 10%.

The use of chemotherapy in an adjuvant/neoadjuvant and metastatic setting has not been sufficiently investigated. Small case series (n <40) have shown that the disease is relatively chemosensitive. Cisplatin, bleomycin, methotrexate and 5-fluorouracil are the agents most commonly studied, but the objective response rates have tends to be low for single agents (<15%) and relatively short lived even for combination regimens with major toxicity, e.g. see Haas *et al.*[10] Overall, there is a lack of data and entry into clinical trials should be encouraged. An EORTC trial of irinotecan and cisplatin has recently closed to recruitment. Results are awaited.

In the case of locally advanced but not metastatic disease, various combined modality techniques have been tried, including intra-arterial and (neo)adjuvant chemotherapy, brachytherapy or external beam radiotherapy with or without surgery. Although there have been individual cases of long-term survival, overall the data are scarce and our current state of knowledge is insufficient to justify advocating a particular form of treatment.

## Conclusion

The recurrence of the cancer in this patient suggests that the only option now is penectomy. The spread to the lymph nodes is a poor prognostic indicator. Treatment options should be discussed with the patient, but there is no reliable evidence on which to base chemotherapeutic regimens.

## Further Reading

1 Greene FL, Page DL, Fleming ID, Fritz A, Balch C, Haller DG, Morrow M. (eds). *AJCC (American Joint Committee on Cancer) Cancer Staging Manual*, 6th edn. Springer-Verlag, New York, 2002: 303.

2 Agrawal A, Pai D, Ananthakrishnan N, Smile SR. The histological extent of the local spread of carcinoma of the penis and its therapeutic implications. *BJU Int* 2000; **85**: 299–301.

3 Brown MD, Zachary CB, Grekin RC, Swanson NA. Penile tumors: their management by Mohs micrographic surgery. *J Dermatol Surg Oncol* 1987; **13**: 1163–7.

4 Azrif M, Logue JP, Swindell R, Cowan RA, Wylie JP, Livsey JE. External-beam radiotherapy in T1–2 N0 penile carcinoma. *Clin Oncol (R Coll Radiol)* 2006; **18**: 320–5.

5 Pandey D, Mahajan V, Kannan RR. Prognostic factors in node-positive carcinoma of the penis. *J Surg Oncol* 2006; **93**: 133–8.

6 McDougal WS, Kirchner FK Jr, Edwards RH, Killion LT. Treatment of carcinoma of the penis: the case for primary lymphadenectomy. *J Urol* 1986; **136**: 38–41.

7 Horenblas S, van Tinteren H, Delemarre JF, Moonen LM, Lustig V, van Waardenburg EW. Squamous cell carcinoma of the penis. III. Treatment of regional lymph nodes. *J Urol* 1993; **149**: 492–7.

8 Wisnescky A, Campos F, de Moraes JR. Surgical treatment of invasive squamous cell carcinoma of the penis: retrospective analysis of 350 cases. *J Urol* 1994; **151**: 1244–9.

9 Ornellas AA, Seixas AL, Marota A. Management of recurrent penile cancer following partial or total penectomy. *Urol Clin North Am* 1994; **21**: 729–37.

10 Haas GP, Blumenstein BA, Gagliano RG, Russell CA, Rivkin SE, Culkin DJ, Wolf M, Crawford ED. Cisplatin, methotrexate and bleomycin for the treatment of carcinoma of the penis: a Southwest Oncology Group study. *J Urol* 1999; **161**: 1823–5.

# Gastrointestinal Cancers

**PROBLEM**

# 23  Oesophageal Cancer

## Case History

A 54-year-old woman with a long-standing history of gastro-oesophageal reflux disease presents with progressive dysphagia and weight loss. An oesophagogastroduodenoscopy confirms a mid-oesophageal tumour and biopsy confirms adenocarcinoma.

**What initial investigations are needed? Outline the immediate management.**

**If there is no evidence of metastatic disease what further staging investigations are needed before deciding to operate?**

**What are the treatment options if, after all investigations, there is no evidence of metastases and the cancer is considered to be operable?**

**How would the management change if the tumour is found to be locally advanced and inoperable?**

**If there is evidence of distant metastatic disease what are the management options?**

# Background

### What initial investigations are needed? Outline the immediate management.

Initial investigations include upper gastrointestinal endoscopy and biopsies and computed tomography (CT).[1] An assessment of the severity of dysphagia is essential. If nutritional intake is severely limited rapid palliation of dysphagia can be achieved by dilatation, stent insertion or palliative radiotherapy.[1] Parenteral nutrition may be required, which can be achieved by nasogastric feeding, percutaneous endoscopic gastroscopy or jejunostomy.

Endoscopic stent insertion is relatively safe and non-invasive providing almost immediate results. Palliative radiotherapy is also usually well tolerated but is not without toxicity, and it can take longer than the other treatments before symptoms improve.

### If there is no evidence of metastatic disease what further staging investigations are needed before deciding to operate?

Prognosis of oesophageal cancer is strongly stage dependent and accurate clinical staging is essential as is an assessment of operability. Endoscopic ultrasound provides the most accurate estimate of disease stage and is superior to CT at detecting lymph node metastases.[1] Laparoscopy is also increasingly being done and is especially helpful in identifying coeliac nodes and subcapsular liver metastases.

Positron emission tomography (PET) scanning with 18F-fluoro-deoxyglucose is used increasingly to detect distant metastases. It is non-invasive and more sensitive than CT, particularly at detecting occult metastases, obviating the need for aggressive treatments. However, evaluation of the primary site and loco-regional nodes is not as accurate.

### What are the treatment options if, after all investigations, there is no evidence of metastases and the cancer is considered to be operable?

Surgery alone as a treatment option for locally advanced disease (T3 or T4) is considered suboptimal with 5-year survival rates of 15–20%. Preoperative and adjuvant treatment strategies are therefore important. Radiotherapy alone is of value in patients with locally advanced disease who are unfit for surgery or chemotherapy. In a study of 101 selected patients with local disease the 3-year and 5-year survival rates were 27% and 21%, respectively.[2] Most patients, however, benefit from preoperative chemotherapy or chemoradiotherapy.

A UK Medical Research Council (MRC) trial randomized 802 patients with operable oesophageal carcinoma to either resection alone or two cycles of preoperative CF (cisplatin and 5-fluorouracil) given every 3 weeks.[3] The results are summarized in Table 23.1. Overall survival was markedly greater in the patient group receiving chemotherapy. Resected specimens from patients who received chemotherapy were smaller, with less frequent extension into the surrounding tissue and less lymph node involvement. There have been many trials in which benefits of preoperative chemotherapy were not seen. One trial reported on 467 patients who were randomized to surgery alone or three cycles of CF-based preoperative chemotherapy.[4] The rates of complete response, median survival and 1-year, 2-year and 3-year survival were not significantly different. As a result of the evidence from the MRC trial, preoperative chemotherapy with CF is widely used in the UK. There is interest in replacing cisplatin with oxaliplatin and trials are ongoing.

**Table 23.1** Results of the Medical Research Council trial comparing surgery alone with preoperative chemotherapy followed by surgery

|  | Surgery alone | Preoperative chemotherapy + surgery |
| --- | --- | --- |
| Patients undergoing surgery (%) | 92 | 97 |
| Patients with R0 resection (%) | 54 | 60 |
| 2-year survival (%) | 34 | 43 |
| Median survival (months) | 13.3 | 16.8 |
| Frequency of local recurrence (%) | 11 | 12 |

**Table 23.2** Results of an Irish study investigating the role of preoperative chemoradiotherapy

|  | Surgery alone | Preoperative chemoradiotherapy |
| --- | --- | --- |
| Median survival (months) | 11 | 16 |
| 3-year survival (%) | 6 | 32 |
| Regional node involvement in surgical specimens (%) | 82 | 42 |

In the USA, combined preoperative chemoradiotherapy is more commonly used. Only one trial has demonstrated a marked survival benefit with preoperative chemoradiotherapy prior to surgery.[5] This Irish study of 113 patients compared surgery alone with preoperative CF-based chemoradiotherapy. Complete pathological response was seen in 25% of patients treated with preoperative chemoradiotherapy and there was less regional node involvement seen in surgical specimens of this group as well (42% versus 82%, $P < 0.001$, respectively). The results are summarized in Table 23.2. Results in the surgery alone arm were inferior to other contemporary series.

## Discussion

### How would the management change if the tumour is found to be locally advanced and inoperable?

In patients with inoperable disease and no distant metastases, the optimum treatment is chemoradiotherapy. The chemotherapy sensitizes the tumour to radiotherapy and therefore there is a greater than additive effect. Almost all randomized trial data have been in squamous cell carcinoma.

A Radiation Therapy Oncology Group (RTOG) trial in which patients with locally advanced disease were randomized to either radiotherapy alone or concurrent chemoradiotherapy (CF based) terminated earlier than planned after 121 patients had been recruited, as an interim analysis showed a marked survival benefit in the chemoradiotherapy arm.[6] An update on this study showed a much improved median survival (14 months with chemoradiotherapy versus 9.3 months with radiotherapy) and 5-year survival (27% versus 0%, respectively).

### If there is evidence of distant metastatic disease what are the management options?

The 5-year survival rate for advanced metastatic adenocarcinoma of the oesophagus is only 2%. The primary emphasis is on palliation of symptoms using a multidisciplinary approach. Palliation of dysphagia is similar to that for patients with locally advanced disease, although the potential risks of parenteral nutrition need to be considered in a patient who may only live for a few months.

Combination chemotherapy is usually given, and, in the UK, first-line treatment involves using the ECF regimen (epirubicin, cisplatin and infusional 5-fluorouracil). The evidence supporting this approach comes from a randomized controlled trial of 274 patients with advanced gastro-oesophageal cancer.[7] This trial compared the ECF regimen with FAMTX (5-fluorouracil, doxorubicin and methotrexate). The results are summarized in Table 23.3. An update of the trial, with a median 27-month follow-up, continues to show a survival advantage for the ECF regimen.[8]

| Table 23.3 | Comparison of the ECF and FAMTX regimens in a randomized trial | |
| --- | --- | --- |
| | ECF | FAMTX |
| Response rate (%) | 45 | 21 |
| Median survival (months) | 8.9 | 5.7 |
| 1-year survival (%) | 36 | 21 |

Early results from a phase III study (REAL-2) are encouraging for oxaliplatin and capecitabine.[9] REAL-2 was a 2 × 2 study that randomized patients with locally advanced or metastatic oesophageal and gastric cancer to one of four regimens:

● ECF (epirubicin, cisplatin and infusional 5-fluorouracil)

● EOF (epirubicin, oxaliplatin and 5-fluorouracil)

● ECX (epirubicin, cisplatin and capecitabine)

● EOX (epirubicin, oxaliplatin and capecitabine).

Approximately 1000 patients were enrolled and median follow-up was 17.1 months. The study concluded that capecitabine was not inferior to 5-FU and that oxaliplatin was not inferior to cisplatin. A superior but not significant response rate was seen with EOX compared with ECF. As expected, there was less nephrotoxicity and haematological toxicity but greater gastrointestinal and neurotoxicity in patients receiving oxaliplatin. On the basis of this trial, it seems feasible to replace 5-FU and cisplatin with capecitabine and oxaliplatin, respectively.

Further randomized trials involving other cytotoxic agents are ongoing as well as those exploring the role of novel biological agents.

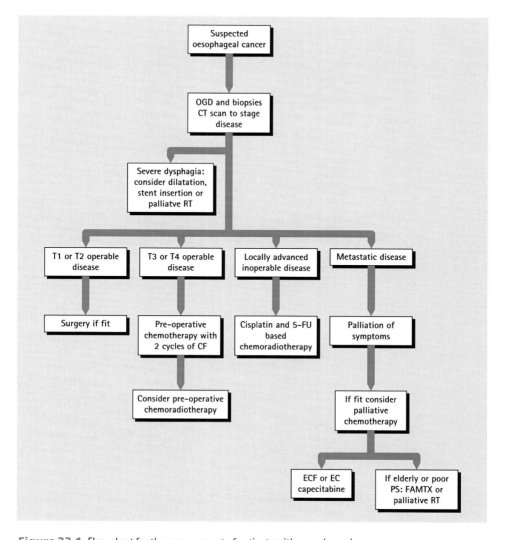

**Figure 23.1** Flow chart for the management of patients with oesophageal cancer.

## Conclusion

 Chemoradiotherapy would be of benefit to this patient, whether or not the tumour is operable. If metastases are found, this indicates a very poor prognosis for the patient. An algorithm summarising the management of all stages of oesophageal cancer is shown in Figure 23.1.

# Further Reading

1   Benhidjeb T, Hohenberger P. Oesophageal cancer. In: Souhami RL, Tannock I, Hohenberger P, Horiot JC. *Oxford Textbook of Oncology*, Vol 2, 2nd edn. New York: Oxford University Press, 2002: 1483–515.

2   Sykes AJ, Burt PA, Slevin NJ, Stout R, Marrs JE. Radical radiotherapy for carcinoma of the esophagus: an effective alternative to surgery. *Radiother Oncol* 1998; **48**: 15–21.

3   Medical Research Council Oesophageal Cancer Working Group. Surgical resection with or without preoperative chemotherapy in oesophageal cancer: a randomised controlled trial. *Lancet* 2002; **359**: 1727–33.

4   Kelsen DP, Ginsberg R, Pajak TF, Sheahan DG, Gunderson L, Mortimer J, Estes N, Haller DG, Ajani J, Kocha W, Minsky BD, Roth JA. Chemotherapy followed by surgery compared with surgery alone for localized esophageal cancer. *N Engl J Med* 1998; **339**: 1979–84.

5   Walsh TN, Noonan N, Hollywood D, Kelly A, Keeling N, Hennessy TP. A comparison of multimodal therapy and surgery for esophageal adenocarcinoma. *N Engl J Med* 1996; **335**: 462–7.

6   Herskovic A, Martz K, al-Sarraf M, Leichman L, Brindle J, Vaitkevicius V, Cooper J, Byhardt R, Davis L, Emami B. Combined chemotherapy and radiotherapy compared with radiotherapy alone in patients with cancer of the esophagus. *N Engl J Med* 1992; **326**: 1593–8.

7   Webb A, Cunningham D, Scarffe JH, Harper P, Norman A, Joffe JK, Hughes M, Mansi J, Findlay M, Hill A, Oates J, Nicolson M, Hickish T, O'Brien M, Iveson T, Watson M, Underhill C, Wardley A, Meehan M. Randomized trial comparing epirubicin, cisplatin, and fluorouracil versus fluorouracil, doxorubicin, and methotrexate in advanced esophagogastric cancer. *J Clin Oncol* 1997; **15**: 261–7.

8   Waters JS, Norman A, Cunningham D, Scarffe JH, Webb A, Harper P, Joffe JK, Mackean M, Mansi J, Leahy M, Hill A, Oates J, Rao S, Nicolson M, Hickish T. Long-term survival after epirubicin, cisplatin and fluorouracil for gastric cancer: results of a randomized trial. *Br J Cancer* 1999; **80**: 269–72.

9   Cunningham D, Rao S, Starling N, Iveson T, Nicolson M, Coxon F, Middleton G, Daniel F, Gates J, Norman A. Randomised multi centre phase III study comparing capecitabine with 5FU and oxaliplatin with cisplatin in patients with advanced oesophagogastric cancer. The REAL2 study. *J Clin Oncol Proc* 2006; **24**: 182–5.

# 24  Gastric Cancer Chemotherapy

## Case History

A 68-year-old man presents with weight loss and persistent abdominal pain and is suspected of having gastric cancer. He undergoes gastric resection for a T3 N1 R0 adenocarcinoma of the stomach and has an uncomplicated postoperative recovery.

**What is initial management?**

**What other investigations would have been done at this time?**

**In the absence of metastatic disease is there a role for preoperative treatment?**

**Are there any postoperative treatment options that may reduce his risk of recurrence?**

A year later he presents with shortness of breath, fatigue and loss of appetite. Investigations reveal hepatic metastases with small-volume lung metastases.

**What options are available for treatment at his second presentation?**

## Background

### What is initial management?

The patient should be resuscitated if necessary. A blood transfusion should be considered for symptomatic anaemia. Oesophagogastroduodenoscopy is usually the diagnostic procedure of choice. It has a higher sensitivity and specificity than double contrast barium meal and allows biopsy. A computed tomography (CT) scan of the chest and abdomen is important in staging the disease.

### What other investigations would have been done at this time?

Endoscopic ultrasound provides greater accuracy in preoperative staging of gastric cancer. Pooled data on more than 2000 patients undergoing endoscopic ultrasound revealed 69% accuracy for nodal stage and 77% for staging the depth of invasion.[1] Laparoscopy is more invasive than CT or endoscopic ultrasound but it is possible to directly visualize the local lymph nodes, peritoneum and liver. It is usually considered in patients in whom definitive surgery is being planned.

# Discussion

### In the absence of metastatic disease is there a role for preoperative treatment?

Preoperative chemotherapy is usually given to 'downstage' a locally advanced tumour before attempted curative resection. Chemotherapy before surgery is usually given to patients whose disease is at a greater risk of metastasizing, i.e. T3 or T4 disease or those with nodal involvement. Most patients will have their disease reassessed radiologically prior to definitive surgery. A small percentage of these patients will still have inoperable disease or will have developed metastases in the interim, sparing them the morbidity of unnecessary gastrectomy.

A small randomized trial in which patients with operable gastric cancer were allocated to receive four cycles of FAMTX (5-fluorouracil [5-FU], doxorubicin and methotrexate) prior to surgery or surgery alone did not find a major benefit from preoperative chemotherapy.[2] A total of 44% of patients could not complete chemotherapy and a greater proportion of curative resections were seen in the surgery-alone arm.

One randomized trial exploring preoperative chemotherapy (MAGIC) found a marked survival benefit (Table 24.1). In all, 503 patients were randomized to surgery alone or preoperative and postoperative chemotherapy;[3] 74% of patients had gastric cancer. The chemotherapy regimen was ECF (epirubicin, cisplatin and 5-FU) and it was planned to give patients three cycles of chemotherapy before and three cycles after surgery. Median follow-up was 3 years. Only 104 patients (42%) were able to complete surgery and all three cycles of postoperative chemotherapy. It would be interesting to compare this regimen with postoperative chemoradiation and trials are ongoing investigating this. However, this treatment is increasingly given in the UK on the basis of the MAGIC trial.

| Table 24.1 | Results of the MAGIC trial | | |
|---|---|---|---|
| | | Surgery alone | Chemotherapy + surgery |
| 5-year survival (%) | | 23 | 36 |
| Patients who underwent curative surgery (%) | | 79 | 70 |
| T1/2 tumour (%) | | 52 | 38 |
| N0/N1 disease (%) | | 84 | 76 |

Preoperative radiotherapy has not been extensively investigated. A Chinese study of 370 patients who were randomly assigned to preoperative radiotherapy (40 Gy) or surgery alone showed a superior 5-year survival rate for the patients treated with radiotherapy (30% versus 20% for surgery alone).[4]

### Are there any postoperative treatment options that may reduce his risk of recurrence?

In the UK there are no recommendations for adjuvant chemotherapy in gastric cancer. A meta-analysis of 19 trials estimated that the risk of death was reduced by 17% with adjuvant chemotherapy and this was even greater when the analysis was limited to

17 trials that required complete resection of disease.[5] Adjuvant chemotherapy is toxic and the planned doses are often not achieved.

In the USA, postoperative adjuvant chemoradiotherapy is usually offered. One of the largest trials that support this was the INT-016 study,[6] in which 556 patients were randomized to observation or adjuvant combined chemoradiotherapy. Chemotherapy (5-FU with leucovorin) and radiotherapy were given (45 Gy in 1.8 Gy fractions). More than two-thirds of tumours were T3 or T4 and 85% of patients had nodal metastases. Table 24.2 summarizes the results. There were significant grade 3/4 toxicities and three patients (1%) died from treatment-related toxicities. The study was criticized for not stipulating that patients should have had an adequate surgical procedure. This factor probably explains the inferior survival seen.

**Table 24.2** Results of the INT–016 trial

|  | Surgery alone | Chemoradiotherapy |
|---|---|---|
| 3-year disease-free survival (%) | 31 | 48 |
| Overall survival (%) | 41 | 50 |
| Median survival (months) | 27 | 36 |

## What options are available for treatment at his second presentation?

Metastatic disease is common at initial presentation with approximately half of patients affected. With regard to further treatment in patients with metastatic disease, the emphasis should be on palliation of symptoms. Simple measures such as pain control with analgesia, blood and/or iron replacement are recommended.

Palliative resection for bleeding or pain should only be considered if symptoms are otherwise uncontrolled. There is no survival benefit for radical gastrectomy in this setting. External beam radiotherapy can give quick relief from pain and bleeding. There are no randomized controlled trials comparing radiotherapy with endoscopic/palliative surgical techniques. Argon plasma coagulation can also be considered for haemorrhage.

In this case, if the patient is stable and has a good performance status then palliative chemotherapy should be considered. Combination chemotherapy is recommended due to better response rates but overall survival rates are similar with single-agent treatments. ECF was compared with FAMTX in a randomized controlled trial involving 274 patients[7] (Table 24.3). More complications were associated with ECF due to the need for central line placement. In the UK this regimen is commonly used as first-line treatment in advanced gastric cancer.

**Table 24.3** Results of a randomized controlled trial comparing ECF and FAMTX

|  | Response rate (%) | Median survival (months) |
|---|---|---|
| ECF | 45 | 8.9 |
| FAMTX | 21 | 5.7 |

### Newer options

Trials involving taxane combinations have yielded interesting results. The results of a multinational trial with 457 patients who received cisplatin + 5-FU with or without docetaxel[8] are summarized in Table 24.4.

| Table 24.4 | Results of a multinational trial of taxane combination treatment | |
|---|---|---|
| | CF | CF + docetaxel |
| Response rate (%) | 25 | 37 |
| Time to progression (months) | 3.7 | 5.6 |
| 2-year survival (%) | 9 | 18 |
| Grade 3/4 diarrhoea (%) | 8 | 20 |

CF, cisplatin + 5-FU.

Early results from a phase III study have demonstrated encouraging results for oxaliplatin and capecitabine.[9] This was a 2 × 2 study that randomized patients with locally advanced or metastatic oesophageal and gastric cancer to one of four regimens as discussed in Chapter 23.

## Conclusion

An algorithm summarising the management of all stages of gastric cancer is shown in Figure 24.1.

## Further Reading

1   Pollack BJ, Chak A, Sivak M Jr. Endoscopic ultrasonography. *Semin Oncol* 1996; **23**: 336–46.

2   Songun I, Keizer HJ, Hermans J, Klementschitsch P, de Vries JE, Wils JA, van der Bijl J, van Krieken JH, van de Velde CJ. Chemotherapy for operable gastric cancer: results of the Dutch randomised FAMTX trial. The Dutch Cancer Group (DGCG). *Eur J Cancer* 1999; **35**: 558–62.

3   Cunningham D, Allum WH, Stenning SP, Thompson JN, van de Velde CJ, Nicolson M, Scarffe JH, Lofts FJ, Falk SJ, Iveson TJ, Smith DB, Langley RE, Verma M, Weeden S, Chua YJ, MAGIC Trial Participants. Perioperative chemotherapy versus surgery alone for resectable gastroesophageal cancer. *N Engl J Med* 2006; **355**: 11–20.

4   Zhang ZX, Gu XZ, Yin WB, Huang GJ, Zhang DW, Zhang RG. Randomized clinical trial on the combination of preoperative irradiation and surgery in the treatment of adenocarcinoma of gastric cardia (AGC) – report on 370 patients. *Int J Radiat Oncol Biol Phys* 1998; **42**: 929–34.

5   Earle C, Maroun J. Adjuvant chemotherapy after curative resection for gastric cancer in non-Asian patients: revisiting a meta-analysis of randomised trials. *Eur J Cancer* 1999; **35**: 1059–64.

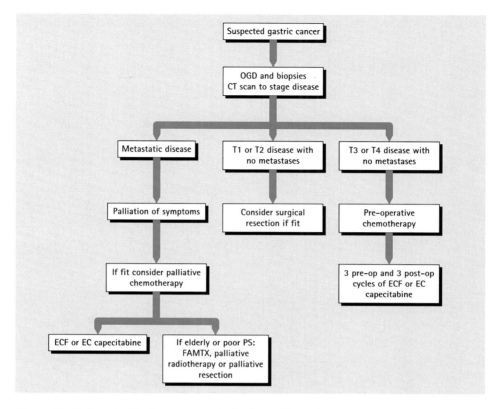

**Figure 24.1** Flow chart for the management of patients with gastric cancer.

6   Macdonald JS, Smalley SR, Benedetti J, Hundahl SA, Estes NC, Stemmermann GN, Haller DG, Ajani JA, Gunderson LL, Jessup JM, Martenson JA. Chemoradiotherapy after surgery compared with surgery alone for adencocarcinoma of the stomach or gastroesophageal junction. *N Engl J Med* 2001; **345**: 725–30.

7   Webb A, Cunningham D, Scarffe JH, Harper P, Norman A, Joffe JK, Hughes M, Mansi J, Findlay M, Hill A, Oates J, Nicolson M, Hickish T, O'Brien M, Iveson T, Watson M, Underhill C, Wardley A, Meehan M. Randomized trial comparing epirubicin, cisplatin, and fluorouracil versus fluorouracil, doxorubicin, and methotrexate in advanced esophagogastric cancer. *J Clin Oncol* 1997; **15**: 261–7.

8   Moiseyenko V, Ajani J, Tjulandin S, Majlis A, Constenla M, Boni C, Anelli A, Yuee A, Van Cutsem E. Final results of a randomized controlled phase III trial (TAX 325) comparing docetaxel (T) combined with cisplatin (C) and 5-fluorouracil (F) to CF in patients (pts) with metastatic gastric adenocarcinoma (MGC). *J Clin Oncol* 2005; **23** (16S): 4002.

9   Cunningham D, Rao S, Starling N, Iveson T, Nicolson M, Coxon F, Middleton G, Daniel F, Gates J, Norman A. Randomised multi centre phase III study comparing capecitabine with 5FU and oxaliplatin with cisplatin in patients with advanced oesophagogastric cancer. The REAL2 study. *J Clin Oncol Proc* 2006; **24**: 182–5.

# 25 Pancreatic Cancer

## Case History

A 74-year-old man presents with weight loss, jaundice, dark urine and pale stools. A computed tomography (CT) scan confirms mass in the head of the pancreas with no evidence of metastatic disease. The patient undergoes a pylorus-preserving pancreaticoduodenectomy. Histological examination confirms adenocarcinoma. A year later he presents with abdominal pain and weight loss. A CT scan confirms liver metastases.

**What are the initial investigations and immediate management?**

**If the patient is fit for a major pancreatic resection what factors determine resectability?**

**What are the important prognostic factors? What advice would you give regarding adjuvant treatment?**

**What treatment options are available in patients with locally advanced disease?**

**What advice would you give the patient on presentation of metastatic disease?**

## Background

### What are the initial investigations and immediate management?

Initial investigations are aimed at obtaining a definitive diagnosis. An ultrasound scan of the liver can detect bile duct dilatation and a mass in the head of the pancreas. CT has better sensitivity than ultrasound and can detect extrapancreatic spread such as liver metastases, lymphadenopathy and ascites. Endoscopic retrograde cholangiopancreatography (ERCP) has high sensitivity and specificity and is of particular use if CT or ultrasound does not reveal a mass. ERCP is useful in patients requiring relief of biliary obstruction. Percutaneous transhepatic cholangiography (PTCA) is an alternative to ERCP for relief of biliary obstruction and is recommended if ERCP fails or cannot be done. Magnetic resonance cholangiopancreatography (MRCP) is the investigation of choice where ERCP/PTCA is not possible as a three-dimensional image can be created of the pancreatic and biliary tree, liver and adjacent vascular structures.

The most important immediate management is relief of biliary obstruction, usually achievable by an endoscopically placed stent. It is considered as effective as a surgical bypass, with lower morbidity and procedure-related mortality.[1] The disadvantages are more frequent readmissions for stent occlusion, recurrent jaundice and cholangitis. Patients with resectable disease should ideally have surgery before relief of biliary obstruction, but in practice this is seldom practical or possible.

In unresectable disease, try to obtain a tissue diagnosis. This can be achieved by percutaneous ultrasound or CT-guided fine-needle aspiration (FNA) or biopsy, endoscopic ultrasound-assisted FNA or biopsy or brushings at ERCP. Once a tissue biopsy is obtained, the patient should be referred to an oncologist for further management.

## Discussion

 **If the patient is fit for a major pancreatic resection what factors determine resectability?**

The factors determining resectability are:

- patient's fitness and willingness to undergo a major pancreatic resection

- lack of major vessel involvement including the portal vein, superior mesenteric artery and vein, coeliac axis and hepatic artery

- absence of metastatic disease.

Three-phase CT scanning provides useful information about major vessel involvement which is essential in determining resectability. Endoscopic ultrasound is also increasingly used in the evaluation of nodal and major vascular involvement. In addition, staging laparoscopy is also increasingly carried out, allowing more accurate staging as well as reducing the rate of cases found to be inoperable at laparotomy. However, whether laparoscopy actually contributes any additional information over triple-phase CT scanning and endoscopic ultrasound remains controversial.

### What are the important prognostic factors? What advice would you give regarding adjuvant treatment?

The important prognostic factors are summarized in Box 25.1. Optimal adjuvant treatment choice remains controversial and current practice is for observation after surgery. A number of adjuvant approaches have been investigated in clinical trials.

---

**Box 25.1 Prognostic factors in pancreatic cancer**

- Nodal status: 5-year survival is 10% for node-positive disease and 25–30% for node-negative disease

- Tumour size: <3 cm confers a favourable prognosis

- Negative margins

- Well-differentiated tumours

- Intraoperative blood loss: <750 ml

The ESPAC-1 trial reported data in two separate publications. In a pooled analysis, 541 patients were randomly assigned to treatment after resection of pancreatic ductal carcinoma.[2] The treatment groups were:

● Postoperative chemoradiotherapy versus none (68 patients)

● Postoperative chemotherapy (5-fluorouracil [5-FU] based) versus none (188 patients)

● 2 × 2 factorial design with four groups (Table 25.1).

| Table 25.1 Design of the ESPAC-1 trial | |
| --- | --- |
| Chemoradiation | Chemotherapy |
| 73 patients | 75 patients |
| Chemoradiotherapy plus chemotherapy | Observation |
| 72 patients | 69 patients |

An initial report of the pooled analysis demonstrated no difference in survival between patients receiving chemotherapy with radiotherapy versus observation (15.5 and 16 months, respectively). A marked survival benefit was seen in patients receiving chemotherapy compared with those on observation (19.7 and 14 months, respectively). The later report focused on patients randomised to the four-arm study[3] (Table 25.2).

| Table 25.2 Summary of the results of the ESPAC trial | Survival (%) | |
| --- | --- | --- |
| | 2-year | 5-year |
| Chemoradiotherapy arm | | |
| No treatment | 41 | 29 |
| Treatment | 20 | 8 |
| Chemotherapy arm | | |
| No treatment | 30 | 8 |
| Treatment | 40 | 21 |

The median overall survival among patients receiving chemotherapy was 20.1 months compared with 15.5 months for the observation arm. The conclusion was that chemoradiotherapy conferred no survival benefit and may even have had a negative impact on survival; the results for adjuvant chemotherapy were more encouraging. The ESPAC-3 study is due to complete accrual and has been designed to test whether postoperative treatment with gemcitabine or 5-FU plus folinic acid improves survival compared with no additional treatment following surgery to remove pancreatic cancer. It will also compare the two regimens.

There is fewer available data for adjuvant chemotherapy alone. In a German study 368 patients with preoperative CA19–9 <2.5 the upper limit of normal were randomized to receive either gemcitabine for 6 months or observation.[4] The median disease-free survival was 14.2 months in the chemotherapy arm and 7.5 months in the observation arm.

### What treatment options are available in patients with locally advanced disease?

Therapeutic options for locally advanced disease include:

- *External beam radiotherapy (EBRT) with concurrent chemotherapy.* This approach has shown a modest survival benefit compared with radiotherapy alone. The Gastrointestinal Tumor Study Group (GITSG) randomly assigned patients with locally advanced pancreatic adenocarcinoma to EBRT (60 Gy) alone or concurrent EBRT (either 40 Gy or 60 Gy) and 5-FU.[5] After 106 patients were enrolled the EBRT alone arm was discontinued when interim analysis showed superior median time to progression and overall survival in the chemoradiation groups. The 1-year survival was 11% in the EBRT alone arm compared with 38% and 36% with 40 Gy and 60 Gy EBRT plus 5-FU, respectively.

- *Palliative chemotherapy with gemcitabine.* This has not been studied extensively in locally advanced disease compared with chemoradiation. The combination of gemcitabine and EBRT has been shown to be toxic but some small studies have been encouraging.[6,7] Randomized trials are needed.

### What advice would you give to the patient on presentation of metastatic disease?

Median survival for patients with metastatic disease is 3–6 months.[8] Emphasis is on palliation of symptoms and improvement in quality of life. Quality-of-life endpoints are more important than tumour measurements in assessing response to treatments or interventions as traditional tumour measurements are often inadequate. In trials, patients who had lacked objective responses to treatment often had reduction of symptoms. The clinical benefit response rate (CBR) is a tool used to assess response to treatments based on quality-of-life endpoints.

Objective response rates to several chemotherapeutic agents tested in the past have been disappointingly low (e.g. 5-FU: 0–9%).[8] A pivotal phase II study on gemcitabine was published in 1996.[9] The response rate was 11% and CBR was 27%. On the basis of this trial, gemcitabine has become the standard of care in advanced pancreatic cancer. This study was followed by a small randomized study in patients with locally advanced or metastatic disease treated with either gemcitabine or 5-FU. A significant CBR in favour of gemcitabine (24% versus 5%) was shown.[10] One-year survival was also considerably better with gemcitabine (18% versus 2%). Many studies have evaluated combining gemcitabine with other agents but none of the regimens were superior to gemcitabine alone. Two trials are worth noting:

- A phase III study of 533 patients compared single-agent gemcitabine with gemcitabine weekly plus capecitabine daily for 21 days every 4 weeks. There was a doubling in response rate (14% versus 7%) and an overall survival benefit (hazard ratio 0.80) for the combination.[11] There was greater haematological toxicity as well as hand–foot syndrome.

- In a phase III trial of gemcitabine plus erlotinib (Tarceva) and gemcitabine with placebo in 569 patients,[12] overall survival was significantly longer in the erlotinib plus gemcitabine arm with an estimated hazard ratio of 0.82 (95% CI, 0.69–0.99; $P = 0.038$), with 1-year survival rates of 23% versus 17% gemcitabine plus erlotinib versus gemcitabine plus placebo, respectively ($P = 0.023$). In the USA, erlotinib has been approved for use in combination with gemcitabine for the treatment of locally advanced, unresectable or metastatic pancreatic cancer.

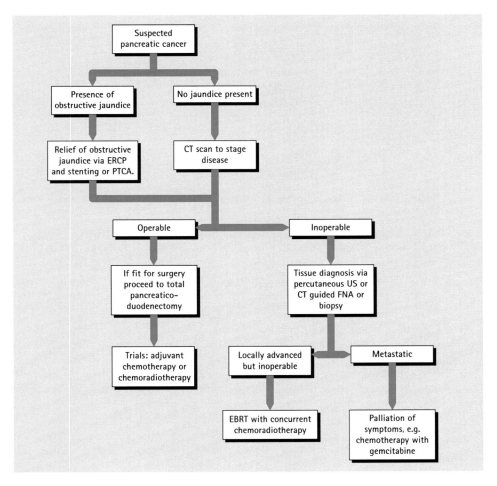

**Figure 25.1** Flow chart for the management of patients with pancreatic cancer.

# Conclusion

CT scanning should be done to evaluate the extent of the lung metastasis and check for metastasis to the liver. Palliative care will be required from a multidisciplinary team. An algorithm summarising the management of all stages of pancreatic cancer is shown in Figure 25.1.

# Further Reading

1 Smith AC, Dowsett JF, Russell RC, Hatfield AR, Cotton PB. Randomized trial of endoscopic stenting versus surgical bypass in malignant low bile duct obstruction. *Lancet* 1994; **344**: 1655–60.

2 Neoptolemos JP, Dunn JA, Stocken DD, Almond J, Link K, Beger H, Bassi C, Falconi M, Pederzoli P, Dervenis C, Fernandez-Cruz L, Lacaine F, Pap A, Spooner D, Kerr DJ, Friess H, Buchler MW; European Study Group for Pancreatic Cancer. Adjuvant chemoradiotherapy and chemotherapy in resectable pancreatic cancer: a randomised controlled trial. *Lancet* 2001; **358**: 1576–85.

3 Neoptolemos JP, Stocken DD, Friess H, Bassi C, Dunn JA, Hickey H, Beger H, Fernandez-Cruz L, Dervenis C, Lacaine F, Falconi M, Pederzoli P, Pap A, Spooner D, Kerr DJ, Buchler MW; European Study Group for Pancreatic Cancer. A randomized trial of chemoradiotherapy and chemotherapy after resection of pancreatic cancer. *N Engl J Med* 2004; **350**: 1200–10.

4 Neuhaus P, Oettle H, Post S, *et al*. A randomized, prospective, multicenter phase III trial of adjuvant chemotherapy with gemcitabine vs observation in patients with resected pancreatic cancer. *J Clin Oncol* 2005; **23**(16S): 4013.

5 Moertel CG, Frytak S, Hahn RG, O'Connell MJ, Reitemeier RJ, Rubin J, Schutt AJ, Weiland LH, Childs DS, Holbrook MA, Lavin PT, Livstone E, Spiro H, Knowlton A, Kalser M, Barkin J, Lessner H, Mann-Kaplan R, Ramming K, Douglas HO Jr, Thomas P, Nave H, Bateman J, Lokich J, Brooks J, Chaffey J, Corson JM, Zamcheck N, Novak JW. Therapy of locally unresectable pancreatic carcinoma: a randomized comparison of high dose (6000 rads) radiation alone, moderate dose radiation (4000 rads + 5-fluorouracil), and high dose radiation + 5-fluorouracil: The Gastrointestinal Tumor Study Group. *Cancer* 1981; **48**: 1705–10.

6 Ammori JB, Colletti LM, Zalupski MM, Eckhauser FE, Greenson JK, Dimick J, Lawrence TS, McGinn CJ. Surgical resection following radiation therapy with concurrent gemcitabine in patients with previously unresectable adenocarcinoma of the pancreas. *J Gastrointest Surg* 2003; **7**: 766–72.

7 Li CP, Chao Y, Chi KH, Chan WK, Teng HC, Lee RC, Chang FY, Lee SD, Yen SH. Concurrent chemoradiotherapy treatment of locally pancreatic cancer: gemcitabine versus 5-fluorouracil, a randomized controlled study. *Int J Radiat Oncol Biol Phys* 2003; **57**: 98–104.

8 Russell R, Ross P, Cunningham D. Cancer of the pancreas. In: *Oxford Textbook of Oncology*, 2nd edn, Vol 2. 1603–26.

9 Rothenberg ML, Moore MJ, Cripps MC, Andersen JS, Portenoy RK, Burris HA 3rd, Green MR, Tarassoff PG, Brown TD, Casper ES, Storniolo AM, Von Hoff DD. A Phase II trial of gemcitabine in patients with 5-FU-refractory pancreas cancer. *Ann Oncol* 1996; **7**: 347–53.

10 Burris HA 3rd, Moore MJ, Andersen J, Green MR, Rothenberg ML, Modiano MR, Cripps MC, Portenoy RK, Storniolo AM, Tarassoff P, Nelson R, Dorr FA, Stephens CD, Von Hoff DD. Improvements in survival and clinical benefit with gemcitabine as first-line therapy for patients with advanced pancreas cancer: a randomized trial. *J Clin Oncol* 1997; **15**: 2403–13.

11 Cunningham D, Chau I, Stocken D, *et al.* Phase III randomized comparison of gemcitabine versus gemcitabine plus capecitabine in patients with advanced pancreatic cancer. *Eur J Cancer Suppl* 2005; **3**: 4.

12 Moore MJ, Goldstein D, Hamm J, Figer A, Hecht JR, Gallinger S, Au HJ, Murawa P, Walde D, Wolff RA, Campos D, Lim R, Ding K, Clark G, Voskoglou-Nomikos T, Ptasynski M, Parulekar W. Erlotinib plus gemcitabine compared to gemcitabine alone in patients with advanced pancreatic cancer: a phase III trial of the National Institute of Canada Clinical Trials Group (NCNC-CTG). *J Clin Oncol* 2005; **23**: 1s (abstract).

**PROBLEM**

# 26 Management of Colorectal Cancer After Surgery

## Case History

A 63-year-old woman had a left hemicolectomy for a Dukes C carcinoma of the descending colon, with 2/12 lymph nodes positive for tumour (pT4 N1 MX). Carcinoembryonic antigen (CEA) was raised preoperatively, but returned to the normal range 4 weeks after the surgery. She is referred for consideration of adjuvant treatment. She has no relevant past medical history.

**How should this patient be further assessed?**

**If no further sites of disease are found, what is her prognosis with no adjuvant treatment, and how is the prognosis altered by 5–fluorouracil?**

**Should this patient be offered adjuvant treatment containing irinotecan, oxaliplatin or monoclonal antibodies (cetuximab or bevacizumab)?**

**How would have the management have differed if the tumour had been a Dukes B carcinoma of the colon (pT4 N0 MX)?**

# Background

## How should this patient be further assessed?

Radiological imaging should be done to exclude the presence of distant metastases and complete tumour staging. The commonest site for distant metastases is the liver and adequate imaging of this site is therefore a priority. Few studies have defined the optimal imaging modality in this situation. Ultrasound and computed tomography (CT) are the most widely available modalities, and both have potential benefits and drawbacks. Current UK guidance suggests that all patients should have a staging CT scan of the abdomen and pelvis.[1] This is largely based on the greater sensitivity (although lower specificity) of CT over ultrasound scanning for the detection of liver metastases.

An elevated preoperative CEA which fails to normalize can be considered a poor prognostic factor. However, it is not an independent prognostic factor due to confounding associations with increasing tumour stage and poor histological differentiation.[2] Routine blood tests and an electrocardiogram (ECG) should also be done to assess for comorbidities.

## If no further sites of disease are found, what is her prognosis with no adjuvant treatment, and how is the prognosis altered by 5–fluorouracil?

Dukes C tumours have a 60% risk of disease recurrence, whereas Dukes B and A tumours have a much lower risk of recurrence of 20% and 10%, respectively. Adjuvant fluoropyrimidine-based chemotherapy is well established for Dukes C tumours, resulting in approximately a 25% reduction in the risk of death.[3–5] This is equivalent to an absolute benefit in 5-year overall survival of 4–12%. Online resources, such as the Mayo clinic database (www.mayoclinic.com/calcs/), allow the estimation of an individual's risk of recurrence and the potential benefit of adjuvant chemotherapy.

The optimal 5-fluorouracil (5-FU) regimen has evolved over the past 15 years. Bolus 5-FU given at a dose of 370–500 mg/m$^2$ is the basis of most adjuvant regimens. A total of 6 months 5-FU modulated by low-dose folinic acid currently appears to be an optimal regimen. Longer periods of treatment or higher doses of folinic acid do not result in superior outcomes.[3,6] Many bolus and infusional 5-FU schedules have been assessed. They seem to have similar efficacy but differ in their convenience and toxicity profiles. Recent evidence also suggests that capecitabine and uracil and tegafur (UFT), oral fluoropyrimidines, are as effective as bolus 5-FU schedules in the adjuvant setting.[7,8]

# Discussion

## Should this patient be offered adjuvant treatment containing irinotecan, oxaliplatin or monoclonal antibodies (cetuximab or bevacizumab)?

Two randomized controlled trials have assessed the use of oxaliplatin in the adjuvant setting. The MOSAIC trial randomized patients to receive infusional 5-FU/leucovorin alone or in combination with oxaliplatin.[9] Patients receiving the oxaliplatin combination regimen had a 5% improvement in 3-year disease-free survival (p=0.002). The NSABP C-07 trial randomized patients similarly to MOSAIC but used bolus chemotherapy regimens. The preliminary efficacy data also show a 5% improvement in 3-year disease-free survival (p=0.004).[10] An improvement in overall survival is usually required before incorporation of a new treatment into the adjuvant setting. The median follow-up of both these trials is currently short and no improvement in overall survival has been detected in either trial.

A striking association has been noted between improvements in 3-year disease-free survival and consequent improvements in 5-year overall survival in previous adjuvant studies.[11] This finding has encouraged the use of oxaliplatin in clinical practice, especially in high-risk Dukes C patients, prior to the demonstration of an overall survival benefit. Grade 3 neurosensory toxicity, characteristic of oxaliplatin, was noted in 8–12% of patients in MOSAIC and C-07; 1–2% of patients had persistent grade 3 symptoms 12 months after completion of chemotherapy. This is a potentially important toxicity in a group of healthy individuals of working age and requires consideration during discussions of the risks and benefits of adjuvant oxaliplatin treatment.

The use of irinotecan, a topoisomerase-1 inhibitor, in the adjuvant setting has been investigated in three randomized controlled trials: CALGB C89803,[12] PETACC3[13] and the FNLCC Accord02 trial.[14] All three trials randomized patients to receive either 5-FU/leucovorin alone or a combination regimen of 5-FU and irinotecan. The CALGB C89803 trial did not show any marked benefit for the addition of irinotecan. Disturbingly, 2.8% of patients receiving the bolus combination chemotherapy schedule died during treatment compared with 1% of patients in the 5-FU/leucovorin arm. The PETACC3 and FNLCC Accord02 trials used similar infusional combination chemotherapy schedules and both trials reported acceptable rates of chemotherapy toxicity and treatment-related mortality. Neither of these trials showed a notable benefit for the addition of irinotecan. Imbalances in the baseline pathological characteristics were noted in both of these trials, with a greater proportion of the patients randomized to receive irinotecan having 'high-risk' features (i.e. T4 and/or N2 disease). Based on current evidence, irinotecan should not be used in the adjuvant setting outside a clinical trial.

Bevacizumab (Avastin) is a humanized monoclonal antibody that binds to and inhibits the activity of the vascular endothelial growth factor (VEGF). Cetuximab (Erbitux) is a chimeric monoclonal antibody that binds to the epidermal growth factor receptor (EGFR, Her-1). Both drugs have shown activity in the metastatic setting, and trials randomizing patients in the adjuvant setting to receive bevacizumab (e.g. QUASAR2, NSABP C-08, AVANT) or cetuximab (PETACC-8, Intergroup 0147) are ongoing. No efficacy or safety data are available as yet and neither drug should be used in the adjuvant setting outside a clinical trial.

### How would the management have differed if the tumour had been a Dukes B carcinoma of the colon (pT4 N0 MX)?

The risk of recurrence for Dukes B tumours is 20%. The UK QUASAR1 trial randomized patients with an uncertain indication for adjuvant chemotherapy, 91% of whom had Dukes B tumours, to receive 6 months of adjuvant 5-FU/leucovorin chemotherapy or the standard policy of observation.[15] Patients receiving chemotherapy had a 4% improvement in recurrence free-survival (relative risk [RR] 0.78 (0.67–0.91), p = 0.001), and a 3% improvement in 5-year overall survival (RR 0.83 (0.71–0.97), p = 0.02). Prior to the presentation of the QUASAR data no adequately powered trials had been conducted in Dukes B cancers. A meta-analysis suggested a similar sized, but non-significant improvement in the outcomes of patients receiving adjuvant chemotherapy.[16,17] The absolute benefit of adjuvant 5-FU chemotherapy for Dukes B tumours is small (3%) and the potential costs and benefits of treatment require discussion on an individual basis.

The Dukes B category encompasses a heterogeneous group of tumours with variable clinical outcomes. Several clinical and pathological prognostic factors have been identified that may help to define patients at a relatively high risk of tumour recurrence. The presence of extramural vascular invasion, involvement of peritoneum or adjacent organs (T4), tumour perforation and a positive surgical margin seem to be particularly important.[18] Patients may be 'under-staged' if relatively few lymph nodes have been assessed. In this situation patients appear to have outcomes similar to Dukes C patients, and for this reason they may be considered for adjuvant chemotherapy. There is no absolute cut-off for the minimum number of lymph nodes required for assessment but UK guidelines suggest that pathologists assess a median of 12 lymph nodes in their practice.[1]

The factors noted above have prognostic value and indicate an increased risk of recurrence that may influence decisions regarding adjuvant treatment. They are not predictive of treatment efficacy, however. Work is ongoing to identify molecular predictors of chemotherapy outcomes but none are currently used in clinical practice.

## Conclusion

After resection of colorectal cancer with curative intent, patients should be staged using radiology. Adjuvant chemotherapy based on 5-FU improves cure rates in Dukes C carcinomas, with a smaller benefit in Dukes B carcinomas. The addition of oxaliplatin to adjuvant chemotherapy appears to reduce recurrence further, but at the cost of neurotoxicity.

## Further Reading

1  National Institute for Clinical Excellence. *Improving Outcomes in Colorectal Cancers.* Guidance on Cancer Services. London: National Institute of Clinical Excellence, 2004.

2  DeVita VT, Hellman S, Rosenberg SA. *Cancer: Principles and Practice of Oncology,* 6th edn. Philadelphia: Lippincott, Williams and Wilkins, 1998.

3  O'Connell MJ, Laurie JA, Kahn M, Fitzgibbons RJ Jr, Erlichman C, Shepherd L, Moertel CG, Kocha WI, Pazdur R, Wieand HS, Rubin J, Vukov AM, Donohue JH, Krook JE, Figueredo A. Prospectively randomized trial of postoperative adjuvant chemotherapy in patients with high-risk colon cancer. *J Clin Oncol* 1998; **16**: 295–300.

4  Moertel CG, Fleming TR, Macdonald JS, Haller DG, Laurie JA, Tangen CM, Ungerleider JS, Emerson WA, Tormey DC, Glick JH, Veeder MH, Mailliard JA. Fluorouracil plus levamisole as effective adjuvant therapy after resection of stage III colon carcinoma: a final report. *Ann Intern Med* 1995; **122**: 321–6.

5  Efficacy of adjuvant fluorouracil and folinic acid in colon cancer. International Multicentre Pooled Analysis of Colon Cancer Trials (IMPACT) investigators. *Lancet* 1995; **345**: 939–44.

6  Comparison of fluorouracil with additional levamisole, higher-dose folinic acid, or both, as adjuvant chemotherapy for colorectal cancer: a randomised trial. QUASAR Collaborative Group. *Lancet* 2000; **355**: 1588–96.

7  Twelves C, Wong A, Nowacki MP, Abt M, Burris H 3rd, Carrato A, Cassidy J, Cervantes A, Fagerberg J, Georgoulias V, Husseini F, Jodrell D, Koralewski P, Kroning H, Maroun J, Marschner N, McKendrick J, Pawlicki M, Rosso R, Schuller J, Seitz JF, Stabuc B, Tujakowski J, Van Hazel G, Zaluski J, Scheithauer W. Capecitabine as adjuvant treatment for stage III colon cancer. *N Engl J Med* 2005; **352**: 2696–704.

8  Lembersky BC, Wieand HS, Petrelli NJ, O'Connell MJ, Colangelo LH, Smith RE, Seay TE, Giguere JK, Marshall ME, Jacobs AD, Colman LK, Soran A, Yothers G, Wolmark N. Oral uracil and tegafur plus leucovorin compared with intravenous fluorouracil and leucovorin in stage II and III carcinoma of the colon: results from National Surgical Adjuvant Breast and Bowel Project Protocol C-06. *J Clin Oncol* 2006; **24**: 2059–64.

9  Andre T, Boni C, Mounedji-Boudiaf L, Navarro M, Tabernero J, Hickish T, Topham C, Zaninelli M, Clingan P, Bridgewater J, Tabah-Fisch I, de Gramont A; Multicenter International Study of Oxaliplatin/5-Fluorouracil/Leucovorin in the Adjuvant Treatment of Colon Cancer (MOSAIC) Investigators. Oxaliplatin, fluorouracil, and leucovorin as adjuvant treatment for colon cancer. *N Engl J Med* 2004; **350**: 2343–51.

10  Wolmark N, Wieand HS, Kuebler JP, Colangelo L, Smith RE. A phase III trial comparing FULV to FU/LV + oxaliplatin in stage II or III carcinoma of the colon: Results of NSABP Protocol C-07. In: Proceedings of the American Society of Clinical Oncology, 2005, Orlando, USA (abstract 3500).

11  Sargent DJ, Wieand HS, Haller DG, Gray R, Benedetti JK, Buyse M, Labianca R, Seitz JF, O'Callaghan CJ, Francini G, Grothey A, O'Connell M, Catalano PJ, Blanke CD, Kerr D, Green E, Wolmark N, Andre T, Goldberg RM, de Gramont A. Disease-free survival versus overall survival as a primary end point for adjuvant colon cancer studies: individual patient data from 20,898 patients on 18 randomized trials. *J Clin Oncol* 2005; **23**: 8664–70.

12  Wang L, Abou-Alfa GK, Liu F, Saltz LB, Kalaigian J, Zhao B, Colville J, Nyoro J, Schwartz B, Schwartz L, Memorial Sloan-Kettering Cancer Center, New York, NY, Bayer Pharmaceuticals, West Haven, CT. Irinotecan plus fluorouracil/leucovorin (IFL) versus fluorouracil/leucovorin alone (FL) in stage III colon cancer (intergroup trial CALGB C89803). In: Proceedings of the American Society of Clinical Oncology, 2004, New Orleans, USA (abstract 3500).

13  Van Cutsem E, Labianca R, Hossfeld D, Bodoky G, Roth A, Aranda E, Nordlinger B, Assadourian S, Wang K, Cunningham D. Randomized phase III trial comparing infused irinotecan/5-fluorouracil (5-FU)/folinic acid (IF) versus 5-FU/FA (F) in stage 3 colon cancer patients: PETACC3. In: Proceedings of the American Society of Clinical Oncology, 2005, Orlando, USA (abstract 8).

14  Ychou M, Raoul J, Douillard J, Bugat R, Mineur L, Viret F, Becouarn Y, Bouche O, Jacobs J, Gourgou-Bourgade S. A phase 3 randomised trial of LV5FU2+CPT-11 vs. LV5FU2 alone in adjuvant high risk colon cancer (FNLCC Accord02/ FFCD9802). In: Proceedings of the American Society of Clinical Oncology, 2005, Orlando, USA.

15  Gray RG, Barnwell J, Hills R, McConkey C, Williams N, Kerr D. QUASAR: A randomised study of adjuvant chemotherapy (CT) vs observation including 3238 colorectal cancer patients. In: Proceedings of the American Society of Clinical Oncology, 2004, New Orleans, USA.

16  Gill S, Loprinzi CL, Sargent DJ, Thome SD, Alberts SR, Haller DG, Benedetti J, Francini G, Shepherd LE, Francois Seitz J, Labianca R, Chen W, Cha SS, Heldebrant MP, Goldberg RM. Pooled analysis of fluorouracil-based adjuvant therapy for stage II and III colon cancer: who benefits and by how much? *J Clin Oncol* 2004; **22**: 1797–806.

17  Efficacy of adjuvant fluorouracil and folinic acid in B2 colon cancer. International Multicentre Pooled Analysis of B2 Colon Cancer Trials (IMPACT B2) Investigators. *J Clin Oncol* 1999; **17**: 1356–63.

18  Petersen VC, Baxter KJ, Love SB, Shepherd NA. Identification of objective pathological prognostic determinants and models of prognosis in Dukes' B colon cancer. *Gut* 2002; **51**: 65–9.

PROBLEM

# 27 Chemotherapy for Metastatic Colorectal Cancer

## Case History

A 76-year-old man presents with an obstructing carcinoma of the sigmoid colon for which he undergoes an emergency Hartmann's procedure. At surgery, multiple peritoneal and liver metastases are noted. He survives the operation, but 4 weeks after surgery is eating poorly, has right upper abdominal pain, and is spending all his time indoors. He has a history of hypertension which is controlled with β blockers. He lives 24 km from the cancer unit with his 74-year-old wife, who is in good health but has partial sight, so does not drive.

**What is his prognosis and how will it be affected by palliative chemotherapy?**

**What are his options for first–line chemotherapy and what factors would influence the recommendation for treatment?**

**For how long should first–line chemotherapy be continued?**

**When should first–line chemotherapy be considered to have failed and what are the options for subsequent lines of treatment?**

## Background

### What is his prognosis and how will it be affected by palliative chemotherapy?

The 5-year survival with metastatic disease is less than 5%. The median survival without treatment is 6–9 months. Current treatments can increase median survival to 18–20 months. Asymptomatic patients have prolonged median survival, longer symptom-free period and longer time to disease progression if chemotherapy is started immediately rather than delaying until symptoms develop. 5-fluorouracil/folinic acid (5-FU/FA) confers survival benefit over supportive care (median survival 11.7 and 8 months; 1-year survival 50% and 34%, respectively).[1] Oxaliplatin or irinotecan in combination with 5-FU/FA have further improved response rates and survival.

### What are his options for first-line chemotherapy and what factors would influence the recommendation for treatment? (Table 27.1)

#### Infusional 5-FU/FA

Infusional 5-FU regimens are costly and often require permanent vascular access and/or admission to hospital. They are superior to bolus regimens in terms of progression-free survival, response rates, toxicity and quality of life, but equally effective in terms of overall survival.

#### Oral fluoropyrimidines

Capecitabine and tegafur/uracil (UFT) mimic protracted venous infusional 5-FU. Potential benefits include convenience, fewer hospital visits, elimination of risks of indwelling central venous catheter, different toxicity profile and fewer treatment-related hospitalizations. Compared with the Mayo regimen, capecitabine has been shown to achieve a markedly superior response rate, superior safety profile, equivalent time to progression and equivalent overall survival.[2] Studies have shown that capecitabine is effective and well tolerated by elderly patients who are ineligible for combination chemotherapy,[3] and that these patients prefer capecitabine to intravenous regimens.[4] Compared with the Mayo regimen, UFT has shown equivalent efficacy but better toxicity profile.[5]

#### Irinotecan in combination with 5-FU/FA

This combination is superior to 5-FU alone in terms of response rate, time to progression and survival.[6–8]

#### Oxaliplatin in combination with 5-FU/FA

This combination has improved efficacy with better response rate, progression-free survival and median survival compared with 5-FU alone.[9–11] Studies comparing the combination of irinotecan and 5-FU/FA with the combination of oxaliplatin and 5-FU/FA have shown mixed results. At present there is not sufficient evidence to suggest that either combination is superior in terms of efficacy.

#### Oxaliplatin in combination with capecitabine

The XELOX regimen has shown similar high activity in younger and older patients with no clinically relevant differences in safety profile.[12] In the context of an ageing population, it provided a highly effective and tolerable treatment option.[13] Patients should be encouraged to participate in ongoing clinical trials.

Factors influencing the choice of treatment include extent of disease, age, performance status, previous treatment, benefits and side effects of treatment, schedule of treatment (inpatient or outpatient, intravenous or oral), convenience, frequency of hospital visits, patients wishes, risks of indwelling central venous catheter, quality of life, comorbidity and cost.

# Discussion

### For how long should first-line chemotherapy be continued?

Usual current practice is to continue first-line chemotherapy for maximum of 6 months if well tolerated, with assessment of response at 3 months and at the end of treatment. There is an ongoing debate whether intermittent use of 5-FU-based chemotherapy is as effective as continuous treatment until disease progression. The ongoing MRC COIN trial may answer this question.

### When should first-line chemotherapy be considered to have failed and what are the options for subsequent lines of treatment?

About 60% of patients experience improvement in their condition or stabilization of disease after first-line 5-FU/FA-based therapy. On progression, the same therapy may be repeated. The chance of response is good if the interval is more than a few months. Eventually, however, patients develop resistance to the drugs. In the remaining 40% of patients, there is primary treatment failure, with progression of disease while on treatment or at the end of it.

Options for subsequent lines of treatment include:

- *Irinotecan.* Compared with best supportive care, irinotecan has shown significant improvement in overall survival and maintained baseline quality of life longer despite causing additional toxicity.[14] Compared with infusional 5-FU, it has again shown increased 1-year survival, median survival and progression-free survival with similar results with quality of life measures.[15]

- *Oxaliplatin in combination with 5-FU/FA.* Compared with 5-FU/FA alone, this combination has shown improved median overall survival, progression-free survival and response rate.

**Table 27.1**  Current (2006) NICE guidelines for first–line and second–line chemotherapy options for metastatic colorectal cancer

| Chemotherapy options | |
| --- | --- |
| First–line | Second–line |
| Infusional 5-FU/folinic acid | Irinotecan |
| Capecitabine or tegafur/uracil | Oxaliplatin and infusional 5-FU/folinic acid |
| Irinotecan and infusional 5-FU/folinic acid | Clinical trials |
| Oxaliplatin and infusional 5-FU/folinic acid | |
| Clinical trials | |

● *Cetuximab.* In patients with metastatic colorectal cancer positive for epidermal growth factor receptor expression, in whom irinotecan and oxaliplatin chemotherapy has failed, cetuximab has shown some activity.[16] It is not approved by National Institute for Health and Clinical Excellence (NICE) for use at present (due for review in 2009). Patients should be encouraged to participate in ongoing clinical trials.

### Treatment sequencing

If a patient has advanced disease and cure is not a goal, and if we plan to use more than one drug, should we give them together from the start or use them sequentially? In the Tournigand study, although the treatment sequences were not markedly different in terms of survival, sequential infusional 5-FU/FA with irinotecan followed by infusional 5-FU/FA with oxaliplatin was better than the opposite sequence.[17] In the FOCUS study, first-line combination treatment was more effective in terms of progression-free survival than first-line 5FU/FA. However, there was no statistically significant difference for overall survival between staged and combination chemotherapy plans.[18]

## Conclusion

In the given scenario the most appropriate chemotherapy option would be capecitabine, provided cardiac function was satisfactory. However, palliative measures should be instituted first, including pain control, steroids to improve appetite and for liver capsule pain, nutritional support, and support from a palliative care team, including a Macmillan nurse. In view of this patient's poor performance status, it is possible that he might never be well enough to benefit from chemotherapy.

## Further Reading

1 Colorectal Cancer Collaborative Group. Palliative chemotherapy for advanced colorectal cancer: systematic review and meta-analysis. *BMJ* 2000; **321**: 531–5.

2 Cassidy J, Twelves C, Van Cutsem E, *et al.* First-line oral capecitabine therapy in metastatic colorectal cancer: a favorable safety profile compared with intravenous 5-fluorouracil/leucovorin. *Ann Oncol* 2002; **13**: 566–75.

3 Feliu J, Escudero P, Llosa F, *et al.* Capecitabine as first line treatment for patients older than 70 years with metastatic colorectal cancer: an Oncopaz Cooperative Group study. *J Clin Oncol* 2005; **23**: 3104–11.

4 Liu G, Franssen E, Fitch MI, *et al.* Patients preference for oral versus intravenous palliative chemotherapy. *J Clin Oncol* 1997; **15**: 110–15.

5 Douillard JY, Hoff PM, Skillings JR, *et al.* Multicenter phase III study of uracil/tegafur and oral leucovorin versus fluorouracil and leucovorin in patients with previously untreated metastatic colorectal cancer. *J Clin Oncol* 2002; **20**: 3605–16.

6  Douillard JY, Cunningham D, Roth AD, *et al*. Irinotecan combined with fluorouracil compared with fluorouracil alone as first-line treatment for metastatic colorectal cancer: a multicentre randomised trial. *Lancet* 2000; **355**: 1041–7.

7  Saltz LB, Cox JV, Blanke C, *et al*. Irinotecan plus fluorouracil and leucovorin for metastatic colorectal cancer. Irinotecan Study Group. *N Engl J Med* 2000; **343**: 905–14.

8  Kohne CH, Van Cutsem E, Wils JA, *et al*. Irinotecan improves the activity of the AIO regimen in metastatic colorectal cancer: Results of EORTC GI Group study 40986. *Proc Am Soc Clin Oncol* 2003; **22**: 254 (abstract 1018).

9  de Gramont A, Figer A, Seymour M, *et al*. Leucovorin and 5-fluorouracil with or without oxaliplatin as first line treatment in advanced colorectal cancer. *J Clin Oncol* 2000; **18**: 2938–47.

10  Giacchetti S, Perpoint B, Zidani R, *et al*. Phase III multicentre randomized trial of oxaliplatin added to chronomodulated fluorouracil-leucovorin as first line treatment of metastatic colorectal cancer. *J Clin Oncol* 2000; **18**: 136–47.

11  Grothey A, Deschler B, Kroening H, *et al*. Phase III study of bolus 5-fluorouracil (5-FU)/ folinic acid (FA) (Mayo) versus weekly high-dose 24h 5-FU infusion/FA + oxaliplatin (OXA) (FUFOX) in advanced colorectal cancer (ACRC). *Proc Am Soc Clin Oncol* 2002; **21**: 129a (abstract 512).

12  Twelves CJ, Butts CA, Cassidy J, *et al*. Capecitabine/Oxaliplatin, a safe and active first line regimen for older patients with metastatic colorectal cancer. Post hoc analysis of a large phase II study. *Clin Colorectal Cancer* 2005; **5**: 101–17.

13  Salud, Escudero P, Feliu J, *et al*. XELOX (capecitabine and oxaliplatin) as 1st line treatment for elderly patients with advanced/metastatic colorectal cancer. *Proc Am Soc Clin Oncol* 2005; **23**: 276 (abstract 3620).

14  Cunningham D, Pyrhonen S, James RD, *et al*. Randomised trial of irinotecan plus supportive care versus supportive care alone after fluorouracil failure for patients with metastatic colorectal cancer. *Lancet* 1998; **352**: 1413–18.

15  Rougier P, Van Cutsem E, Bajetta E, *et al*. Randomised trial of irinotecan versus fluorouracil by continuous infusion after fluorouracil failure in patients with metastatic colorectal cancer. *Lancet* 1998; **352**: 1407–12.

16  Cunningham D, Humblet Y, Siena S, *et al*. Cetuximab (C225) alone or in combination with irinotecan (CPT-11) in patients with epidermal growth factor receptor (EGFR)-positive, irinotecan-refractory metastatic colorectal cancer (MCRC). *Proc Am Soc Clin Oncol* 2003; **22**: 252 (abstract 1012).

17  Tournigand C, Andre T, Achille E, *et al*. FOLFIRI followed by FOLFOX6 or the reverse sequence in advanced colorectal cancer: a randomized GERCOR study. *J Clin Oncol* 2004; **22**: 229–37.

18  Seymour M. Fluorouracil, Oxaliplatin and CPT-11 (irinotecan), use and Sequencing (MRC FOCUS): a 2135-patient randomized trial in advanced colorectal cancer (ACRC). American Society of Clinical Oncology Annual Meeting, 2005 (abstract 3518).

## Additional Further Reading

Gallego R, Sanchez N, Maurel J. Chemotherapy for elderly patients with advanced colorectal carcinoma. *Expert Rev Anticancer Ther* 2006; **6**: 795–800.

Golfinopoulos V, Pentheroudakis G, Pavlidis N. Treatment of colorectal cancer in the elderly: a review of the literature. *Cancer Treat Rev* 2006; **32**: 1–8.

Goyle S, Maraveyas A. Chemotherapy for colorectal cancer. *Dig Surg* 2005; **22**: 401–14.

National Institute for Clinical Excellence. Technology Appraisal 61, 2003.

National Institute for Clinical Excellence. Technology Appraisal 93, 2005.

Pasetto LM, Monfardini S. The role of capecitabine in the treatment of colorectal cancer in the elderly. *Anticancer Res* 2006; **26**: 2381–6.

Terstriep S, Grothey A. First- and second-line therapy of metastatic colorectal cancer. *Expert Rev Anticancer Ther* 2006; **6**: 921–30.

**PROBLEM**

# 28 Liver Resection for Metastatic Colorectal Cancer

## Case History

A 70-year-old man has rising levels of carcinoembryonic antigen (CEA) 3 years after a left hemicolectomy for Dukes C carcinoma of the descending colon. An abdominal ultrasound scan is suggestive of liver metastases. The patient is fit and asymptomatic and is offered a work-up for liver resection.

**What further assessment should this patient have?**

**What factors determine tumour resectability?**

**Assuming the liver can be cleared of tumour, what is the immediate and long–term prognosis?**

**What are the patient's options if the liver is the only site of disease, but the tumours are not resectable?**

# Background

### What further assessment should this patient have?

All patients with suspected or diagnosed liver metastases which might be amenable to resection should be referred to specialist liver surgeons for evaluation.[1] Patients who may be undergoing a liver resection require a full medical assessment to ensure fitness for major surgery. If there are doubts about existing comorbidities, the patient should have an anaesthetic review or be referred to the appropriate specialist prior to surgery. Blood tests that should be done before surgery include a full blood count, clotting screen, urea and electrolytes, tumour markers and liver function tests. It is important to check the synthetic function of the liver as people with steatosis, fibrosis or cirrhosis will not tolerate a major liver resection.

Staging computed tomography (CT) of the chest, abdomen and pelvis should be done. Magnetic resonance imaging (MRI) of the liver is done as it has a higher sensitivity in detecting and characterizing smaller lesions (Figure 28.1). Precise anatomical imaging and tumour mapping is essential, to assess the feasibility of a safe oncological liver resection and to determine the presence of extra-hepatic metastases.[2] The radiological assessment is completed with intraoperative ultrasound. Intraoperative ultrasound helps in detecting hitherto unknown lesions and in the localization of deep lesions that are difficult to palpate.

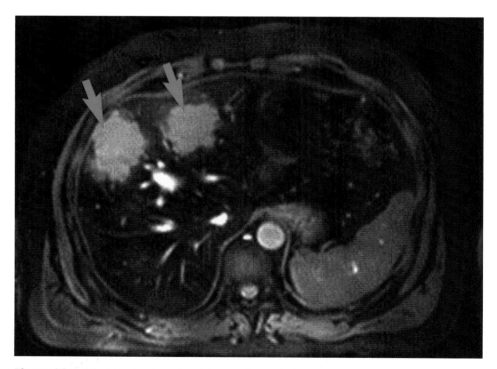

**Figure 28.1** MR image showing colorectal cancer liver metastases.

### What factors determine tumour resectability?

Surgical resection is currently the gold standard, potentially curative treatment for liver metastases (Figure 28.2 – *see inside back cover*). However, less than 30% of patients are suitable due to the extent and distribution of the disease or concurrent medical disability.[3]

Most patients with liver metastases do not require extended surgery. However, central tumours, tumours near the major vessels or multiple tumours spread over three segments necessitate extended resections to obtain adequate oncological clearance. Previously, extended resections were not usually considered due to associated morbidity and a high risk of perioperative mortality. With advances in surgical and anaesthetic techniques, the mortality from hepatic resection has reduced from as much as 20% to less than 5%.[1,4,5] The lower mortality and improved long-term survival has pushed towards more aggressive surgery.

Surgery is indicated if metastases can be resected leaving sufficient liver parenchyma, regardless of the number or size of the lesions. More than 20% of functional liver should be left to reduce the risk of hepatic insufficiency following resection.[6] The percentage of residual liver should be higher following chemotherapy. This is due to the occurrence of chemotherapy-associated steatohepatitis and sinusoidal obstruction syndrome.[7,8]

Strategies have evolved to increase the functional reserve of the liver prior to resection. These include preoperative portal vein embolization and a two-stage hepatectomy. The objective of portal vein embolization is to block the portal venous flow to the hemi-liver containing the metastases, thereby inducing contralateral hypertrophy and increasing the size of the remnant liver.[1,6,9]

Extrahepatic metastases, excluding resectable pulmonary metastases, indicate a poor prognosis and are a relative contraindication to hepatic resection. They are not an absolute contraindication if the extrahepatic metastases can be resected simultaneously.[10]

Repeated liver resections should be considered if a patient presents with hepatic recurrence. The same criteria should be followed as applied to the first operation. Repeat hepatic resections are technically challenging due to adhesions and the distortion and anatomical disorientation of the liver architecture that accompanies regeneration. However, surgery is the treatment of choice for patients with resectable recurrent disease.[10,11]

### Assuming the liver can be cleared of tumour, what is the immediate and long-term prognosis?

Liver metastases are the main cause of death in patients with colorectal cancer. They are present in 15–25% patients when diagnosed with the primary tumour and will develop in another 40–50% patients following treatment of the colorectal primary.[11-13]

The 5-year survival rate for patients undergoing a curative liver resection is about 40%. The mean survival for untreated metastases is 6–12 months, which can be extended to 12–18 months with the newer chemotherapy regimens.[1,5,11,13] The two factors clearly associated with poorer outcome are positive resection margins and the presence of extrahepatic disease at the time of liver resection.[5,14]

After a curative liver resection, 50–70% of patients will develop local, regional or distant recurrence, 50% will have recurrent disease in the liver remnant and 30% will have disease isolated to the liver.[2] Of these patients, 10% will be suitable for a second hepatectomy.[10,11] After a second liver resection, a third of patients who develop a recurrence in the liver will be suitable for a further hepatectomy.[15] The morbidity from repeat liver resections is now similar to that of the first resection and there is no difference in overall survival.[2,11] There is no difference in survival between synchronous and metachronous metastases.[1,14]

## Discussion

 **What are the patient's options if the liver is the only site of disease, but the tumours are not resectable?**

The aim of treatment for unresectable liver metastases is to prolong survival and to maintain a good quality of life.[16] Neoadjuvant chemotherapy is often offered with modern regimens incorporating oxaliplatin or irinotecan besides 5-fluorouracil and leucovorin. Patients should be re-evaluated after neoadjuvant chemotherapy as metastases may have adequately downsized to allow resection.[16] The extent of resection (residual disease versus all involved areas) is not generally agreed, and is governed by technical considerations. The 5-year survival for patients undergoing resection after a good response to chemotherapy is now approaching that of those undergoing resection first.[1,17] However, patients whose disease progresses despite neoadjuvant chemotherapy have a poor prognosis and surgical intervention cannot be justified.

Hepatic artery infusion is an alternative to prolonged systemic chemotherapy. The aim is to treat known metastases in the liver, plus suspected micro-metastases, with high chemotherapy concentrations, while minimizing systemic toxicity. Chemotherapy is infused into the hepatic artery, the main blood supply to liver metastases; the portal vein supplies most of the normal liver cells.[6,12,18] The hepatic artery catheter must be surgically placed; regional perfusion chemotherapy can be technically difficult to deliver. Some studies have shown considerable radiological response, allowing patients to subsequently undergo surgical resection.[18]

Cryosurgical ablation (CSA) and radiofrequency ablation (RFA) are techniques used for the localized destruction of liver metastases in patients unsuitable for surgery. The intention is to destroy the whole tumour plus an adjacent cuff of normal tissue to create a tumour-free margin.[19] In CSA, very low temperatures cause tumour cell destruction via protein denaturation and cellular dehydration. The freeze–thaw cycles destroy the cells.[19] However, CSA is associated with a high rate of complications and has been overtaken by RFA.

RFA is a novel technique. It is an optional treatment for patients who are unsuitable for resection, and it is an important complement to surgical resection in patients with small, deep-set, contralateral lesions. RFA works by converting electromagnetic energy into thermal injury within the target tissue. Over 60 °C, coagulative necrosis occurs[11] and at higher temperatures, the cell membrane, nucleus and whole architecture is damaged.[3,20,21] The current is produced by a generator connected to a needle electrode with a movable hub that advances and retracts a curved electrode from its tip (Figure 28.3). RFA can be performed via a percutaneous image-guided approach, laparoscopically or during open laparotomy. It is considered a safe technique with low mortality and morbidity.[22,23]

Although initially RFA showed favourable results,[24] recent studies have shown a high

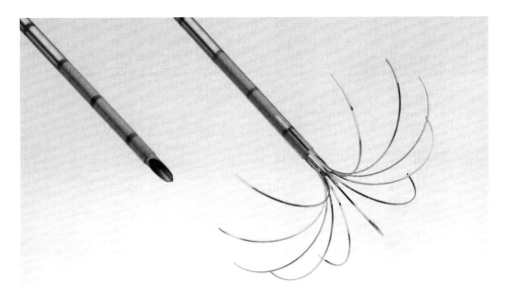

**Figure 28.3** Electrode used in radiofrequency ablation.

rate of local recurrence, up to 40%.[20] This correlates with the failure to ablate lesions completely. Careful selection of tumours can decrease the local recurrence rate nearer to that of surgical resection, while minimizing the morbidity and mortality accompanying an operation.[3] It has been established that RFA provides a survival benefit over chemotherapy alone in patients. Therefore although survival after RFA is not comparable with that after resection it should be considered when surgery is not possible.[3]

## Conclusion

The size and location of the metastases and liver function should be evaluated by CT scan, to assess whether the patient is suitable for liver resection. If the tumours are not resectable neoadjuvant chemotherapy and local ablation could be discussed.

## Further Reading

1 McLoughlin JM, Jenson EH, Malafa M. Resection of colorectal liver metastases: current perspectives. *Cancer Causes Control* 2006; **13**: 32–41.

2 Chu QD, Vezeridis MP, Avradopoulos KA, Wanebo HJ. Repeat hepatic resection for recurrent colorectal cancer. *World J Surg* 1997: **21**: 292–6.

3 Feliberti EC, Wagman LD. Radiofrequency ablation of liver metastases from colorectal cancer. *Cancer Causes Control* 2006; **13**: 48–51.

4 Capussotti L, Polastri R. Operative risks of major hepatic resections. *Hepatogastroenterology* 1998; **45**: 184–90.

5   Scheele J, Stang R, Altendorf-Hofmann A, Paul M. Resection of colorectal liver metastases. *World J Surg* 1995; **19**: 59–71.

6   Selzner N, Pestalozzi BC, Kadry Z, Selzner M, Wildermuth S, Clavien PA. Downstaging colorectal liver metastases by concomitant unilateral portal vein ligation and selective intra-arterial chemotherapy. *Br J Surg* 2006; **93**: 587–92.

7   Karoui M, Penna C, Amin-Hashem M, Mitry E, Benoist S, Franc B, Rougier P, Nordlinger B. Influence of preoperative chemotherapy on the risk of major hepatectomy for colorectal liver metastases. *Ann Surg* 2006; **243**: 1–7.

8   Fernandez FG, Ritter J, Goodwin JW, Linehan DC, Hawkins WG, Strasberg SM. Effect of steatohepatitis associated with irinotecan or oxaliplatin pretreatment on resection of hepatic colorectal metastases. *J Am Coll Surg* 2005; **200**: 845–53.

9   Simmonds PC, Primrose JN, Colquitt JL, Garden OJ, Poston GJ, Rees M. Surgical resection of hepatic metastases from colorectal cancer: A systemic review of published studies. *Br J Cancer* 2006; **94**: 982–99.

10  Muratore A, Polastri R, Bouzari H, Vergara V, Ferrero A, Capussotti L. Repeat hepatectomy for colorectal metastases: a worthwhile operation? *J Surg Oncol* 2001; **76**: 127–32.

11  Shaw IM, Rees M, Welsh FK, Bygrave S, John TG. Repeat hepatic resection for recurrent colorectal liver metastases is associated with favourable long-term survival. *Br J Surg* 2006; **93**: 457–64.

12  Kemeny N, Huang Y, Cohen AM, Shi W, Conti JA, Brennan MF, Bertino JR, Turnbull AD, Sullivan D, Stockman J, Blumgart LH, Fong Y. Hepatic artery infusion of chemotherapy after resection of hepatic metastases from colorectal cancer. *N Engl J Med* 1999; **341**: 2039–48.

13  Bennett JJ, Cao D, Posner MC. Determinants of unresectability and outcome of patients with occult colorectal hepatic metastases. *J Surg Oncol* 2005; **92**: 64–9.

14  Memon MA, Beckingham IJ. Surgical resection of colorectal liver metastases. *Colorect Dis* 2001; **3**: 361–73.

15  Tanaka K, Shimada H, Mitsuyoshi O, Togo S, Saitou S, Yamaguchi S, Endo I, Sekido H. Procedures for choice for resection of primary and recurrent liver metastases from colorectal cancer. *World J Surg* 2004; **28**: 482–7.

16  Benoist S, Pautrat K, Mitry E. Treatment strategy for patients with colorectal cancer and irresectable liver metastases. *Br J Surg* 2005; **92**: 1155–60.

17  Capussotti L, Muratore A, Mulas MM, Massucco P, Aglietta M. Neoadjuvant chemotherapy and resection for initially irresectanle colorectal liver metastases. *Br J Surg* 2006; **93**: 1001–6.

18  Homsi J, Garrett CR. Hepatic arterial infusion of chemotherapy for hepatic metastases from colorectal cancer. *Cancer Causes Control* 2006; **13**: 42–7.

19  Joosten J, Jager G, Oyen W, Wobbes T, Ruers T. Cryosurgery and radiofrequency ablation for unresectable colorectal liver metastases. *Eur J Surg Oncol* 2005; **31**: 1152–9.

20  van Duijnhoven FH, Jansen MC, Junggeburt JM, van Hillegersberg R, Rijken AM, van Coevorden F, van der Sijp JR, van Gulik TM, Slooter GD, Klaase JM, Putter H, Tollenaar RA. Factors influencing the local failure rate of radiofrequency ablation of colorectal liver metastases. *Ann Surg Oncol* 2006; **13**: 651–8.

21  Siperstien AE, Gitomirski A. History and technological aspects of radiofrequency thermoablation. *Cancer J* 2000; **5**: 293–303.

22 Livraghi T, Solbiati L, Meloni MF, Gazelle GS, Halpern EF, Goldberg SN. Treatment of focal liver tumours with percutaneous radio-frequency ablation: complications encountered in a multicentre study. *Radiology* 2003; **226**: 441–51.

23 Casaril A, Abu-Hilal M, Ciola M, Invernizzi L, Campagnaro T, Nicoli N. One death after radiofrequency thermal ablation for hepatocellular carcinoma in a cirrhotic patient. *Surgery* 2003; **133**: 598.

24 Oshowo A, Gillams A, Harrison E, Lees WR, Taylor I. Comparison of resection and radiofrequency ablation for treatment of solitary colorectal liver metastases. *Br J Surg* 2003; **90**: 1240–3.

25 Abdalla EK, Vauthey JN, Ellis LM, Ellis V, Pollock R, Broglio KR, Hess K, Curley SA. Recurrence and outcomes following hepatic resection, radiofrequency ablation, and combined resection/ablation for colorectal liver metastases. *Ann Surg* 2004; **239**: 818–25.

# Melanoma

# 29 Management of Primary Melanoma

## Case History

A 50-year-old man presents with an ulcerated lesion on his shoulder and an axillary mass. Excision biopsy of the lesion reveals a 5 mm Breslow thickness nodular melanoma, and axillary dissection reveals 4/15 lymph nodes positive for melanoma, with no extracapsular spread. He has been referred for consideration of adjuvant treatment.

What is the recommended excision margin for the primary melanoma?

What are the surgical considerations regarding wider excision of this lesion?

If there is no disease elsewhere, what is this patient's prognosis?

What is the evidence for activity of low-dose, medium-dose and high-dose interferon in melanoma?

What are the short-term and long-term side effects of high-dose interferon?

Should this patient have adjuvant axillary radiotherapy?

## Background

**What is the recommended excision margin for the primary melanoma?**

The recommended excision margin is 2 cm. Two trials were conducted in patients with melanomas <2 mm, the World Health Organization (WHO) trial[1] compared margins of 1 cm and 3 cm and the Swedish Melanoma Group trial[2] compared margins of 2 cm and

5 cm. The Intergroup trial[3] randomized patients with 1–4 mm melanomas to 2 cm and 4 cm margins. There were no differences in local recurrence, disease-free survival and overall survival between the narrow and wide excision groups. A UK-MSG trial[4] compared 1 cm and 3 cm margins for melanomas >2 mm and showed higher rates of local recurrence in the 1 cm margin arm but no difference in overall survival. Therefore, a 1 cm margin is adequate for melanomas <2 mm and a 2 cm margin for melanomas >2 mm.

### What are the surgical considerations regarding wider excision of this lesion?

Wide excision of the shoulder lesion with a 2 cm margin may risk cosmetic morbidity and functional loss, and require skin grafting. Similarly, the axillary dissection may result in lymphoedema, cosmetic disfigurement and functional loss.

### If there is no disease elsewhere, what is this patient's prognosis?

The patient has T4 N3 M0 stage IIIc disease and the corresponding 5-year and 10-year overall survival rates are 26.7% ± 2.5% and 18.4% ± 2.5% (Table 29.1).[5]

## Discussion

### What is the evidence for activity of low-dose, medium-dose and high-dose interferon in melanoma?

Four randomized controlled trials of high-dose interferon[6–9] have been published and with a fifth trial in abstract form only. Updated analysis from the landmark Eastern Cooperative Oncology Group (ECOG) 1684 trial[6] comparing HDI and observation showed an improvement in relapse-free survival but not in overall survival. The confirmatory trial ECOG 1690[7] showed a trend to improvement in relapse-free survival but not in overall survival. The ECOG 1694 trial[8] showed the benefit of high-dose interferon in relapse-free survival and overall survival compared with a ganglioside vaccine, but the vaccine may not have been an appropriate control. The NCCTG trial[9] compared intramuscular high-dose interferon and observation and noted no difference in survival. Pooled results from the three ECOG studies[10] revealed a difference in relapse-free survival but not in overall survival.

Medium-dose interferon was investigated in a large European Organisation for Research and Treatment of Cancer (EORTC) trial. There was a trend towards benefit in the treatment arms for disease-free survival but no notable differences overall.[11] Five randomized controlled trials comparing low-dose interferon with observation have not shown a disease-free survival or overall survival advantage with the drug.[12] Finally, two meta-analyses of all randomized controlled trials comparing interferon and observation have shown a marked difference in relapse-free survival but not in overall survival.[13,14]

### What are the short-term and long-term side effects of high-dose interferon?

Sixty-seven percent of patients in the ECOG 1684 trial[6] experienced severe (grade ≥3) toxicity including constitutional and neurological symptoms, myelosuppression and hepatotoxicity, with 9% of patients developing life-threatening toxicities. There were two

## Table 29.1 Survival rates for melanoma TNM and staging categories

| Pathologic stage | TNM | Thickness (mm) | Ulceration | No.+ nodes | Nodal size | Distant metastasis | No. of patients | Survival ± SE | | | |
|---|---|---|---|---|---|---|---|---|---|---|---|
| | | | | | | | | 1-Year | 2-Year | 5-Year | 10-Year |
| IA | T1a | 1 | No | 0 | – | – | 4510 | 99.7 ± 0.1 | 99.0 ± 0.2 | 95.3 ± 0.4 | 87.9 ± 1.0 |
| IB | T1b | 1 | Yes or level IV, V | 0 | – | – | 1380 | 99.8 ± 0.1 | 98.7 ± 0.3 | 90.0 ± 1.0 | 83.1 ± 1.5 |
| | T2a | 1.01–2.0 | No | 0 | – | – | 3285 | 99.5 ± 0.1 | 97.3 ± 0.3 | 89.0 ± 0.7 | 79.2 ± 1.1 |
| IIA | T2b | 1.01–2.0 | Yes | 0 | – | – | 958 | 98.2 ± 0.5 | 92.9 ± 0.9 | 77.4 ± 1.7 | 64.4 ± 2.2 |
| | T3a | 2.01–4.0 | No | 0 | – | – | 1717 | 98.7 ± 0.3 | 94.3 ± 0.6 | 78.7 ± 1.2 | 63.8 ± 1.7 |
| IIB | T3b | 2.01–4.0 | Yes | 0 | – | – | 1523 | 95.1 ± 0.6 | 84.8 ± 1.0 | 63.0 ± 1.5 | 50.8 ± 1.7 |
| | T4a | >4.0 | No | 0 | – | – | 563 | 94.8 ± 1.0 | 88.6 ± 1.5 | 67.4 ± 2.4 | 53.9 ± 3.3 |
| IIC | T4b | >4.0 | Yes | 0 | – | – | 978 | 89.9 ± 1.0 | 70.7 ± 1.6 | 45.1 ± 1.9 | 32.3 ± 2.1 |
| IIA | N1a | Any | No | 1 | Micro | – | 252 | 95.9 ± 1.3 | 88.0 ± 2.3 | 69.5 ± 3.7 | 63.0 ± 4.4 |
| | N2a | Any | No | 2–3 | Micro | – | 130 | 93.0 ± 2.4 | 82.7 ± 3.8 | 63.3 ± 5.6 | 56.9 ± 6.8 |
| IIB | N1a | Any | Yes | 1 | Micro | – | 217 | 93.3 ± 1.8 | 75.0 ± 3.2 | 52.8 ± 4.1 | 37.8 ± 4.8 |
| | N2a | Any | Yes | 2–3 | Micro | – | 111 | 92.0 ± 2.7 | 81.0 ± 4.1 | 49.6 ± 5.7 | 35.9 ± 7.2 |
| | N1b | Any | No | 1 | Macro | – | 122 | 88.5 ± 2.9 | 78.5 ± 3.7 | 59.0 ± 4.8 | 47.7 ± 5.8 |
| | N2b | Any | No | 2–3 | Macro | – | 93 | 76.8 ± 4.4 | 65.6 ± 5.0 | 46.3 ± 5.5 | 39.2 ± 5.8 |
| IIIC | N1b | Any | Yes | 1 | Macro | – | 98 | 77.9 ± 4.3 | 54.2 ± 5.2 | 29.0 ± 5.1 | 24.4 ± 5.3 |
| | N2b | Any | Yes | 2–3 | Macro | – | 109 | 74.3 ± 4.3 | 44.1 ± 4.9 | 24.0 ± 4.4 | 15.0 ± 3.9 |
| | N3 | Any | Any | 4 | Micro/macro | – | 396 | 71.0 ± 2.4 | 49.8 ± 2.7 | 26.7 ± 2.5 | 18.4 ± 2.5 |
| IV | M1a | Any | Any | Any | Any | Skin, SQ | 179 | 59.3 ± 3.7 | 36.7 ± 3.6 | 18.8 ± 3.0 | 15.7 ± 2.9 |
| | M1b | Any | Any | Any | Any | Lung | 186 | 57.0 ± 3.7 | 23.1 ± 3.2 | 6.7 ± 2.0 | 2.5 ± 1.5 |
| | M1c | Any | Any | Any | Any | Other visceral | 793 | 40.6 ± 1.8 | 23.6 ± 1.5 | 9.5 ± 1.1 | 6.0 ± 0.9 |
| Total | | | | | | | 17600 | | | | |

Source: Balch et al., 2001.[5]

early deaths from hepatotoxicity. Similar toxicities were encountered in ECOG 1690,[7] but there were no treatment-related deaths. In the induction phase, dose reductions and delays due to toxicity occurred in 44% and 37% of patients in ECOG 1684[6] and ECOG 1690,[7] respectively. Similarly, in the maintenance phase, dose reductions and delays due to toxicity occurred in 36% and 52% of the patients, respectively. Long-term side effects include hypothyroidism and hyperlipidaemia.

### Should this patient have adjuvant axillary radiotherapy?

Adjuvant radiotherapy following lymphadenectomy is controversial and generally not recommended. Small randomized and non-randomized studies have shown improved loco-regional control among patients with high-risk features such as multiple positive nodes, extracapsular extension or recurrent nodal disease. Most of these studies have included patients with cervical, axillary or inguinal adjuvant radiotherapy, and, in general, the 5-year loco-regional control rates range from 84% to 95% compared with rates of 50–80% with surgery alone. However, the 5-year overall survival remains unchanged ranging from 22% to 50%,[15–18] and adjuvant radiotherapy is associated with moderate toxicity. The reported rates of lymphoedema following axillary radiotherapy range from 17.1% to 41%.[15,16] Adjuvant radiotherapy cannot be recommended as there is still a lack of large randomized controlled studies and insufficient data on long-term toxicity.

## Conclusion

This patient's melanoma should be excised with a margin of 2 cm, and the axillary lymph node also excised. Long-term survival for this stage of disease is low. Interferon does not seem to improve survival and can cause toxicity, so its use would not be recommended in this case. Radiotherapy is also not recommended for this patient.

## Further Reading

1  Veronesi U, Cascinelli N, Adamus J, Balch C, Bandiera D, Barchuk A, Bufalino R, Craig P, De Marsillac J, Durand JC. Thin stage I primary cutaneous malignant melanoma. Comparison of excision margins of 1 or 3 cm. *N Engl J Med* 1988; **318**: 1159.

2  Cohn-Cedermark G, Rutqvist LE, Andersson R, Breivald M, Ingvar C, Johansson H, Jonsson PE, Krysander L, Lindholm C, Ringborg U. Long-term results of a randomised study by the Swedish Melanoma Study Group on 2 cm versus 5 cm resection margins for patients with cutaneous melanoma with a tumour thickness of 0.8–2.0 mm. *Cancer* 2000; **89**: 1495–501.

3  Balch CM, Soong SJ, Smith T, Ross MI, Urist MM, Karakousis CP, Temple WJ, Mihm MC, Barnhill RJ, Jewell WR, Wanebo HJ, Desmond R. Long-term results of a prospective surgical trial comparing 2 cm vs 4 cm excision margins for patients with 1–4 mm melanomas. *Ann Surg Oncol* 2001; **8**: 101–8.

4  Thomas JM, Newton-Bishops J, A'Hern R, Coombes G, Timmons M, Evans J, Cook M, Theaker J, Fallowfield M, O'Neill T, Ruka W, Bliss JM. Excision margins in high-risk malignant melanoma. *N Engl J Med* 2004; **350**: 757–66.

5  Balch CM, Buzaid AC, Soong SJ, Atkins MB, Cascinelli N, Coit DG, Fleming ID, Gershenwald JE, Houghton A Jr, Kirkwood JM, McMasters KM, Mihm MF, Morton DL, Reintgen DS, Ross MI, Sober A, Thompson JA, Thompson JF. Final version of the American Joint Committee on Cancer Staging System for cutaneous melanoma. *J Clin Oncol* 2001; **19**: 3635–48.

6  Kirkwood JM, Strawderman MH, Ernstoff MS, Smith TJ, Borden EC, Blum RH. Interferon alfa-2b adjuvant therapy of high-risk resected cutaneous melanoma: the Eastern Cooperative Oncology Group Trial EST 1684. *J Clin Oncol* 1996; **14**: 7–17.

7  Kirkwood JM, Ibrahim JG, Sondak VK, Richards J, Flaherty LE, Ernstoff MS, Smith TJ, Rao U, Steele M, Blum RH. High- and low-dose interferon alfa-2b in high-risk melanoma: first analysis of Intergroup Trial E1690/S9011/C9190. *J Clin Oncol* 2000; **18**: 2444–58.

8  Kirkwood JM, Ibrahim JG, Sosman JA, Sondak VK, Agarwala SS, Ernstoff MS, Rao U. High dose interferon alfa-2b significantly prolongs relapse-free and overall survival compared with the GM2-KLH/QS-21 vaccine in patients with resected Stage IIB-IV melanoma: results of the IntergroupTrial E1694/ S9512/ C509801. *J Clin Oncol* 2001; **19**: 2370–80.

9  Creagan ET, Dalton RJ, Ahmann DL, Jung SH, Morton RF, Langdon RM Jr, Kugler J, Rodrigue LJ. Randomised surgical adjuvant clinical trial of recombinant interferon alfa-2b in selected patients with malignant melanoma. *J Clin Oncol* 1995; **13**: 2776–83.

10  Kirkwood J, Manola J, Ibrahim J, Sondak VK, Ernstoff MS, Rao U. A pooled analysis of Eastern Cooperative Oncology Group and Intergroup trials of high-dose adjuvant interferon for melanoma. *Clin Cancer Res* 2004; **10**: 1670–7.

11  Eggermont AM, Suciu S, Mackie R, Ruka W, Testori A, Kruit W, Punt CJ, Delauney M, Sales F, Groenewegen G, Ruiter DJ, Jagiello I, Stoitchkov K, Keilholz U, Lienard D; EORTC Melanoma Group. Post-surgery adjuvant therapy with intermediate doses of interferon alfa 2b versus observation in patients with stage IIb/III melanoma (EORTC 18952): randomised controlled trial. *Lancet* 2005; **366**: 1189–96.

12  Verma S, Quirt I, McCready D, Bak K, Charette M, Iscoe N. Systematic review of systemic adjuvant therapy for patients at high-risk for recurrent melanoma. *Cancer* 2006; **106**: 1431–42.

13  Wheatley K, Ives N, Hancock B, Gore M, Eggermont A, Suciu S. Does adjuvant interferon-alpha for high-risk melanoma provide a worthwhile benefit? A meta-analysis of the randomised trials. *Cancer Treat Rev* 2003; **29**: 241–52.

14  Pirard D, Heenen M, Melot C, Vereecken P. Interferon-alpha as adjuvant postsurgical treatment of melanoma. *Dermatology* 2004; **208**: 43–8.

15  Strom EA, Ross MI. Adjuvant radiotherapy after axillary lymphadenectomy for metastatic melanoma: toxicity and local control. *Ann Surg Oncol* 1995; **2**: 445–9.

16  Ballo MT, Strom EA, Zagars GK, Bedikian AY, Prieto VG, Mansfield PF, Lee JE, Gershenwald JE, Ross MI. Adjuvant irradiation for axillary metastases from malignant melanoma. *Int J Radiat Oncol Biol Phys* 2002; **52**: 964–72.

17  Ballo MT, Merrick IR, Cormier JN, Myers JN, Lee JE, Gershenwald JE, Hwu P, Zagars GK. Combined-modality therapy for patients with regional nodal metastases from melanoma. *Int J Radiat Oncol Biol Phys* 2006; **64**: 106–13.

18  Fuhrmann D, Lippold A, Borrrosch F, Ellwanger U, Garbe C, Suter L. Should adjuvant radiotherapy be recommended following resection of regional lymph node metastases of malignant melanomas? *Br J Dermatol* 2001; **144**: 66–70.

# 30  Melanoma in Pregnancy

## Case History

A 28-year-old woman who is 14 weeks pregnant with her first child presents with an enlarging pigmented lesion on her lower leg which has bled on several occasions. Excision biopsy under local anaesthetic reveals an ulcerated nodular malignant melanoma of 3.6 mm Breslow thickness, with excision margins of less than 3 mm.

**What should be the further surgical management?**

**What staging investigations should she have?**

**What are the implications for her pregnancy?**

**How will her pregnancy influence her prognosis?**

## Background

### What should be the further surgical management?

This patient has a T3b primary lesion. Although she is pregnant, appropriate surgery at the site of the primary lesion should not be delayed. She requires a wide local excision (WLE) of the primary lesion. Wide excision minimizes the risk of leaving behind malignant cells that may locally recur or metastasize. Risk factors for local recurrence are thick primaries, ulceration and head and neck primaries.[1] Inappropriately large excisions may lead to cosmetic disfigurement, functional deficits and require major surgery with skin grafting, therefore a minimal (but appropriate) excision margin is essential. The recommended excision margin in this case is 2 cm (see Chapter 29) to the level of the deep fascia with a split skin graft or flap. This may be done under local anaesthestic.

The management of the lymph node basin for T2–3 lesions remains an area of controversy. The rationale that early removal of subclinically involved nodes is superior to removal once obvious nodal disease develops is supported by several retrospective studies showing that 5-year survival rates improved in patients with intermediate thickness lesions. Subsequent prospective studies including the World Health Organization (WHO) trial,[2] the Intergroup Melanoma trial[3] and a systematic review[4] have shown that elective lymph node dissection (ELND) compared with delayed node dissection had no effect on survival.

ELND is associated with considerable morbidity with overall reported rates of wound morbidity, infection, lymphoedema and delayed healing between 35% and 51% in the axilla and 25–90% in the inguinal region. A post hoc subgroup analysis in the WHO trial showed that patients with positive nodes on ELND had a marked survival advantage over the group with positive nodes and a delayed LND but 80% of patients who received ELND did not have nodal metastases and therefore only 20% receiving ELND may have benefited. These findings support use of sentinel node biopsy (SNB) to identify patients with a high risk of nodal disease. Several small studies have shown that SNB is a highly sensitive and specific test for nodal staging and SLN status is a powerful independent factor predicting survival.[5]

Several confirmatory randomized trials of SNB are ongoing. The MSLT-1 trial compared WLE/SNB with WLE alone; patients with positive SNB underwent immediate LND and the WLE-alone arm underwent delayed LND after clinical detection of nodal disease. After 59.5 months of follow-up, interim results showed a significant improvement in 5-year disease-free survival ($P = 0.01$) but no overall survival advantage in the WLE/SNB arm (87% versus 86% in the WLE-alone arm).[6] The 5-year survival was significantly higher after immediate LND for SN-positive patients than delayed LND for clinical nodal recurrence (71% and 55%, respectively) but this was not a strictly randomized comparison as the latter group may have been a biologically unfavourable group of patients. MSLT-II is investigating the therapeutic benefit of LND compared with SNB alone in SN-positive patients. SNB is not without morbidity but the overall postoperative complication rate of 5% is lower than observed in ELND.[7] As there is currently no evidence of a therapeutic benefit form SNB, patients with lesions >1 mm should be offered SNB in a setting of a clinical trial. This pregnant patient will not be eligible for a trial.

### What staging investigations should she have?

UK guidelines recommend that patients with stage IIb (see Table 29.1)[5] and over should have the following staging investigations: full blood count; liver function tests; lactate dehydrogenase; chest radiograph and liver ultrasound or computed tomographic scan with contrast of the chest, abdomen and/or pelvis.[8] In this patient's case, imaging investigations with risk of radiation exposure must be avoided. Pregnancy-related changes in blood tests will have to be considered when interpreting the results of the blood test.

## Discussion

### What are the implications for her pregnancy?

A comprehensive MEDLINE database search from 1966 to 2002 revealed 27 reported cases of metastatic melanoma in pregnancy affecting the placenta and/or fetus. The fetus was affected in six of these cases and five of the six infants died of the disease.[9] However, a large epidemiological study in which there were only a few women with regional and distant disease, and women who terminated their pregnancies prior to 20 weeks were excluded, showed that there were no differences in the rates of caesarean delivery, length of hospital stay, risk of low birth weight, prematurity and neonatal death in 148 pregnant women with melanoma compared with pregnant women without melanoma.[10] This patient appears to have early-stage disease and therefore should carry the pregnancy to full term. There are no data justifying the termination of pregnancy as a therapeutic intervention to improve survival (see below).

### How will her pregnancy influence her prognosis?

Her pregnancy should not influence her prognosis. Initial concerns were raised when case reports and small retrospective studies from the 1950–70s reported a poorer prognosis in pregnant women with melanoma and two small epidemiological studies reported shorter disease-free intervals in pregnant women compared to non-pregnant women with melanoma.[11,12] However, recent larger epidemiological studies[10,13,14] have shown that pregnancy does not have an adverse effect on survival. Compared to non-pregnant women with melanoma, there were no differences with regard to tumour location, histological subtype, tumour ulceration, vascular invasion or disease stage. Although these studies showed no statistically significant difference in tumour thickness, two studies[13,14] showed a trend towards thicker melanomas in pregnant women.

## Conclusion

Despite being pregnant, this patient should have further surgery, to ensure that an excision margin of 2 cm is achieved. During the work-up for staging, physiological changes due to her pregnancy must be considered. There is no current evidence to suggest that her prognosis is affected by the pregnancy and there is no medical need for termination of pregnancy.

## Further Reading

1 Balch CM, Soong SJ, Smith T, Ross MI, Urist MM, Karakousis CP, Temple WJ, Mihm MC, Barnhill RJ, Jewell WR, Wanebo HJ, Desmond R. Long-term results of a prospective surgical trial comparing 2 cm vs 4 cm excision margins for patients with 1–4 mm melanomas. *Ann Surg Oncol* 2001; **8**: 101–8.

2 Cascinelli N, Morabito A, Santinami M, Mackie RM, Belli F. Immediate or delayed dissection of regional nodes in patients with melanoma of the trunk: a randomised trial. WHO Melanoma Programme. *Lancet* 1998; **351**: 793–6.

3 Balch CM, Soong SJ, Bartolucci AA, Urist MM, Karakousis CP, Smith TJ, Temple WJ, Ross MI, Jewell WR, Mihm MC, Barnhill Rl, Wanebo HJ. Efficacy of an elective regional lymph node dissection of 1 to 4 mm thick melanomas for patients 60 years of age and younger. *Ann Surg* 1996; **224**: 255–63.

4 Lens MB, Dawes M, Goodacre T, Newton- Bishop JA. Elective lymph node dissection in patients with melanoma: systematic review and meta-analysis of randomised controlled trials. *Arch Surg* 2002; **137**: 458–61.

5 Balch CM, Buzaid AC, Soong SJ, Atkins MB, Cascinelli N, Coit DG, Fleming ID, Gershenwald JE, Houghton A Jr, Kirkwood JM, McMasters KM, Mihm MF, Morton DL, Reintgen DS, Ross MI, Sober A, Thompson JA, Thompson JF. Final version of the American Joint Committee on Cancer Staging System for cutaneous melanoma. *J Clin Oncol* 2001; **19**: 3635–48.

6 Morton DL, Thompson JF, Cochran AJ, Essner R, Elashoff R; Multicenter Selective Lymphadenectomy Trial Group. Interim results of the Multicenter Selective Lympadenectomy Trial (MSLT-1) in clinical stage 1 melanoma. American Society of Clinical Oncology Annual Meeting, 2005 (abstract 7500).

7   McMasters KM, Noyes RD, Reintgen DS, Goydos JS, Beitsch PD, Davidson BS, Sussman JJ, Gershenwald J, Ross MI; Sunbelt Melanoma Trial. Lessons learnt from the Sunbelt melanoma trial. *J Surg Oncol* 2004; **86**: 212–23.

8   Roberts DLL, Anstey AV, Barlow RJ, Cox NH on behalf of the British Association of Dermatologists and Newton-Bishop JA, Corrie PG, Evans J, Gore ME, Hall PN, Kirkham N on behalf of the Melanoma Study Group. UK guidelines for the management of cutaneous melanoma. *Br J Dermatol* 2002; **146**: 7–17.

9   Alexander A, Samlowski WE, Grossman D, Bruggers CS, Harris RM, Zone JJ, Noyes RD, Bowen GM, Leachman SA. Metastatic melanoma in pregnancy: risk of transplacental metastases in the infant. *J Clin Oncol* 2003; **21**: 2179–86.

10  O'Meara AT, Cress R, Xing G, Danielsen B, Smith LH. Malignant melanoma in pregnancy. *Cancer* 2005; **103**: 1217–26.

11  Houghton AM, Flannery J, Viola MV. Malignant melanoma of the skin occurring in pregnancy. *Cancer* 1981; **48**: 407–10.

12  Reintgen DS, McCarty KS Jr, Vollmer R, Cox E, Seigler HF. Malignant melanoma and pregnancy. *Cancer* 1985; **55**: 1340–4.

13  Daryanani D, Plukker JT, De Hullu JA, Kuiper H, Nap RE, Hoekstra HJ. Pregnancy and early stage melanoma. *Cancer* 2003; **97**: 2248–53.

14  Lens MB, Rosdahl I, Ahlbom A, Farahmand BY, Synnerstad I, Boeryd B, Newton Bishop JA. Effect of pregnancy on survival in women with cutaneous malignant melanoma. *J Clin Oncol* 2004; **22**: 4369–75.

PROBLEM

# 31  Medical Management of Metastatic Melanoma

## Case History

A 60-year-old man had a melanoma resected from his back 5 years ago, and had an axillary dissection with 3/16 nodes positive for melanoma 2 years later. On routine follow-up, a chest radiograph shows multiple bilateral coin lesions.

**How should this patient be further imaged?**

**Is a tissue diagnosis necessary, and why?**

**Assuming no other sites of disease, and that the patient is asymptomatic, what would be the initial management options?**

**What palliative medical treatments could be considered for this patient?**

# Background

### How should this patient be further imaged?

Prior to further imaging, the patient should have a physical examination paying particular attention to possible regional recurrence. Blood tests including lactate dehydrogenase, urea and electrolytes, liver function tests, calcium and full blood count should be done.

The most reliable method for evaluating lung metastasis is contrast computed tomography (CT). The accuracy of CT scan was compared with chest radiograph in a study of 42 patients with high-risk melanoma.[1] Unequivocal nodules were revealed by CT scan in 20 patients but in only 11 by chest radiograph. CT scan is also superior for assessing mediastinal and hilar adenopathy and the presence of lymphangitis, which is particularly important in assessing a patient with a potentially resectable isolated pulmonary metastasis. If CT scan confirms multiple pulmonary metastases, then the patient can be followed by chest radiograph to assess his progression or his response to systemic treatment.

The liver is a common site of metastatic disease (in as many as 58% of patients with metastatic melanoma[2]), and can be assessed by ultrasound or CT. Liver metastases are usually multiple, but solitary lesions may be considered for resection, radiofrequency ablation or cryotherapy, in which case further assessment by magnetic resonance imaging (MRI) is advisable. Small-bowel metastasis in melanoma is not uncommon.[3] Brain imaging in asymptomatic patients is controversial. Up to 25% of patients with metastatic melanoma have asymptomatic brain metastases, but it is unclear whether these lesions require intervention. Some clinicians therefore advocate imaging to look for central nervous system (CNS) involvement only in symptomatic patients,[4] in which case MRI is the study of choice.

### Is a tissue diagnosis necessary, and why?

Tissue diagnosis is important when there are doubts about the diagnosis and when the disease is not typically following its natural history. In early melanoma most studies indicate that about 80% of recurrences occur within first 3 years. However, up to 16% of first recurrences have been reported to occur after 5 years.[5]

Thus, in this patient, distant metastasis occurring 3 years after node dissection is not surprising, and it would be safe to omit a biopsy. However, if the history were less typical, lung biopsy should be considered.

# Discussion

### Assuming no other sites of disease, and that the patient is asymptomatic, what would be the initial management options?

Once melanoma is unresectable, the prognosis is extremely poor and management should be aimed at symptom palliation. Unresectable stage IV melanoma is refractory to most standard systemic therapy. Response rates of up to 20% may be achieved, but there is no associated increase in median survival and less than 5% of patients survive 5 years. In a meta-analysis of 83 studies with 6322 patients, the median survival of patients treated for metastatic disease was 8.9 months in studies published since 1985.[6] Long-term survival was 13.6% at 2 years and 2.3% at 5 years.

Patients should be involved in making decisions about their management. They should be made aware of the poor prognosis and should be encouraged to consider clinical trials. In this case, watchful waiting would be a reasonable initial management. The patient should be reviewed regularly, and disease progression monitored with blood tests and chest radiographs.

## What palliative medical treatments could be considered for this patient?

### Palliative chemotherapy

The standard off-trial systemic treatment of unresectable stage IV melanoma is with dacarbazine (DTIC). DTIC is considered to be the most active single agent with a response rate of 10–20%.[7] The vast majority of responses are partial and the median response duration is only 4–6 months. Other agents with modest single agent activity include vinca alkaloids, platinum compounds and taxanes.

The single-agent activity of DTIC has led to its use in combination with a variety of other agents. Although response rates may be higher, multiple drug regimens do not improve survival compared with single-agent DTIC and are not recommended outwith clinical trials.[8]

### Biological treatment and biochemotherapy

The two biological treatments that appear most active against melanoma are interferon-$\alpha$ and interleukin-2 (IL-2). Response rates for interferon-$\alpha$ range from 8% to 22% and long-term administration on a three times per week basis appears superior to once a week or more intermittent schedules.[9] Response to IL-2 is similar and is in the 10–20% range. IL-2 in high doses is used by some centres for unresectable stage IV melanoma. Side effects include capillary leak syndrome, cardiac arrhythmias and renal complications.[10]

Combination of chemotherapy and interferon-$\alpha$ or IL-2 has failed to produce appreciably better response rates, durations or overall survival.[8] Toxicity is greater with biochemotherapy and for these reasons it is not considered a standard of care.

### Palliative care

Patients with advanced melanoma require a coordinated multiprofessional approach with input from the specialist palliative care team. Patients may need rehabilitative, functional, social and financial support services. A patient may be referred at any point in the cancer journey, and especially if he or she has poorly controlled symptoms.

### Clinical trials and novel approaches

A combined phase I/II study of sorafenib, a signal transduction inhibitor, plus carboplatin and paclitaxel in refractory melanoma has shown some promise, with 14/36 partial responses and 17 patients with prolonged periods of stable disease.[11] Sorafenib plus DTIC was also studied in 30 patients with advanced metastatic melanoma;[12] 5 patients (16%) had partial response and 13 patients (43%) had stable disease. First- and second-line trials are ongoing. Other approaches include immunomodulation (e.g. with the MDX-010 anti-CTLA-4 antibody) and gene therapy.

## Conclusion

CT scanning should be done to evaluate the extent of the lung metastasis and check for metastasis to the liver. Palliative care will be required, from a multidisciplinary team.

## Further Reading

1  Heaston DK, Putman CE, Rodan BA, Nicholson E, Ravin CE, Korobkin M, Chen JT, Seigler HF. Solitary pulmonary metastasis in high risk melanoma patients: a prospective comparison of conventional and computed tomography. *Am J Roentgenol* 1983; **141**:169–74.

2  Shirkhoda A, Albin J. Malignant melanoma: correlating abdominal and pelvic CT with clinical staging. *Radiology* 1987; **165**: 75.

3  Reintgen DS, Thompson W, Garbutt J, Seigler HF. Radiologic, endoscopic, and surgical considerations of melanoma metastatic to the gastrointestinal tract. *Surgery* 1984; **95**: 635–9.

4  Kuvshinoff BW, Kurtz C, Coit DG. Computed tomography in evaluation of patients with stage III melanoma. *Ann Surg Oncol* 1997; **4**: 252–8.

5  McCarthy WH, Shaw HM, Thompson JF, Milton GW. Time and frequency of recurrence of cutaneous stage 1 malignant melanoma with guidelines for follow up. *Surg Gynecol Obstet* 1988; **166**: 497–502.

6  Lee ML, Tomsu K, Von Eschen KB. Duration of survival for disseminated malignant melanoma: results of a meta-analysis. *Melanoma Res* 2000; **10**: 81–92.

7  Crosby T, Fish R, *et al.* Systemic treatments for metastatic cutaneous melanoma. In: *Cochrane Library*, issue 4, Update Software, Oxford, 2002.

8  Hernberg M, *et al.* Regimens with or without interferon-alpha as treatment for metastatic melanoma and renal cell carcinoma: an overview of randomized trials. *J Immunother* 1999; **22**: 145–54.

9  Agarwala SS, Kirkwood JM. Interferons in melanoma. *Curr Opin Oncol* 1996; **8**: 167–174.

10  Atkins MB, Lotze MT, Dutcher JP, Fisher RI, Weiss G, Margolin K, Abrams J, Sznol M, Parkinson D, Hawkins M, Paradise C, Kunkel L, Rosenberg SA. High dose recombinant interleukin-2 therapy for patients with metastatic melanoma: analysis of 270 patients treated between 1985 and 1993. *J Clin Oncol* 1999; **17**: 2105.

11  Flaherty KT, Brose M, Schuchter L, Tuveson D, Lee R, Schwartz B, Lathia C, Weber B, O'Dwyer P. Phase I/II trial of BAY 43–9006, carboplatin and paclitaxel demonstrates preliminary antitumour activity in the expansion cohort of patients with metastatic melanoma. *J Clin Oncol* 2004; **22** (Suppl) (abstract 7507).

12  Lorigan P, Corrie D, Chao P. Phase II trial of sorafenib combined with dacarbazine in metastatic melanoma patients. *J Clin Oncol* 2006; **24** (Suppl) (abstract 8012).

# Lung Cancer

**PROBLEM**

## 32 Lung Cancer: Initial Diagnosis and Work-up

## Case History

A reasonably fit 62-year-old smoker presents with persistent cough. Bronchoscopy reveals an obstructing endobronchial tumour in the right middle lobe bronchus, 1 cm from the subcarina. Biopsy confirms squamous cell carcinoma. A computed tomography (CT) staging scan shows collapse/consolidation in the right middle lobe distal to a 2.5 cm tumour and several 1.5–2 cm lymph nodes in the mediastinum in the N1 and N2 positions. No metastatic nodules are visualized within the other lobes of the lung, and there are no distant metastases.

**What is the bronchoscopic and radiological stage of this tumour?**

**What are the implications for management?**

## Background

**What is the bronchoscopic and radiological stage of this tumour?**

Accurate staging in patients with non-small cell lung cancer (NSCLC) has a critical role in determining optimal therapy (Tables 32.1 and 32.2). It reflects the nature and extent of disease and provides important prognostic information. Surgery remains the treatment

**Table 32.1**   TNM staging of non–small cell lung cancer

**Primary tumour (T)**

| | |
|---|---|
| Tx | Primary tumour cannot be assessed or tumour proven by the presence of malignant cells in sputum or bronchial washings but not visualized by imaging or bronchoscopy |
| T0 | No evidence of primary tumour |
| Tis | Carcinoma *in situ* |
| T1 | Tumour <3 cm in greatest dimension, surrounded by lung or visceral pleura, without bronchoscopic evidence of invasion more proximal than the lobar bronchus |
| T2 | Tumour with any of the following features of size or extent:<br>● >3 cm in greatest dimension<br>● involves main bronchus >2 cm distal to the carina<br>● invades the visceral pleura<br>● associated with atelectasis or obstructive pneumonitis that extends to the hilar region but does not involve the entire lung |
| T3 | Tumour of any size that directly invades the following: chest wall (including superior sulcus tumours), diaphragm, mediastinal pleura, parietal pericardium; or tumour in the main bronchus <2 cm distal to the carina but without involvement of the carina; or associated atelectasis or obstructive pneumonitis of the entire lung |
| T4 | Tumour of any size that involves any of the following: mediastinum, heart, great vessels, trachea, oesophagus, vertebral body, carina; or tumour with a malignant pleural or pericardial effusion, or with satellite tumour nodule(s) within the ipsilateral primary tumour lobe of the lung |

**Regional lymph nodes (N)**

| | |
|---|---|
| Nx | Regional lymph nodes cannot be assessed |
| N0 | No regional lymph node metastases |
| N1 | Metastases to ipsilateral peribronchial and/or ipsilateral hilar lymph nodes and intrapulmonary nodes involved by direct extension of primary tumour |
| N2 | Metastases to ipsilateral mediastinal and/or subcarinal lymph nodes |
| N3 | Metastases to contralateral mediastinal, contralateral hilar, ipsilateral or contralateral |

**Distant metastases (M)**

| | |
|---|---|
| Mx | Presence of distant metastases cannot be assessed |
| M0 | No distant metastases |
| M1 | Distant metastases present |

of choice for early-stage NSCLC, and the likelihood of curative surgery depends on the local extent of the primary tumour and presence of any distant metastases.[1,2]

Bronchoscopy is both a diagnostic and staging investigation, in this case revealing a T1 tumour. CT is used to define the extent of disease and determine whether the primary tumour is resectable. Magnetic resonance imaging (MRI) of the chest does not offer improvement in the accuracy of primary tumour staging[3] and is not routinely done.

# Discussion

## What are the implications for management?

Figure 32.1 provides an algorithm for the management of NSCLC.

| Table 32.2 | Staging of non–small cell lung cancer |
|---|---|
| **Stage grouping** | **TNM subsets** |
| 0 | Carcinoma *in situ* |
| IA | T1 N0 M0 |
| IB | T2 N0 M0 |
| IIA | T1 N1 M0 |
| IIB | T2 N1 M0<br>T3 N0 M0 |
| IIIA | T3 N1 M0<br>T1 N2 M0<br>T2 N2 M0<br>T3 N2 M0 |
| IIIB | T4 N0 M0<br>T4 N1 M0<br>T1 N3 M0<br>T2 N3 M0<br>T3 N3 M0<br>T4 N3 M0 |
| IV | Any T Any N M1 |

This patient's primary lesion is amenable to lobectomy. However, he has abnormally enlarged nodes in the N1 and N2 positions, i.e. radiological stage IIIA disease. Nodal staging is important in patients with NSCLC as it has important implications for suitability for curative surgery.[4] Patients who have stage IIIA disease with N2 node involvement have a poorer prognosis and are unlikely to be cured by surgery alone.[4,5] The survival rate for N2 disease, however, depends on whether this is a radiological, mediastinoscopic or postoperative histological finding. Some postoperative survival statistics include patients in whom preoperatively unsuspected N2 disease was diagnosed only microscopically in a few N2 nodes resected at operation. These patients' survival, clearly, is superior to that of most stage IIIA patients. Patients with N3 node-positive disease are not suitable for curative surgery.[5]

Nodal disease assessment is difficult, as enlarged nodes on chest radiograph or CT scan do not necessarily imply nodal metastases. Accuracy of CT for nodal staging is not high, with sensitivity and specificity of 60–65% and 60–70%, respectively.[5] Nodes may be enlarged due to inflammatory or other benign processes and conversely, normal-sized nodes may contain malignant cells. The large N1 and N2 nodes in this case may be due to malignant involvement or because of inflammation reactive to the obstructive pneumonitis.

Mediastinoscopy or, occasionally, transcarinal bronchoscopic fine needle aspiration (FNA) may be done to obtain histological or cytological confirmation of intrathoracic lymph node involvement. Mediastinoscopy remains the most accurate method of nodal staging but may be associated with a small but important morbidity and mortality.[6–8] Some surgical centres offer one-step staging and definitive surgery, i.e. mediastinoscopy

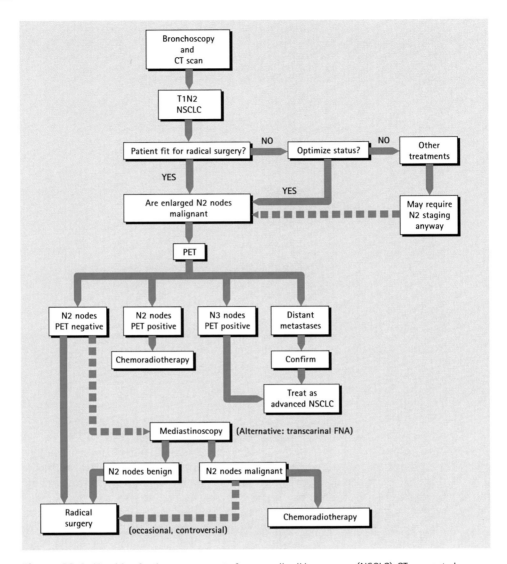

**Figure 32.1** Algorithm for the management of non-small cell lung cancer (NSCLC). CT, computed tomography; PET, positron emission tomography; FNA, fine needle aspiration.

and frozen section of lymph nodes, proceeding to thoracotomy and definitive surgery if nodes are reactive rather than malignant.

There has been increasing interest in non-invasive staging using whole-body positron emission tomography (PET) with 18-FDG ([18F] fluoro-2-deoxyglucose), which has a higher rate of detection of mediastinal nodes as well as extrathoracic metastases.[8–10] Studies have shown PET scan to be consistently more accurate than CT for mediastinal node staging with negative predictive values >90%.[9] It has been suggested that in some cases mediastinoscopy is not necessary if the mediastinum is PET negative.[11] Incorporating PET into conventional staging also upstages approximately 25% of patients, detecting unsuspected extrathoracic metastases in around 10%.[10,12] The cost of PET may be compensated by more appropriate patient selection and avoidance of futile surgery.[13,14]

PET has some limitations. 18-FDG is taken up by muscles and by areas of active inflammation, which may give false-positive results. Furthermore, precise location of focal abnormalities is difficult to determine on PET, needing visual correlation with CT. Integrated PET-CT has been shown to be superior in determining stage of NSCLC compared with other radiological modalities.[15] However, PET-CT is not widely available. If the PET scan in the case study patient did not reveal unsuspected distant metastases, it is likely that mediastinoscopy and pathological staging of the lymph nodes would be indicated in any case, as the only radiological contraindication for potentially curative surgery is presence of 'radiologically abnormal nodes'.

If clinical assessment or PET suggests metastatic disease not revealed on staging CT then additional site-specific tests, such as isotope bone scan and CT/MRI of the brain could be useful. However, in general, these are not indicated in asymptomatic patients. Some centres, however, are adopting the practice of a CT brain scan for lung adenocarcinoma before resection, because of the relatively high rate of unsuspected brain metastases in this subset of patients. Others advocate that patients with N2 nodes undergo ultrasound of the supraclavicular area and FNA of any nodes thus revealed, as this yields a positive result in a subset of patients for whom radical surgery is therefore not appropriate.

Finally, we must also take into account the patient's fitness for surgery. Patients with poor performance status and those with history of marked weight loss are more likely to have advanced disease and should be staged particularly carefully. Many patients with NSCLC have coexisting smoking-related chronic obstructive airways disease and/or atherosclerotic cardiovascular disease, so careful preoperative assessment of their pulmonary function and cardiovascular risk factors is necessary.[1,2]

## Conclusion

Surgery remains the treatment of choice for early-stage NSCLC. In this case, the decision whether the patient has surgery or not will depend on whether the N2 nodes, enlarged on CT, prove malignant or not.

## Further Reading

1  British Thoracic Society; Society of Cardiothoracic Surgeons of Great Britain and Ireland Working Party. Guidelines on the selection of patients with lung cancer for surgery. *Thorax* 2001; **56**: 89–108.

2  Beckles MA, Spiro SG, Colice GL, Rudd RM. The physiologic evaluation of patients with lung cancer being considered for resectional surgery. *Chest* 2003; **123**: 105–14.

3   Webb WR, Gatsonis C, Zerhouni EA, Heelan RT, Glazer GM, Francis IR, McNeil BJ. CT and MR imaging in non small cell bronchogenic carcinoma: report of the radiologic Diagnostic Oncologic Group. *Radiology* 1991; **178**: 705–13.

4   Mountain CF, Dresler CM. Regional lymph node classification for lung cancer staging. *Chest* 1997; **111**: 1718–23.

5   McLoud TC, Bourgoin PM, Greenberg RW, Kosiuk JP, Templeton PA, Shepard JA, Moore EH, Wain JC, Mathisen DJ, Grillo HC. Bronchogenic carcinoma: analysis of staging in the mediastinum with CT by correlative lymph node mapping and sampling. *Radiology* 1992; **182**: 319–23.

6   Hammoud ZT, Anderson RC, Meyers BF, Guthrie TJ, Roper CL, Cooper JD, Patterson GA. The current role of mediastinoscopy in the evaluation of thoracic disease. *J Thorac Cardiovasc Surg* 1999; **118**: 894–9.

7   Schimmer C, Neukam K, Elert O. Staging of non small cell lung cancer; clinical value of positron emission tomography and mediastinoscopy. *Interact Cardiovasc Thorac Surg* 2006; **5**: 418–23.

8   Kelly RF, Tran T, Holmstrom A, Murar J, Sequrola RJ Jr. Accuracy and cost-effectiveness of [18F]-2-fluoro-deoxy-D-glucose-positron emission tomography scan in potentially resectable non-small cell lung cancer. *Chest* 2004; **125**: 1413–23.

9   Toloza EM, Harpole L, McCrory DC. Noninvasive staging of non-small cell lung cancer: a review of the current evidence. *Chest* 2003; **123**: 137–46.

10  Reed CE, Harpole DH, Posther KE, Woolson SL, Downey RJ, Meyers BF, Heelan RT, MacApinlac HA, Jung SH, Silvestri GA, Siegel BA, Rusch VW; American College of Surgeons Oncology Group Z0050 trial. Results of American College of Surgeons Oncology Group Z0050 Trial: The utility of positron emission tomography in staging potentially operable non-small cell lung cancer. *J Thorac Cardiovasc Surg* 2003; **126**: 1943–51.

11  Kernstine KH, Mclaughlin KA, Menda Y, Rossi NP, Kahn DJ, Bushnell DL, Graham MM, Brown CK, Madsen MT. Can FDG-PET reduce the need for mediastinoscopy in potentially resectable nonsmall cell lung cancer? *Ann Thorac Surg* 2002; **73**: 394–402.

12  Pieterman RM, Van Putten JWG, Meuzelaar JJ, Mooyaart EL, Vaalburg W, Koëter GH, Fidler V, Pruim J, Groen HJ. Preoperative staging of non-small cell lung cancer with positron-emission tomography. *N Engl J Med* 2000; **343**: 254–61.

13  Verboom P, Tinteren HV, Hoekstra OS, Smit EF, van den Bergh JH, Schreurs AJ, Stallaert RA, van Velthoven PC, Comans EF, Diepenhorst FW, van Mourik JC, Postmus PE, Boers M, Grijseels EW, Teule GJ, Uyl-de Groot CA; PLUS study group. Cost-effectiveness of FDG-PET in staging non-small cell lung cancer: the PLUS study. *Eur J Nucl Med Mol Imaging* 2003; **30**: 1444–9.

14  Dietlein M, Weber K, Gandjour A, Moka D, Theissen P, Lauterbach KW, Schicha H. Cost-effectiveness of FDG-PET for the management of potentially operable non-small cell lung cancer: priority for a PET-based strategy after nodal-negative CT results. *Eur J Nucl Med* 2000; **27**: 1598–609.

15  Lardinois D, Weder W, Hany TF, Kamel EM, Korom S, Seifert B, von Schulthess GK, Steinert HC. Staging on non-small-cell lung cancer with integrated positron-emission tomography and computed tomography. *N Engl J Med* 2003; **348**: 2500–7.

# 33 Adjuvant Treatment for Resected Non-small Cell Lung Cancer

## Case History

A 69-year-old man is referred by a thoracic surgeon following complete resection of T2 N1 squamous cell carcinoma of the lung. Resection margins are clear.

**What trials form the evidence base for adjuvant chemotherapy in this situation?**

**What factors would you take into account when deciding whether to offer this patient adjuvant chemotherapy?**

**What will you tell the patient?**

**If you and the patient decide that chemotherapy should be given, what regimen(s) and duration would you choose and why?**

## Background

### What trials form the evidence base for adjuvant chemotherapy in this situation?

In 1995, a meta-analysis of updated data from 52 randomized clinical trials (1394 patients) indicated that adjuvant chemotherapy in surgically resected stage IB, II and IIIA non-small cell lung cancer (NSCLC) did not appreciably improve overall survival. There was, however, a trend in favour of chemotherapy regimens that included cisplatin. This analysis led to the development of several subsequent adjuvant chemotherapy trials with improved patient selection and refined drug regimens.

The International Adjuvant Lung Cancer Trial (IALT) showed that adjuvant cisplatin-based chemotherapy improved relapse-free survival by 5.1% and overall survival by 4.1% at 5 years. The IALT included 1867 patients and investigated stage IA–IIIA disease, comparing three or four cycles of adjuvant combination chemotherapy including cisplatin combined with either etoposide, vinorelbine, vinblastine or vindesine, against observation.[1] The National Cancer Institute of Canada (NCIC) JBR.10 trial showed a 15% improvement in overall survival in the chemotherapy-treated group at 5 years. This trial included 482 patients and investigated stage IB–II disease, comparing four cycles of a combination of vinorelbine and cisplatin against observation.[2] The Adjuvant Navelbine International Trialist Association (ANITA) trial (including 840 patients, again comparing a combination of vinorelbine and cisplatin against observation in patients with stage IB–IIIA disease) showed an improvement in overall survival of 8.6% at 5 years, maintained at 7 years.[3]

On the other hand, early reports of the Cancer and Leukaemia Group B (CALGB)

9633 trial indicated a marked 12% improvement in overall survival, but a 2006 update showed only a non-significant trend in favour of treatment at 5 years. That trial included 344 patients with stage IB disease only, comparing four cycles of a combination of pacli-taxel and carboplatin against observation. The Adjuvant Lung Cancer Project Italy (ALPI) study also found no significant difference between adjuvant cisplatin-based chemotherapy and observation in completely resected NSCLC.

However, the Lung Adjuvant Cisplatin Evaluation (LACE) meta-analysis concluded there was benefit of adjuvant cisplatin-based chemotherapy – of the order of 5%. In keeping with the updated CALGB results, the LACE meta-analysis failed to substantiate benefit in stage IB patients.[4]

# Discussion

 **What factors would you take into account when deciding whether to offer this patient adjuvant chemotherapy?**

The main curative therapeutic approach for stage IA–IIB NSCLC is surgery. The ratio-nale for the use of systemic therapy in completely resected NSCLC is based on, first, knowledge that distant metastatic disease is the primary cause of death for most patients with early-stage NSCLC and, second, that evidence of micrometastasis at the time of surgery corresponds with reduced survival.[5]

It is important to appreciate that toxicity secondary to chemotherapy is important (in the IALT trial there was a 23% risk of grade 4 toxicity, primarily neutropenia, and a 0.8% risk of treatment-related death[2]), and it must be considered whether or not such clinical risk is worthwhile for small improvements in survival. Lung cancer patients often have comorbidities, which should be taken into account when deciding whether a patient will be able to tolerate a particular chemotherapy regimen. Presumably the case study patient is a relatively fit man with good physiological reserves, as he was a candidate for surgical resection in the first place. A physical assessment should be done to ensure that a full postoperative recovery has been made and that his performance status is good enough to tolerate chemotherapy (0–2).

More than 50% of lung cancer patients are diagnosed at 65 years or older. The patients included in the adjuvant trials mentioned above were not representative of this age group: the median patient age in the ANITA trial was 59 years[3] and in the CALGB trial it was 61 years. Elderly patients may not tolerate treatment as well as younger patients because of reduced organ function and increased comorbidities associated with increas-ing age (see references in Chapters 9 and 38). Patients who are older will probably not complete a full course of chemotherapy. However, even with reduced doses a survival benefit in favour of adjuvant cisplatin-based chemotherapy has been seen.[3]

## What will you tell the patient?

It is important that the patient understands that he may well have been cured by surgery. However, patients with NSCLC have a high risk of recurrent disease, and this often occurs at sites distant to the primary tumour. One of the ways of reducing the risk of recurrence is adjuvant chemotherapy. This man falls into the group of patients who may benefit from adjuvant chemotherapy. However, it must be made clear that chemotherapy does not eliminate the risk of recurrence, and that there are also major toxicities associated with chemotherapy.

A recent subanalysis has suggested that the levels of ERCC1 gene expression in the tumour may help to predict which patients will probably benefit, but this is not routinely assayed in clinical practice.[6] It is possible that in the not too distant future, such patient discussions will be better informed by knowledge of the molecular pathology of the tumour and its relationship to benefit from adjuvant therapy.

### If you and the patient decide that chemotherapy should be given, what regimen(s) and duration would you choose and why?

Given that the three trials discussed above, which showed a considerable survival advantage in favour of adjuvant chemotherapy used vinorelbine and cisplatin, this is the combination we would recommend. It appears that four cycles of adjuvant chemotherapy are sufficient. Close examination of the data from the ANITA trial shows that most patients did not receive their chemotherapy as planned, resulting in reduced dose intensity (and yet a survival benefit was still demonstrated).[3] The question about optimum dose intensity therefore remains somewhat open.

## Conclusion

Recent trials suggest that cisplatin-based chemotherapy improves overall survival of surgically resected NSCLC by about 5%, when delivered as adjuvant treatment. This can be discussed with the patient, provided he has recovered well from the surgery and is medically fit for chemotherapy.

## Further Reading

1   Arriagada R, Bergman B, Dunant A, Le Chevalier T, Pignon JP, Vansteenkiste J; International Adjuvant Lung Cancer Trial Collaborative Group. Cisplatin-based adjuvant chemotherapy in patients with completely resected non-small-cell lung cancer. *N Engl J Med* 2004; **350**: 351–60.

2   Winton T, Livingston R, Johnson D, Rigas J, Johnston M, Butts C, Cormier Y, Goss G, Inculet R, Vallieres E, Fry W, Bethune D, Ayoub J, Ding K, Seymour L, Graham B, Tsao MS, Gandara D, Kesler K, Demmy T, Shepherd F; National Cancer Institute of Canada Clinical Trials Group; National Cancer Institute of the United States Intergroup JBR.10 Trial Investigators. Vinorelbine plus cisplatin vs. observation in resected non-small-cell lung cancer. *N Engl J Med* 2005; **352**: 2589–97.

3   Douillard JY, Rosell R, De Lena M, Carpagnano F, Ramlau R, Gonzales-Larriba JL, Grodzki T, Pereira JR, Le Groumellec A, Lorusso V, Clary C, Torres AJ, Dahabreh J, Souquet PJ, Astudillo J, Fournel P, Artal-Cortes A, Jassem J, Koubkova L, His P, Riggi M, Hurteloup P. Adjuvant vinorelbine plus cisplatin versus observation in patients with completely resected stage IB-IIIA non-small-cell lung cancer (Adjuvant Navelbine International Trialist Association [ANITA]): a randomised controlled trial. *Lancet Oncol* 2006; **7**: 719–27.

4   Pignon JP, Tribodet H, Scagliotti GV, *et al.* Lung Adjuvant Cisplatin Evaluation (LACE): A pooled analysis of five randomized clinical trials including 4,584 patients. *J Clin Oncol* 2006; 24(Suppl 18S) (abstract 7008).

5   Passlick B, Kubuschok B, Izbicki JR, Thetter O, Pantel K. Isolated tumor cells in bone marrow predict reduced survival in node-negative non-small cell lung cancer. *Ann Thoracic Surg* 1999; **68**: 2053–8.

6   Olaussen KA, Dunant A, Fouret P, Brambilla E, Andre F, Haddad V, Taranchon E, Filipits M, Pirker R, Popper HH, Stahel R, Sabatier L, Pignon JP, Tursz T, Le Chevalier T, Soria JC; IALT Bio Investigators. DNA repair by ERCC1 in non-small-cell lung cancer and cisplatin-based adjuvant therapy. *N Engl J Med* 2006; **355**: 983–91.

**PROBLEM**

# 34  Advanced Non-small Cell Lung Cancer

## Case History

You are asked to see a 54-year-old woman with advanced non-small cell lung cancer (NSCLC), staged as T4 N2 M1 (lung metastases). Taking a careful history, you decide her performance status is 1.

**What is the predicted survival for such patients?**

**What therapeutic options will you discuss with her?**

**If you and she reach a decision to try chemotherapy, what regimen(s) could you choose and on what evidence would this choice be based?**

There is a good partial response on the end-of treatment scan but 3 months later a computed tomography (CT) scan shows asymptomatic progression in the primary lesion (T4). Her performance status remains very good.

**How will you approach the management now?**

## Background

### What is the predicted survival for such patients?

With rare exceptions, patients with advanced NSCLC die from their disease. The overall median survival ranges from less than 6 months for patients with poor performance status to 2 years for fit patients with stage IIIB disease. The proportion of patients who are alive 1 year after diagnosis has increased slightly over the past decade with about a third of patients with stage IIIB or IV disease being alive at 1 year and 10–21% alive 2 years after diagnosis. The most important factor predicting survival is the performance status. Patients with

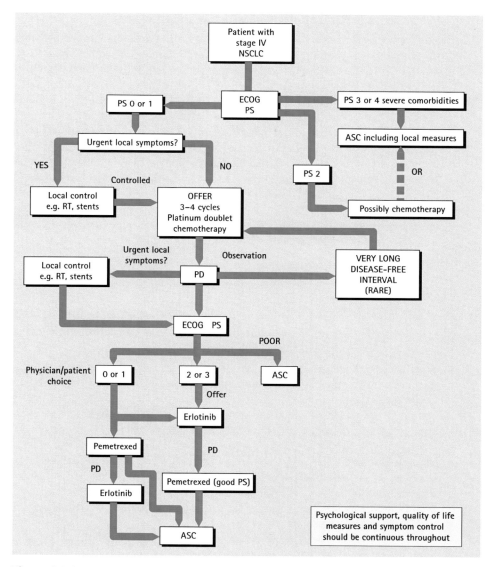

**Figure 34.1** Algorithm for management of patients with advanced non-small cell lung cancer (NSCLC). ECOG, Eastern Cooperative Oncology Group; PS, performance status; ASC, active supportive care; PD, progressive disease; RT, radiotherapy.

advanced NSCLC who are compromised by their disease have much poorer survival compared with those less compromised. This stark contrast was first documented by Finkelstein *et al.* in a landmark analysis of 893 patients with stage IV NSCLC. In that study, the 1-year survival rate was 36% for patients with performance status 0, 16% for performance status 1, and 9% for performance status 2 (*P* <0.001). In the era of modern chemotherapy, performance status is still predictive of survival, as well as of toxicity of treatment.[1,2]

### What therapeutic options will you discuss with her?

The goal of treatment of all patients with advanced NSCLC is to improve symptoms and delay disease progression while maintaining the quality of life (Figure 34.1). A meta-analysis and at least 1 randomized trial have shown a modest but marked survival advantage in favour of best supportive care (BSC) with chemotherapy compared with BSC alone in patients with good performance status.[3,4] An improvement in the median survival time of 6–8 weeks is expected for those advanced NSCLC patients who are receiving platinum-based chemotherapy, translating to a 10% improvement in the 1-year survival rate. Therefore, a 54-year-old woman with performance status 1 should be offered combination chemotherapy with a clear explanation of the benefits and the associated risks. Equally important is good supportive care, addressing symptoms such as superior vena cava obstruction, haemoptysis, upper airway obstruction and bone pain. As the objective response rate to chemotherapy is less than 50%, symptoms such as these are usually treated urgently with local measures such as stents or radiotherapy before chemotherapy is considered.

## Discussion

 **If you and she reach a decision to try chemotherapy, what regimen(s) could you choose and on what evidence would this choice be based?**

Large clinical trials comparing a doublet regimen of platinum (carboplatin or cisplatin) have failed to show a major advantage of one of any of the doublets containing platinum and one of the other 'new' chemotherapy agents, e.g. a taxane, vinorelbine or gemcitabine, over another doublet. There are of course differences in toxicity, need for intravenous hydration, etc., which should be taken into account when individualizing the choice of chemotherapy for the patient. If there is any suspicion that a patient might need urgent radiotherapy if there is no response to chemotherapy, it is best to avoid radiosensitizing agents such as gemcitabine which may complicate its delivery. Acceptable doublets in current clinical use include paclitaxel/carboplatin, gemcitabine/cisplatin, docetaxel/cisplatin, vinorelbine/cisplatin and gemcitabine/carboplatin.[2,5,6] It appears that there is no advantage of giving six cycles of combination chemotherapy compared with three to four cycles.[7]

There is a good partial response on the end-of treatment scan but 3 months later a computed tomography (CT) scan shows asymptomatic progression in the primary lesion (T4). Her performance status remains very good.

### How will you approach the management now?

The therapeutic options in relapse of NSCLC after first-line chemotherapy are active supportive care (ASC) with or without second-line chemotherapy or an epidermal growth factor receptor (EGFR) inhibitor (Figure 34.1). The systemic treatments do confer some survival advantages and may improve quality of life. However, objective response rates are even more modest than for first-line chemotherapy. Therefore it is crucial to know whether the progressive primary lesion looks as if it may cause symptoms, e.g. imminent bronchial compression. If so, the focus should be on control of this, for example with radiotherapy or stenting, before considering systemic treatment.

Shepherd *et al.* first showed, with docetaxel, that second-line chemotherapy can improve outcomes in patients who have received cisplatin therapy.[8] More recently, a study of more than 500 patients with advanced disease showed that pemetrexed, a multi-targeted antifolate, had similar efficacy to docetaxel but with less toxicity.[9] In that study, the median survival time was 8.3 months in the pemetrexed treatment arm and 7.9 months in the docetaxel arm, with similar objective response rates, progression-free survival and time to progressive disease. There is no evidence that combining cytotoxic drugs in second-line treatment confers any additional benefit.

The BR.21 study was a phase 3 trial of erlotinib in patients who had progressed after standard first-line and/or second-line chemotherapy. A total of 731 patients were randomly assigned in a 2:1 ratio to receive 150 mg of erlotinib daily or placebo. The primary endpoint was overall survival. The response rate was 8.9% in the erlotinib group and less than 1% in the placebo group ($P$ <0.001). The overall survival was 6.7 months and 4.7 months, respectively ($P$ <0.001) in favour of erlotinib. This trial included patients with much poorer performance status than the second-line trials of cytotoxic agents.[10]

Therefore there is now a choice of second-line and possibly even third-line agents for our patient. Although the chances of response to erlotinib are much greater in patients whose cancer carries certain mutations in the EGFR pathway, statistical modelling of the BR.21 study indicate that even patients without detectable mutations may benefit from erlotinib. Mutation testing has not entered routine practice to select for treatment, although this may be imminent. In the absence of predictive mutation testing, the immediate choice between pemetrexed and erlotinib depends on patient preference and the presence of clinical factors that are associated with erlotinib response, such as female sex, absence of smoking history and adenocarcinoma histology.

## Conclusion

The prognosis and long-term survival prospects of this patient are poor, therefore symptomatic treatment is the most important. Chemotherapy does confer a modest survival advantage, but the relatively small benefits must be discussed with the patient.

## Further Reading

1 Finkelstein DM, Ettinger DS, Ruckdeschel JC. Long-term survivors in metastatic non-small cell lung cancer: an Eastern Cooperative Oncology Group study. *J Clin Oncol* 1986; **4**: 702–9.

2 Schiller JH, Harrington D, Belani CP, Langer C, Sandler A, Krook J, Zhu J, Johnson DH; Eastern Cooperative Oncology Group. Comparison of four chemotherapy regimens for advanced non-small-cell lung cancer. *N Engl J Med* 2002; **346**: 92–8.

3 Non-Small Cell Collaborative Group. Chemotherapy in non-small cell lung cancer: a meta analysis using updated data on individual patients from 52 randomized clinical trials. *BMJ* 1995; **311**: 899–909.

4 Stephens RJ, Fairlamb D, Gower N, Maslove L, Milroy R, Napp V, Peake MD, Rudd RM, Spiro S, Thorpe H, Waller D; on behalf of all participants, CRC and UCL Cancer Trials Centre, London, UK. The Big Lung Trial (BLT): determining the value of cisplatin-based

chemotherapy for all patients with non-small cell lung cancer: preliminary results in the supportive care setting. *Proc Am Soc Clin Oncol* 2002; **21**: 291a (Abstract 1161).

5 Fossella F, Pereira JR, von Pawel J, Pluzanska A, Gorbounova V, Kaukel E, Mattson KV, Ramlau R, Szczesna A, Fidias P, Millward M, Belani CP. Randomized, multinational, phase III study of docetaxel plus platinum combinations versus vinorelbine plus cisplatin for advanced non-small-cell lung cancer: the TAX 326 Study Group. *J Clin Oncol* 2003; **21**: 3016–24.

6 Danson S, Middleton MR, O'Byrne KJ, Clemons M, Ranson M, Hassan J, Anderson H, Burt PA, Fairve-Finn C, Stout R, Dowd I, Ashcroft L, Beresford C, Thatcher N. Phase III trial of gemcitabine and carboplatin versus mitomycin, ifosfamide, and cisplatin or mitomycin, vinblastine, and cisplatin in patients with advanced nonsmall cell lung carcinoma. *Cancer* 2003; **98**: 542–53.

7 Smith IE, O'Brien ME, Talbot DC, Nicolson MC, Mansi JL, Hickish TF, Norton A, Ashley S. Duration of chemotherapy in advanced non-small-cell lung cancer: a randomized trial of three versus six courses of mitomycin, vinblastine, and cisplatin. *J Clin Oncol* 2001; **19**: 1336–43.

8 Shepherd FA, Dancey J, Ramlau R, Mattson K, Gralla R, O'Rourke M, Levitan N, Gressot L, Vincent M, Burkes R, Coughlin S, Kim Y, Berille J. Prospective randomized trial of docetaxel versus best supportive care in patients with non-small-cell lung cancer previously treated with platinum-based chemotherapy. *J Clin Oncol* 2000; **18**: 2095–103.

9 Hanna N, Shepherd FA, Fossella FV, Pereira JR, De Marinis F, von Pawel J, Gatzemeier U, Tsao TC, Pless M, Muller T, Lim HL, Desch C, Szondy K, Gervais R, Shaharyar, Manegold C, Paul S, Paoletti P, Einhorn L, Bunn PA Jr. Randomized phase III trial of pemetrexed versus docetaxel in patients with non-small-cell lung cancer previously treated with chemotherapy. *J Clin Oncol* 2004; **22**: 1589–97.

10 Shepherd FA, Pereira JR, Ciuleanu T, *et al.* Erlotinib in previously treated non-small-cell lung cancer. *N Engl J Med* 2005; **353**: 123–32.

PROBLEM

# 35 Small Cell Carcinoma of the Lung

## Case History

A 65-year-old ex-smoker presents with a right upper lobe mass and enlarged ipsilateral hilar lymph nodes on computed tomography (CT) scan. Full radiological staging reveals no other metastases. Bronchoscopy shows that he has an endobronchial abnormality in the right upper lobe bronchus that on biopsy shows small cell lung cancer (SCLC).

**How will you stage this cancer?**

**What factors influence prognosis in this disease?**

**If this patient has no adverse prognostic factors, what treatment(s) would you recommend and on what evidence would that be based?**

**What are the 2–year and 5–year survival rates for patients like him who have optimum treatment?**

## Background

### How will you stage this cancer?

On the basis of the Veterans' Administration Lung Cancer Study Group staging, this patient has limited disease, defined as tumour confined to one hemi-thorax and/or that which can be encompassed within a radiotherapy field.[1] SCLC is an aggressive form of lung cancer which is often widespread at presentation. Even where radiological staging is negative for metastases, disseminated micro-metastases are often present. Therefore minor differences in tumour stage do not alter prognosis. Reflecting this, there are only two broad stage groupings in clinical use, limited disease or extensive disease. Treatment decisions rely on the distinction of limited disease from extensive disease and on other prognostic factors (see below).

There is some variation in the definition of limited disease. Additional features which may still allow a patient to be staged as having limited disease include ipsilateral pleural effusion, left recurrent laryngeal nerve palsy and superior vena cava obstruction. Extensive disease, as implied by its name, involves disease beyond that defined by limited disease. Extensive disease includes patients with bilateral pleural effusions, pericardial effusions and metastatic disease. Common sites of metastasis are the liver, adrenals, bone and brain.

### What factors influence prognosis in this disease?

As well as stage grouping, performance status, sex and biochemical variables affect prognosis. As would be expected, patients with limited disease, good performance status

(0–1) and normal biochemical variables fare better. The prognosis for women is better than that for men.

A prognostic scoring system, the Manchester Prognostic Score,[2] is used clinically and consists of a five-point system:

- performance status 2 or worse = +1
- extensive disease = +1
- sodium below lower limit of normal = +1
- alkaline phosphatase >1.5 × upper limit of normal = +1
- lactate dehydrogenase >upper limit of normal = +1.

A patient can be assessed as having a good, intermediate or poor prognosis based on a score of 0–1, 2–3 and 4–5, respectively.

# Discussion

 **If this patient has no adverse prognostic factors, what treatment(s) would you recommend and on what evidence would that be based?**

In the absence of adverse prognostic factors and significant comorbidity, optimum treatment of limited disease should include a combination of chemotherapy and radiotherapy. SCLC is an initially chemosensitive, usually disseminated disease, and therefore chemotherapy is the first line of treatment. In limited disease it can induce responses in most patients and complete responses in approximately 50–75% of patients. Despite excellent initial responses to chemotherapy being common, long-term cure is unusual and relapses are often resistant to treatment, hence the addition of radiotherapy. Combination treatment with cisplatin and etoposide (PE) is considered the standard option for patients with a good performance status (0–1). Cisplatin is a nephrotoxic drug, requiring considerable intravenous hydration so it is essential that patients have adequate renal function (glomerular filtration rate >60 ml/min) and that there is no history of cardiac failure. This is a practical issue for SCLC patients who often have cardiovascular disease as a result of long-term smoking. Other common side effects of cisplatin include marked nausea and vomiting, peripheral neuropathy and renal wasting of $K^+$ and $Mg^{2+}$. This regimen can also cause myelosuppression with neutropenic sepsis, mucositis, diarrhoea and alopecia.

Outcomes are marginally inferior when carboplatin is substituted for cisplatin. However, carboplatin offers the advantage that it may be used relatively safely in patients with renal or cardiac impairment and is generally well tolerated, even in patients with poor performance status. As most SCLC patients have extensive disease and/or comorbidities, carboplatin is widely used. Substitution of etoposide with irinotecan initially seemed promising, but another randomized controlled trial has not supported a change in practice.[3]

Another question which has arisen in the treatment of this initially chemosensitive cancer is whether increasing dose density in good prognosis patients can improve outcomes. Recently, ICE (ifosfamide, platinum and etoposide) given 2-weekly with granulocyte-colony stimulating factor (G-CSF) and autologous blood support was compared with 4-weekly standard ICE in patients with a good prognosis. The trial showed a reduction in the rate of neutropenic sepsis and reduced duration of chemotherapy, but there was no improvement in overall survival for the dose dense arm.[4] Therefore, there is no strong evidence that any other regimen would be superior to PE for this patient.

The addition of thoracic radiotherapy to chemotherapy improves the outcome in limited disease SCLC. Meta-analyses suggest a 5% improvement in overall survival at 3 years.[5,6] This benefit is probably limited to patients under 65 years – this needs to be borne in mind, considering this patient is 65 years old. There remains controversy regarding the timing and scheduling of thoracic irradiation. A meta-analysis examining the timing of radiotherapy showed that early thoracic radiotherapy (concurrent with the first or second cycle of chemotherapy) provided a survival advantage at 2 years.[7] However, this survival benefit was not maintained at 3 years. A Cochrane review also suggests benefit for early thoracic radiotherapy; but, in contrast, benefit was not apparent at 2 years but at 5 years.[8] Another meta-analysis identified the time from the start of any treatment to the end of radiotherapy to be inversely related to survival,[9] again suggesting that the timing of radiotherapy is biologically important.

Many patients who achieve a complete response to their initial treatment have a reasonable disease-free interval of months but then have a relapse. These relapses often involve the central nervous system, which severely affects both survival and quality of remaining life. Prophylactic cranial irradiation[10] has been shown to improve disease-free survival and overall survival (approximately 5%), and to decrease the incidence of brain metastases by 15% at three years.

### What are the 2–year and 5–year survival rates for similar patients who have optimum treatment?

The general outlook for SCLC is poor but there is a proportion of long-term survivors who are usually patients like this patient with limited disease, who receive optimum treatment. Such patients' 5-year survival figures vary considerably from 10% to 25%.[11] Patients enrolled in clinical trials are reported as having 2-year survival rates of 20–70% but, as for all cancers, the outcome for SCLC patients eligible for and participating in clinical trials does not necessarily reflect that for SCLC in the general population.

## Conclusion

To summarize, if this patient is of good performance status and has adequate cardiac and renal function the treatment should be chemotherapy with cisplatin and etoposide (4–6 cycles) with concurrent thoracic radiotherapy. If a good response is achieved the patient should receive prophylactic cranial irradiation.

## Further Reading

1  American Joint Committee on Cancer. Lung. In: *AJCC Cancer Staging Manual*, 6th edn. Springer, New York, 2002: 167–81.

2  Cerny T, Blair V, Anderson H, Bramwell V, Thatcher N. Pretreatment prognostic factors and scoring system in 407 small-cell lung cancer. *Int J Cancer* 1987; **39**: 146–9.

3 Hanna N, Bunn PA Jr, Langer C, Einhorn L, Guthrie T Jr, Beck T, Ansari R, Ellis P, Byrne M, Morrison M, Hariharan S, Wang B, Sandler A. Randomized phase III trial comparing irinotecan/cisplatin with etoposide/cisplatin in patients with previously untreated extensive-stage disease small-cell lung cancer. *J Clin Oncol* 2006; **24**: 2038-43.

4 Lorigan P, Woll PJ, O'Brien ME, Ashcroft LF, Sampson MR, Thatcher N. Randomized phase III trial of dose-dense chemotherapy supported by whole-blood hematopoietic progenitors in better-prognosis small-cell lung cancer. *J Natl Cancer Inst* 2005; **97**: 666–74.

5 Pignon JP, Arriagada R, Ihde DC, Johnson DH, Perry MC, Souhami RL, Brodin O, Joss RA, Kies MS, Lebeau B, *et al.* A meta-analysis of thoracic radiotherapy for small-cell lung cancer. *N Engl J Med* 1992; **327**: 1618–24.

6 Warde P, Payne D. Does thoracic irradiation improve survival and local control in limited-stage small-cell carcinoma of the lung? A meta-analysis. *J Clin Oncol* 1992; **10**: 890–5.

7 Fried DB, Morris DE, Poole C, Rosenman JG, Halle JS, Detterbeck FC, Hensing TA, Socinski MA. Systematic review evaluating the timing of thoracic radiation therapy in combined modality therapy for limited-disease small-cell lung cancer. *J Clin Oncol* 2004; **22**: 4837–45.

8 Pijls-Johannesma MC, de Ruysscher DK, Dekker AL, Lambin P. Early versus late chest radiotherapy for limited stage small cell lung cancer. *Cochrane Database Syst Rev* 2005; **2**: CD004700.

9 De Ruysscher D, Pijls-Johannesma M, Bentzen SM, Minken A, Wanders R, Lutgens L, Hochstenbag M, Boersma L, Wouters B, Lammering G, Vansteenkiste J, Lambin P. Time between the first day of chemotherapy and the last day of chest radiation is the most important predictor of survival in limited-disease small-cell lung cancer. *J Clin Oncol* 2006; **24**: 1057–63.

10 Auperin A, Arriagada R, Pignon JP, Le Pechoux C, Gregor A, Stephens RJ, Kristjansen PE, Johnson BE, Ueoka H, Wagner H, Aisner J. Prophylactic cranial irradiation for patients with small cell lung cancer in complete remission. Prophylactic Cranial Irradiation Overview Collaborative Group. *N Engl J Med* 1999; **341**: 476–84.

11 Hahn NM, Hanna N. Combined chemoradiotherapy in small cell lung cancer. *Hematol Oncol Clin North Am* 2005; **19**: 321–42.

# Breast and Gynaecological Cancer

**PROBLEM**

# 36 Indications for Adjuvant Chemotherapy in Breast Cancer

## Case Histories

Today three new patients with recently diagnosed breast cancer are due at the clinic. As the oncologist who will be seeing them for a decision about adjuvant chemotherapy, you review the notes and histology. The salient features are as follows:

Patient 1: age 42, premenopausal, no comorbidity, 3.5 cm, G3 tumour, no lymph node (LN) positive, oestrogen receptor (ER) and progesterone receptor (PR) negative, HER-2 negative

Patient 2: age 56, postmenopausal, no comorbidity. Screen-detected tumour, 1 cm, G2 tumour, no LN positive, ER negative, PR positive, HER-2 negative

Patient 3: age 61, postmenopausal, obese, previous small inferior myocardial infarction, currently asymptomatic on medical treatment; 2 cm G2 tumour, 5/15 LN positive, ER and PR positive, HER-2 negative

**What is each woman's risk of recurrence and death from breast cancer?**

**How might these be influenced by the use of chemo- and/or hormone therapy?**

**What specific short-term and long-term issues will you take into account when deciding on treatment and follow-up?**

# Background

The strongest prognostic factors that predict for future recurrence and death from breast cancer are age, comorbidity, tumour size and grade, number of involved lymph nodes and HER-2/neu status (Table 36.1). Adjuvant!Online (www.adjuvantonline.com) is an example of a computer-based model that uses algorithms to estimate 10-year disease-free and overall survival. It incorporates all of the above prognostic factors, except for HER-2/neu level of expression. The risk estimate, derived from Surveillance, Epidemiology and End Results registry data, has been independently validated and is consistent with the published literature.[1] This tool is a great resource to the clinician, as it facilitates the objective estimation of outcome with local treatment alone and of the absolute benefits expected from systemic adjuvant hormonal therapy and/or chemotherapy. These estimates can be used by the clinician and patient in shared decision-making regarding the risks and benefits of systemic adjuvant therapy. With the development of DNA microarrays, there have been many attempts to subclassify breast cancers further by gene expression profiles, stratifying patients into prognostic subsets. Although certain 'molecular signatures' have been identified as strongly predictive of outcome, these differ between studies. There is no prospective clinical data yet proving the utility of these techniques, or their superiority over pathological and clinical parameters, in guiding the choice of adjuvant treatment in breast cancer patients.

| Table 36.1 Definition of risk categories for patients with breast cancer* | |
|---|---|
| Low risk | Node-negative and all of the following<br>    Tumour ≤2 cm<br>    Grade 1<br>    No peritumoural vascular invasion<br>    HER-2/neu negative<br>    Age ≥35 years |
| Intermediate risk | Node-negative and ≥1 of the following<br>    Tumour >2 cm<br>    Grade 2–3<br>    Peritumoral vascular invasion<br>    HER-2/neu gene overexpressed or amplified<br>    Age <35 years<br>    Node positive (1–3) and HER-2/neu negative |
| High risk | Node positive (1–3) and HER-2/neu gene overexpressed or amplified<br>Node positive (≥4) |

*International Consensus Guidelines (St Gallen, Switzerland, 2005).

# Discussion

## Patient 1

This woman is premenopausal with a T2 N0, stage IIA, intermediate risk breast cancer. For women with lymph-node negative hormone-receptor-negative tumours >1 cm, adjuvant chemotherapy is recommended (category 1 evidence).

With local treatment alone, she has a theoretical 64% chance of being alive at 10 years (35% chance of dying of breast cancer and 1% from other causes). As her tumour is not endocrine responsive, there is no role for tamoxifen or gonadotrophin-releasing hormone (goserelin). There is a wide range of chemotherapeutic options, and treatment should be targeted to the individual patient. First-generation regimens, such as six cycles of cyclophosphamide, methotrexate and fluorouracil (CMF), fluorouracil, epirubicin and cyclophosphamide (FE(50)C) or four cycles of Adriamycin and cyclophosphamide (AC), seem equi-efficacious and reduce the risk of death by a relative 5–10% over local treatment alone.

Second-generation regimens reduce the hazard of death or recurrence by an additional relative 15–20%. Some of these regimens have only been studied in the node-positive populations but one might in theory also extrapolate these results to node-negative patients. These regimens generally use greater than four cycles of therapy and more than two agents, including an anthracycline. Choosing AC/T (sequential addition of paclitaxel (T) to AC) over a CMF-like regimen translates into a 16% proportional improvement relative to CMF-like regimens in the risk of relapse and breast cancer related death. However, this benefit may be partially offset by the increased toxicity of these regimens.

Third-generation regimens, such as TAC × 6, FE(100)C × 3 followed by docetaxel × 3 (FEC/D) and dose-dense (2-weekly) AC × 4 followed by T × 4 regimens have been shown to confer a relative 15–20% superior efficacy to second generation regimens (35% when compared to CMF). However, increased fatigue, mucositis and dermatological side effects are associated with these regimens. The rate of febrile neutropenia is up to 25% unless filgrastim is incorporated. Although the data shows a survival advantage with the third-generation regimens, there is a concern about the lack of long-term toxicity data on dose-dense regimens and the possibility of higher risk of secondary leukaemia. The accelerated paclitaxel-containing regimens may be more beneficial in the ER-negative versus ER-positive subgroups. In our patient's case the addition of adjuvant CMF, AC/T, FEC(100) would add an additional 9%, 14% and 17% increment, respectively, in overall survival.

An important consideration to bear in mind with this patient (see Chapter 39) is the increased risk of BRCA mutations associated with triple-negative breast tumours, especially in younger patients and/or those with a strong family history of breast cancer. These patients are at increased risk for a new primary breast or ovarian cancer.

## Patient 2

This postmenopausal woman has T1 N0, stage I, intermediate-risk breast cancer. Because of screening, her presentation is among the most common nowadays. Of 100 patients with similar histology, 91% will be alive at 10 years with five dying of cancer and four from other causes.

The current National Comprehensive Cancer Network (NCCN) guidelines recommend not administering adjuvant systemic therapy to women with tumours <0.5 cm because their prognosis is favourable without adjuvant therapy. For tumours such as this – 0.6–1 cm – the guidelines advise consideration of other prognostic features such as angiolymphatic invasion, high nuclear grade, HER-2/neu overexpression or negative hormone receptor status when deciding whether to offer adjuvant systemic therapy (category 2B evidence). The use of chemotherapy in these relatively lower risk subsets of women must be based on balancing the expected absolute risk reduction and the individual patient's willingness to experience toxicity to achieve that incremental risk reduction.

The addition of chemotherapy will save one extra life at 10 years per hundred women treated with CMF, and a further life with second generation/third generation regimens. In this case the absolute benefits of chemotherapy are exceptionally modest. This poses the challenge of communicating the realistic risks and benefits of treatment to patients, in ways that are both easily understood and clinically meaningful.

However, there is some benefit from chemotherapy. In the Early Breast Cancer Triallists' Collaborative Group's overview of polychemotherapy, they demonstrated a 30% proportional risk reduction of cancer recurrence which translated into an absolute risk reduction of 5.7% in patients 50–69 years old with node-negative tumours and a 2% absolute risk reduction in mortality.[2] The National Surgical Adjuvant Breast and Bowel Project (NSABP) B20 trial shown a trend towards survival advantage with the addition of CMF to tamoxifen over tamoxifen alone in patients with hormone-responsive cancer.[3] Although studies suggest that many patients will accept adjuvant chemotherapy for small degrees of benefit, women differ in the amount of benefit that they feel to be worthwhile in order to make taking adjuvant systemic chemotherapy beneficial.[4] Patient preferences should be considered and a thorough discussion of the benefits and risks of each therapeutic option is required for each individual.

The NCCN guidelines recommend that all patients with invasive cancers that are ER- or PR-positive should be considered for adjuvant endocrine therapy. In women with ER-positive breast cancer, adjuvant tamoxifen decreased the annual odds of recurrence by 39% and the annual odds of death by 31% irrespective of chemotherapy, patient age, menopausal status or axillary lymph node status. In 2004, the American Society of Clinical Oncology committee stated that in postmenopausal women with hormone receptor-positive breast cancer an aromatase inhibitor may be substituted for tamoxifen, as initial adjuvant therapy, which reduces the risk of recurrence.[5] The effects of treatment with an aromatase inhibitor for longer than 5 years have not been studied. There are no data to recommend taking tamoxifen after an aromatase inhibitor. The major adjuvant aromatase inhibitor trials include the 68-month completed treatment analysis of the ATAC trial,[6] the first report from the BIG-1-98 trial[7] and the combined analysis of data from the ABCSG/ARNO trials. So far, only the data from the relatively small ARNO study have shown an improvement in overall survival in women who switched to an aromatase inhibitor after tamoxifen, although longer follow-up of the larger trials may confirm this effect.[8]

In this case, it would be appropriate to opt for hormonal treatment alone, probably with an aromatase inhibitor.

## Patient 3

This patient has hormone-responsive T1 N2, stage IIIA, high-risk breast cancer. Of 100 similar patients, 48% will be alive in 10 years; 28.6% dying secondary to cancer and 23% secondary to other causes. The two major North American guidelines both suggest that this patient should get both hormone therapy and chemotherapy (category 1 evidence).[9] The addition of tamoxifen will potentially save seven extra lives and chemotherapy an additional two lives. For node-positive patients anthracycline-containing regimens are preferred. There is data supporting A–CMF for patients with four or more positive lymph nodes. However, retrospective analysis of several clinical trials suggests that the superiority of an anthracycline-containing regimen may be limited to those tumours that over express HER-2/neu.[10] The results of two randomized trials

comparing anthracycline-containing chemotherapy with or without sequential paclitaxel in women with axillary node-positive breast cancer suggest improved disease-free
rates and, in one, improved overall survival, with the addition of paclitaxel. A randomized trial comparing docetaxel, doxorubicin and cyclophosphamide (TAC) with fluorouracil, doxorubicin and cyclophosphamide (FAC) in node-positive breast cancer
showed that TAC is superior to FAC.[11] Dose intensity may be important. A trial examining the intensity and sequencing of paclitaxel-containing chemotherapy showed a
26% reduction in the hazard of recurrence and a 31% reduction in the hazard of death
for the dose-dense regimens.[12]

In this patient it is important to consider the cardiotoxic effects of anthracyclines, left
breast radiotherapy and the possible incremental risk of coronary artery disease and
hypercholesterolaemia associated with an aromatase inhibitor. Left ventricular ejection
fraction (LVEF) must be calculated at baseline using either echocardiography or MUGA
scanning and closely monitored throughout treatment. If the patient has symptomatic
heart failure or the baseline LVEF is <50%, one would consider avoiding anthracyclines.
Anthracyclines exert their antitumour effect by interfering with mammalian DNA topoisomerase II and forming a ternary complex. Overexpression of topoisomerase II appears
to predict response to anthracycline-based therapy.[13] Therefore, in patients who do not
over express topoisomerase II one might consider omitting an anthracycline, but including a taxane, if the patient has relative contraindications.

Results of the Intergroup trial 0100 suggest that delaying initiation of tamoxifen until
after completion of chemotherapy should be the preferred therapy sequence. Treatment
of advanced disease is not known to be favourably influenced by early detection of covert
disease. After completion of local and systemic adjuvant therapies, routine follow-up in
asymptomatic women should be limited to regular clinical examination and imaging of
the breast, avoiding other elective imaging.

## Conclusion

These three histories highlight the importance of tailoring treatment to the individual.

Consensus guidelines suggest that Patient 1 should receive adjuvant chemotherapy,
probably a second-generation regimen. Consideration should be given to referring her
for genetic screening, as she has an increased likelihood of carrying a BRCA mutation.

Patient 2 has hormone-responsive breast cancer, with a good prognosis. The absolute
benefits of chemotherapy are small; therefore, adjuvant hormone therapy alone is a reasonable choice.

Patient 3 has the poorest prognosis of the group. Ideally, she should receive chemotherapy and hormone therapy, with careful attention to minimising cardiotoxicity.

## Further Reading

1 Olivotto IA, Bajdik CD, Ravdin PM, Speers CH, Coldman AJ, Norris BD, Davis GJ, Chia SK,
  Gelmon KA. Population-based validation of the prognostic model ADJUVANT! for early
  breast cancer. *J Clin Oncol* 2005; **23**: 2716–272.

2 Early Breast Cancer Trialists' Collaborative Group. Effects of chemotherapy and hormonal therapy for early breast cancer on recurrence and 15-year survival: an overview of the randomized trials. *Lancet* 2005; **365**: 1687–717.

3 Fisher B, Jeong JH, Bryant J, Anderson S, Dignam J, Fisher ER, Wolmark N; National Surgical Adjuvant Breast and Bowel Project randomised clinical trials. Treatment of lymph node-negative, oestrogen receptor-positive breast cancer: long-term findings from National Surgical Adjuvant Breast and Bowel Project randomised clinical trials. *Lancet* 2004; **364**: 858–68.

4 Ravdin PM, Siminoff LA, Harvey JA, *et al.* Survey of breast cancer patients concerning their knowledge and expectations of adjuvant therapy. *J Clin Oncol* 1998; **16**: 515–21.

5 Winer E, Hudis C, Burstein H. American Society of Clinical Oncology technology assessment on the use of aromatase inhibitors as adjuvant therapy for postmenopausal women with hormone receptor-positive breast cancer: status report 2004. *J Clin Oncol* 2005; **23**: 619–29.

6 ATAC Trialists' Group. Results of the ATAC (Arimidex, Tamoxifen, Alone or in Combination) trial after completion of 5 years' adjuvant treatment for breast cancer. *Lancet* 365: 60–2.

7 Thurlimann B, Keshaviah A, Mouridsen H, *et al.* BIG 1-98: Randomized double-blind phase III study to evaluate letrozole (L) vs. tamoxifen (T) as adjuvant endocrine therapy for postmenopausal women with receptor-positive breast cancer. *Proceedings ASCO* 2005 (abstract no. 511).

8 Jakesz R, Jonat W, Gnant M, Mittlboeck M, Greil R, Tausch C, Hilfrich J, Kwasny W, Menzel C, Samonigg H, Seifert M, Gademann G, Kaufmann M, Wolfgang J; ABCSG and the GABG. Switching of postmenopausal women with endocrine-responsive early breast cancer to anastrozole after 2 years' adjuvant tamoxifen: combined results of ABCSG Trial 8 and ARNO 95 Trial. *Lancet* 2005; **366**: 455–62.

9 Goldhirsch A, Glick JH, Gelber RD, Coates AS, Thurlimann B, Senn HJ; Panel members. Meeting highlights: International expert consensus on the primary therapy of early breast cancer 2005. *Ann Oncol* 2005; **16**: 1669–83.

10 Pritchard KI, Shepherd LE, O'Malley FP, Andrulis IL, Tu D, Bramwell VH, Levine MN; National Cancer Institute of Canada Clinical Trials Group. HER2 and responsiveness of breast cancer to adjuvant chemotherapy. *N Engl J Med* 2006; **354**: 2103–11.

11 Martin M, Pienkowski T, Mackey J, Pawlicki M, Guastalla JP, Weaver C, Tomiak E, Al-Tweigeri T, Chap L, Juhos E, Guevin R, Howell A, Fornander T, Hainsworth J, Coleman R, Vinholes J, Modiano M, Pinter T, Tang SC, Colwell B, Prady C, Provencher L, Walde D, Rodriguez-Lescure A, Hugh J, Loret C, Rupin M, Blitz S, Jacobs P, Murawsky M, Riva A, Vogel C; Breast Cancer International Research Group 001 Investigators/Adjuvant docetaxel for node-positive breast cancer. *N Engl J Med* 2005; **352**: 2302–13.

12 Citron ML, Berry DA, Cirrincione C, Hudis C, Winer EP, Gradishar WJ, Davidson NE, Martino S, Livingston R, Ingle JN, Perez EA, Carpenter J, Hurd D, Holland JF, Smith BL, Sartor CI, Leung EH, Abrams J, Schilsky RL, Muss HB, Norton L. Randomized trial of dose-dense versus conventionally scheduled and sequential versus concurrent combination chemotherapy as postoperative adjuvant treatment of node-positive primary breast cancer: first report of Intergroup Trial C9741/Cancer and Leukemia Group B Trial 9741. *J Clin Oncol* 2003; **21**: 1431–9.

13 Martin-Richard M, Munoz M, Albanell J, Colomo L, Bellet M, Rey MJ, Tabernero J, Alonso C, Cardesa A, Gascon P, Fernandez PL. Serial topoisomerase II expression in primary breast cancer and response to neoadjuvant anthracycline-based chemotherapy. *Oncology* 2004; **66**: 388–94.

**PROBLEM**

# 37  Management of HER-2 Positive Breast Cancer

## Case History

A 50-year-old woman had a left-sided modified mastectomy and axillary lymph node clearance for a 2 cm grade II invasive ductal carcinoma. Lymphovascular invasion was present and two out of 15 lymph nodes were positive for metastatic carcinoma. The deep margin was closest at 2 mm. The tumour was oestrogen receptor (ER) and progesterone receptor (PR) negative and HER-2/neu 2+ on immunohistochemistry. Her medical history included a myocardial infarction 5 years ago and subsequent endovascular coronary artery stenting. She has a 20 pack-year smoking history and drinks 30 units of alcohol per week. She is taking aspirin, carvedilol, ramipril and atorvastatin. She is asymptomatic and routine bloods are all normal.

**Before considering adjuvant therapy in this patient what further work-up is required?**

**What is the current thinking on immunohistochemistry and fluorescence *in-situ* hybridization (FISH) analysis for HER-2/neu status?**

**If this patient's cancer is deemed definitely HER2-positive, what is the evidence for adjuvant trastuzumab?**

**What are the safety issues with trastuzumab and how should you monitor for trastuzumab toxicity?**

## Background

**Before considering adjuvant therapy in this patient what further work up is required?**

Anthracycline-containing chemotherapy is the standard of care for lymph node negative breast cancer with any risk of recurrence. Lymph node positive patients may be given doxorubicin/cyclophosphamide followed by a taxane.[1] Before this patient starts such a regimen, her baseline left ventricular ejection fraction (LVEF) needs to be assessed with echocardiography or multiple-gated acquisition scanning (MUGA). Her medical history and smoking history have particular relevance in view of the effect of anthracyclines on the heart. The sample should be sent for FISH analysis of HER-2/neu status (see below).

A radiation oncology opinion should be sought in view of the close deep margins and lymph node spread. This referral could be made during chemotherapy, as the final decision on radiotherapy does not change the plan for chemotherapy. As always (see Chapter 39) a detailed family history of malignancy is important. A liver ultrasound is often done but there are scant data to support its usefulness in this setting. There is no documented role for full body computed tomography (CT) scanning or isotope bone scanning in this scenario.

## Discussion

### What is the current thinking on immunohistochemistry and FISH analysis for HER-2/neu status?

It is important to evaluate accurately the HER-2/neu status of invasive breast cancer. There can be significant inter-observer variability in immunohistochemistry analyses. However, when an automated cellular imaging system (ACIS), which is not routine, is used with immunohistochemistry it has been shown that when the score is <1.5 and >2.6 the correlation between FISH and immunohistochemistry is good (Figure 37.1 – *see inside front cover*). Current thinking suggests that all immunohistochemistry reported as 2+ should be sent for FISH. When the ACIS is used FISH may not be required with scores of <1.5 and >2.6.[2]

### If this patient's cancer is deemed definitely HER-2 positive, what is the evidence for adjuvant trastuzumab?

HER2-positive tumours account for approximately 20% of all breast cancers. These cancers have an aggressive course, often being lymph node positive. Relapse after a short disease-free interval is common. A few data show that they may be resistant to some chemotherapy, although they may be sensitive to anthracyclines. Five randomized trials have shown that adjuvant trastuzumab decreases the risk of recurrence of HER-2 positive breast cancer by approximately 50%. These trials are the HERA, NASBP B31 and NCCTG N9831, BCIRG 006 and Finnish (FinHER) studies.[3–6] The HERA study randomized patients to observation, trastuzumab 3-weekly for 1 year or trastuzumab 3-weekly for 2 years after any adjuvant or neoadjuvant chemotherapy. In NSABP B31, patients were given doxorubicin/cyclophosphamide × four cycles 3-weekly followed by paclitaxel × four cycles 3-weekly, randomizing patients to receive that chemotherapy alone or to receive trastuzumab for 1 year starting concurrently with paclitaxel. NCCTG N9831 was similar except for a treatment arm where trastuzumab for a year followed paclitaxel rather than being started concomitantly. BCIRG 006 used doxorubicin/cyclophosphamide followed by docetaxel rather than paclitaxel and included a non-anthracycline arm. Finally, the FinHER study evaluated vinorelbine or docetaxel with or without 9 weeks of trastuzumab followed by three cycles of fluorouracil/epirubicin and cyclophosphamide.

Hazard ratios for disease-free survival in all the above mentioned studies range from 0.4 to 0.54 and *P*-values were highly significant. There is no universal consensus about the optimal schedule (weekly or 3-weekly) or timing (concurrent versus post chemotherapy, earlier versus later) of adjuvant trastuzumab. In fact, scheduling may not be crucial as trastuzumab has a long half-life and the adjuvant trial results suggest that taxanes given 3 weekly or weekly result in a similar disease-free survival advantage. However, timing and duration are a different matter. It is possible that trastuzumab given prior to anthracycline in the FinHER study persisted during anthracycline administration and resulted anthracycline/trastuzumab synergy. Even more important, the only study in which over-all survival advantage reached significance was the NSABP study, strongly suggesting that trastuzumab is more effective when started early and continued for at least a year.

### What are the safety issues with trastuzumab and how should you monitor for trastuzumab toxicity?

Cardiotoxicity (principally congestive cardiac failure) is the most important adverse effect of trastuzumab. Its incidence is about 1.4% in women receiving the drug as a single agent. From the big trastuzumab adjuvant trials the following can be concluded:

● concomitant administration of trastuzumab with a non-anthracycline-based regimen, e.g. docetaxel or carboplatin brings a very low risk of cardiotoxicity (0–0.3%)

● administration of anthracyclines and taxanes followed by trastuzumab is associated with an increased risk of cardiac dysfunction – up to 1.4%

● administration of trastuzumab and a taxane after four cycles of doxorubicin/cyclophosphamide is associated with an increased risk of severe congestive cardiac failure (1.5–3.4%).

Thus it appears that trastuzumab can act as a molecular modifier of anthracycline-induced cardiotoxic effects and associated congestive cardiac failure.[7] The question arises whether patients (such as the case study patient) who will benefit from adjuvant trastuzumab but are at particularly high risk of cardiotoxicity, may be spared anthracy-cline therapy. The BCIRG 006 trial suggested that the topoisomerase gene is overex-pressed in about a third of HER-2 positive patients who may benefit from anthracycline-based chemotherapy. However, HER-2 positive tumours with no co-amplification of this gene may only need non-anthracycline based regimens.[5] Baseline cardiac function should be assessed with echocardiography or MUGA scanning prior to chemotherapy exposure. LVEF is the most important variable (Table 37.1). Identification of pre-existing risk factors and assessment of LVEF are vital before trastuzumab is started. LVEF should be assessed at least every 3 months during treat-ment. There is evidence suggesting that trastuzumab-related cardiotoxicity is reversible.[8] The mean time to recovery is about 6 weeks. However, if the LVEF fails to recover suffi-ciently after a second consecutive measurement, trastuzumab should be discontinued.

**Table 37.1** Surveillance of left ventricular ejection fraction (LVEF) in patients on trastuzumab and appropriate action

| LVEF | Drop in LVEF <10% | Drop in LVEF 11–15% | Drop in LVEF >15% |
|---|---|---|---|
| >50% | Continue trastuzumab | Continue trastuzumab | Hold trastuzumab, repeat LVEF in 4 weeks |
| 45–50% | Continue trastuzumab | Hold trastuzumab, repeat LVEF in 4 weeks | Hold trastuzumab, repeat LVEF in 4 weeks |
| <45% | Hold trastuzumab. repeat LVEF in 4 weeks | Hold trastuzumab, repeat LVEF in 4 weeks | Hold trastuzumab, repeat LVEF in 4 weeks |

Trastuzumab is to be permanently discontinued if it is held after two consecutive evaluations of LVEF.
Trastuzumab is to be permanently discontinued if it is held after three non-consecutive evaluations.

## Conclusion

This patient has a HER-2 positive cancer with a high chance of recurrence, which can be reduced by the use of adjuvant trastuzumab. Given her cardiac history, one must consider carefully which cytotoxic drugs she receives, as well as ensuring her LVEF is monitored before and during treatment.

## Further Reading

1   Dang CT. Drug treatments for adjuvant chemotherapy in breast cancer: recent trials and future directions. *Expert Rev Anticancer Ther* 2006; **6**: 427–36.

2   Ciampa A, Xu B, Ayata G, Baiyee D, Wallace J, Wertheimer M, Edmiston K, Khan A. HER2 status in breast cancer: correlation of gene amplification by FISH with IHC expression using advanced cellular systems. *Appl Immunohistochem Mol Morphol* 2006; **14**: 132–7.

3   Piccart-Gebhart MJ, Procter M, Leyland-Jones B, Goldhirsch A, Untch M, Smith I, Gianni L, Baselga J, Bell R, Jackisch C, Cameron D, Dowsett M, Barrios CH, Steger G, Huang CS, Andersson M, Inbar M, Lichinitser M, Lang I, Nitz U, Iwata H, Thomssen C, Lohrisch C, Suter TM, Ruschoff J, Suto T, Greatorex V, Ward C, Straehle C, McFadden E, Dolci MS, Gelber RD; Herceptin Adjuvant (HERA) Trial Study Team. Trastuzumab after adjuvant chemotherapy in HER2 positive breast cancer. *N Engl J Med* 2005; **353**: 1659–72.

4   Romond EH, Perez EA, Bryant J, Suman VJ, Geyer CE Jr, Davidson NE, Tan-Chiu E, Martino S, Paik S, Kaufman PA, Swain SM, Pisansky TM, Fehrenbacher L, Kutteh LA, Vogel VG, Visscher DW, Yothers G, Jenkins RB, Brown AM, Dakhil SR, Mamounas EP, Lingle WL, Klein PM, Ingle JN, Wolmark N. Trastuzumab plus adjuvant chemotherapy for operable HER2-positive breast cancer. *N Engl J Med* 2005; **353**: 1673–84.

5   Slamon D, Eiermann W, Robert N, *et al.* Phase III randomised study comparing doxorubicin and cyclophosphamide followed by docetaxel with doxorubicin and cyclophosphamide followed by docetaxel and trastuzumab in HER2 positive early breast cancer patients: BCIRG 006 study. *Breast Cancer Res Treat* 2005; **94**(Suppl 1): S5.

6   Joensuu H, Kellokumpu-Lehtinen PL, Bono P, Alanko T, Kataja V, Asola R, Utriainen T, Kokko R, Hemminki A, Tarkkanen M, Turpeenniemi-Hujanen T, Jyrkkio S, Flander M, Helle L, Ingalsuo S, Johansson K, Jaaskelainen AS, Pajunen M, Rauhala M, Kaleva-Kerola J, Salminen T, Leinonen M, Elomaa I, Isola J; FinHer Study Investigators. Trastuzumab in combination with docetaxel or vinorelbine as adjuvant treatment of breast cancer. The FinHer trial. *Breast Cancer Res Treat* 2005; **94**(Suppl 1): S5.

7   Chien KR. Herceptin and the heart – a molecular modifier of cardiac failure. *N Engl J Med* 2006; **354**: 789–90.

8   Ewer MS, Vooletich MT, Durand JB, Woods ML, Davis JR, Valero V, Lenihan DJ. Reversibility of trastuzumab-related cardiotoxicity: new insights based on clinical course and response to medical treatment. *J Clin Oncol* 2005; **23**: 7820–6.

## PROBLEM

# 38 Advanced Breast Cancer in the Elderly

## Case History

A previously fit 80-year old woman presents with a self-detected 4.5 cm mass in the upper outer quadrant of the left breast. The skin is red, thickened and puckered but there is no ulceration. On full history she complains of pain in her right leg over the past 3 weeks. A plain radiograph shows a large lytic lesion in the proximal third of the right femur. An isotope bone scan suggests several other rib lesions and a large hot spot in the right femur. The chest radiograph is clear of metastases although it shows slight cardiomegaly. Liver ultrasound shows no abnormality.

**What steps would you consider in the management of this patient?**

**Which other specialties will you involve in her care?**

**Discuss how you will arrive at a decision about systemic management of this patient.**

## Background

**What steps would you consider in the management of this patient?**

This woman has a clinical and radiological diagnosis of metastatic breast cancer. Although this is an incurable condition with a quoted median life expectancy in the order of 20 months, survival may be considerably longer in the absence of visceral metastases.[1] The priorities in this setting should be palliation of symptoms and extension of survival while maintaining quality of life. A history should be sought of current symptoms, general health and past medical problems. At this age a social history, taking into account any impairment in activities of daily living and instrumental activities of daily living, will be particularly important as these sensitive measures of functional status are useful in guiding treatment (see Chapter 9). Examination should seek to identify other possible sites of disease (e.g. axillary lymphadenopathy) and comorbidities.

To confirm the diagnosis, a needle core biopsy of the breast mass should be done (Figure 38.1). This should be tested for hormone receptor expression and HER-2/neu overexpression, to guide systemic treatment and give prognostic information. Further staging investigations, i.e. a computed tomography (CT) scan of chest and abdomen, could be done to identify possible unidentified lung, liver or nodal metastases, but it may not lead to a change in current management. Routine haematological and biochemical tests also guide treatment and exclude major bone marrow or liver dysfunction, which would alter management.

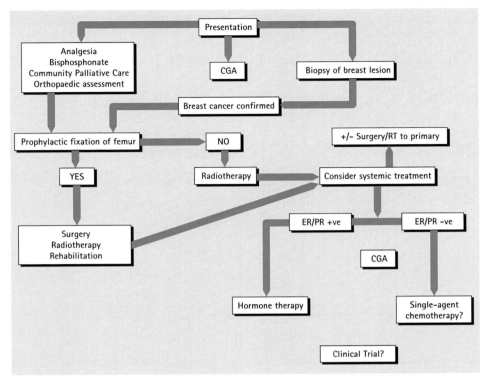

**Figure 38.1** Algorithm for management of advanced breast cancer in the case study patient. CGA, comprehensive geriatric assessment; RT, radiotherapy; ER, oestrogen receptor; PR, progesterone receptor.

Symptomatic management of the bone pain should be a priority. Administration of analgesics should follow the World Health Organization (WHO) ladder. The addition of a bisphosphonate may add to pain control, and will reduce the risk of bone complications.[2]

## Discussion

### Which other specialties will you involve in her care?

An urgent step in the management of this patient should be an opinion from an orthopaedic surgeon about the benefit of prophylactic fixation of the femur, to avoid fracture and improve pain. There are multiple case series aiming to identify risk factors for fracture, including pain, the lytic nature of lesions, their size and associated cortical destruction. These have been the basis of the development of the widely used Mirels' score, although there is no absolute agreement.[3,4] Palliative radiotherapy should be discussed with a clinical oncologist, either as primary treatment or following fixation.

Current guidelines recommend referral for surgical treatment of the primary tumour (toilette mastectomy) if there are pending or currently troublesome symptoms such as bleeding, infection or pain. Radiotherapy is an alternative form of local control. There is no symptomatic indication in this case for urgent local control measures, but there could be the potential to combine surgical procedures, and emerging evidence suggests that complete removal of the primary tumour in metastatic disease may improve survival.[5]

After treatment of the femoral lesion, physiotherapy and occupational therapy will be crucial to help the patient return to independent functioning, particularly as she may live quite long. A social worker can advise about available benefits and support for activities of daily living, as she may have residual disability. Involvement of a community palliative care team would be beneficial for ongoing symptom control and psychological support.

### Discuss how you will arrive at a decision about systemic management of this patient

Options for systemic treatment depend on the molecular pathology of the tumour and the fitness of the patient. If, as is likely, the tumour expresses oestrogen receptor (ER) and/or progesterone receptor (PR), hormone treatment should be the first-line consideration. It is a simple, effective, well-tolerated first-line treatment in postmenopausal women. In large studies, both anastrozole and letrozole have been shown to have superior response rates and progression-free survival compared with tamoxifen.[6–8] The exception to using hormones as first-line treatment is the presence of life-threatening visceral disease (not evident in this case), where it may not provide a swift enough response. In those clinical situations, cytotoxic chemotherapy becomes the first-line treatment of choice. There are no trials comparing the benefits of first-line hormone treatment to chemotherapy, but there is good evidence that concurrent therapy is of no additional benefit. Trials comparing aromatase inhibitors with or without a selection of novel targeted drugs are recruiting worldwide, and participation of elderly patients with breast cancer, who have been under-represented in previous trials, should be encouraged.

Systemic chemotherapy can be given safely to patients in later life. Though there remains debate about the merits of combination chemotherapy versus sequential single-agent treatments in advanced breast cancer, the latter is usually recommended in the elderly, because of concerns for toxicity. Where chemotherapy for the elderly has been considered extensively, Eastern Cooperative Oncology Group (ECOG) performance status and functional status, rather than chronological age, are felt to be useful predictors of toxicity and benefit from chemotherapy[9] (see also Chapter 9).

Anthracyclines are usually recommended as first-line chemotherapy in advanced breast cancer. However, advanced age and underlying heart disease, along with hypertension and diabetes, are recognized risk factors for dose-related anthracycline-induced cardiac toxicity – and this patient already has cardiomegaly. Other agents include taxanes, vinorelbine or capecitabine. Weekly paclitaxel or vinorelbine are both reasonable choices for the elderly.[10] Although capecitabine may be preferred by some clinicians and patients because of its oral administration, caution is advised. Capecitabine, as a pro-drug, has the potential to cause unexpected toxicity due to alterations in metabolism in the elderly, particularly in the presence of concurrent medications. If the tumour over expresses HER-2/neu, there are some data to support the use of trastuzumab in older patients. In the reference study of single-agent treatment (median age 50), the response did not alter with advancing age; however, a decrease in left ventricular ejection fraction was more common.[10] Elderly women, like our patient, may have underlying cardiac dysfunction, which is a clear risk factor for trastuzumab cardiac toxicity. Data about combining trastuzumab with chemotherapy are lacking for patients over 65.

## Conclusion

This patient's initial management should focus on establishing the diagnosis of breast cancer and treating the femoral metastasis. If the cancer is hormone-responsive, adjuvant hormone treatment in combination with bisphosphonate therapy should follow.

## Further Reading

1 Briasoulis E, Karavasilis V, Kostadima L, Ignatiadis M, Fountzilas G, Pavlidis N. Metastatic breast carcinoma confined to bone: portrait of a clinical entity. *Cancer* 2004; **101**: 1524–8.

2 Hillner BE, Ingle JN, Chlebowski RT, Gralow J, Yee GC, Janjan NA, Cauley JA, Blumenstein BA, Albain KS, Lipton A, Brown S; American Society of Clinical Oncology. American Society of Clinical Oncology 2003 update on the role of bisphosphonates and bone health issues in women with breast cancer. *J Clin Oncol* 2003; **21**: 4042–57.

3 Mirels H. Metastatic disease in long bones: a proposed scoring system for diagnosing impending pathologic fractures. *Clin Orthop Relat Res* 2003; (**415 Suppl**): S4–13.

4 Ward WG, Spang J, Howe D. Metastatic disease of the femur. Surgical management. *Orthop Clin North Am* 2000; **31**: 633–45.

5 Rapiti E, Verkooijen HM, Vlastos G, Fioretta G, Neyroud-Caspar I, Sappino AP, Chappuis PO, Bouchardy C. Complete excision of primary breast tumor improves survival of patients with metastatic breast cancer at diagnosis. *J Clin Oncol* 2006; **24**: 2743–9.

6 Nabholtz JM, Buzdar A, Pollak M, Harwin W, Burton G, Mangalik A, Steinberg M, Webster A, von Euler M. Anastrozole is superior to tamoxifen as first-line therapy for advanced breast cancer in postmenopausal women: results of a North American multicenter randomized trial. Arimidex Study Group. *J Clin Oncol* 2000; **18**: 3758–67.

7 Bonneterre J, Thurlimann B, Robertson JF, Krzakowski M, Mauriac L, Koralewski P, Vergote I, Webster A, Steinberg M, von Euler M. Anastrozole versus tamoxifen as first-line therapy for advanced breast cancer in 668 postmenopausal women: results of the Tamoxifen or Arimidex Randomized Group Efficacy and Tolerability study. *J Clin Oncol* 2000; **18**: 3748–57.

8 Mouridsen H, Gershanovich M, Sun Y, Perez-Carrion R, Boni C, Monnier A, Apffelstaedt J, Smith R, Sleeboom HP, Jaenicke F, Pluzanska A, Dank M, Becquart D, Bapsy PP, Salminen E, Snyder R, Chaudri-Ross H, Lang R, Wyld P, Bhatnagar A. Phase III study of letrozole versus tamoxifen as first-line therapy of advanced breast cancer in postmenopausal women: analysis of survival and update of efficacy from the International Letrozole Breast Cancer Group. *J Clin Oncol* 2003; **21**: 2101–9.

9 Gridelli C, Aapro M, Ardizzoni A, Balducci L, De Marinis F, Kelly K, Le Chevalier T, Manegold C, Perrone F, Rosell R, Shepherd F, De Petris L, Di Maio M, Langer C. Treatment of advanced non-small-cell lung cancer in the elderly: results of an international expert panel. *J Clin Oncol* 2005; **23**: 3125–37.

10 Cobleigh MA, Vogel CL, Tripathy D, Robert NJ, Scholl S, Fehrenbacher L, Wolter JM, Paton V, Shak S, Lieberman G, Slamon DJ. Multinational study of the efficacy and safety of humanized anti-HER2 monoclonal antibody in women who have HER2-overexpressing metastatic breast cancer that has progressed after chemotherapy for metastatic disease. *J Clin Oncol* 1999; **17**: 2639–48.

# 39 Approach to a Breast Cancer Patient with a Positive Family History

## Case History

A 30-year-woman has been referred following a wide local excision and axillary clearance of a 2 cm grade III invasive ductal carcinoma. The tumour shows lymphovascular invasion and 2 of 11 lymph nodes are involved. Immunohistochemistry is negative for oestrogen receptor (ER), progesterone receptor (PR) and HER-2. The patient starts adjuvant chemotherapy.

A detailed family history reveals the pedigree shown in Figure 39.1.

**Should the patient be referred to a clinical genetics service?**

**What are the implications for the management of the patient's recently diagnosed breast cancer and for her personal risk of developing further cancers?**

**What are the implications for the patient's family members including her sister, brother and niece?**

**How would the patient's management have changed if the germline BRCA1/2 mutation screen had not identified a mutation?**

## Background

Refer to the patient's pedigree as shown in Figure 39.1.

## Discussion

### Should the patient be referred to a clinical genetics service?

All patients presenting to an oncology clinic should have their family history recorded, including at least first- and second-degree relatives. Ideally this should also include the age of cancer diagnosis, tumour site, any multiple cancers and any Jewish ancestry (as there are three founder mutations particularly common among patients of Ashkenazi Jewish descent). It is important to remember to differentiate and separate maternal and paternal relatives. Breast cancer is common, however, so most women even with a family history of breast cancer do not fall into a high-risk category.[1]

The National Institute of Health and Clinical Excellence (NICE) defines three risk groups:

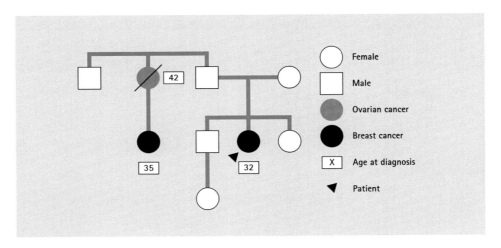

**Figure 39.1** The patient's pedigree.

- Near population risk (lifetime risk of developing breast cancer <17%)
- Moderate risk (lifetime risk of developing breast cancer 17–30%)
- High (lifetime risk of developing breast cancer >30%, or a greater than 20% chance of an abnormal BRCA1, BRCA2 or p53 gene in the family).

Any person judged as having a moderate or high risk of developing breast cancer should be seen by a clinical geneticist.[2]

On the basis of the family history provided, there is enough evidence that this patient should be referred to a clinical genetics service. Patients being considered for genetic testing should be referred to tertiary care for genetic counselling regarding their risks and options. The possible value of the test must be discussed, including the meaning of a positive and negative result. BRCA1/2 mutations account for the majority of multiple-case families with both breast and ovarian cancers, and/or male and female breast cancers. However, they account for less than a third of the inherited component in families where the only cancer is female breast cancer. Overall BRCA1/2 mutations account for less than 5% of breast cancers.

During her adjuvant chemotherapy the patient is referred to a clinical genetics service. After receiving appropriate genetic counselling, she chooses to undergo a germline BRCA1/2 screen. She is found to have inherited a BRCA1 mutation.

### What are the implications for the management of the patient's recently diagnosed breast cancer and for her personal risk of developing further cancers?

As this patient has BRCA1 mutation she should be cared for in a tertiary centre. Current recommendations, however, do not suggest that her actual breast cancer should be treated differently from that in a patient without a BRCA1/2 mutation. Management decisions should be made in a multidisciplinary setting and should take into account the ongoing cancer risks.

To reduce her risk of developing a second primary breast cancer, screening or surgical prophylaxis (bilateral mastectomy) should be discussed. There is evidence from several studies that surveillance is effective in detecting breast cancers in high-risk patients, but there is no evidence that it reduces breast cancer mortality. Mammography in younger women is less effective as a breast cancer screening tool due to the increased density of younger breasts. A study of 1900 women with moderate or high-risk family histories (20% with BRCA1/2 mutations) showed increased sensitivity but reduced specificity for magnetic resonance imaging (MRI) compared with mammography (80% and 33%, respectively).[3] Mammography was better than MRI at detecting ductal carcinoma *in situ*. A UK study also supported these findings.[4] A recent revision of NICE guidelines has recommended yearly MRI for women aged 30–49 with BRCA1 and BRCA2 mutations, as well as certain other subgroups of women at risk. An alternative to screening in this patient is to consider bilateral mastectomy. However, it is recognized that this is only appropriate for a few women. Mastectomy has been shown in one observational study to reduce breast cancer risk in BRCA1/2 mutation carriers by 95% (50% versus 2% risk).[5] Most women cope with prophylactic mastectomy, but a small minority do develop long-term psychological difficulties. Women considering this must be aware of the potential for breast cancer to be diagnosed incidentally, and also that there are case reports of breast cancer developing despite prophylactic mastectomies. Trials to assess the efficacy of chemoprevention in high-risk women, using drugs such as tamoxifen and aromatase inhibitors, are ongoing.

As yet there is no evidence supporting ovarian cancer screening, even in high-risk populations; again trials are ongoing. Bilateral salpingo-oophorectomy (BSO) has been shown to be effective at reducing ovarian cancer incidence (96%),[6] but there does remain a small risk of developing primary peritoneal carcinoma. A 50% reduction in the risk of breast cancer in BRCA1 carriers was also demonstrated in the same study, despite most BRCA1 associated cancers being ER negative. The optimum timing of BSO is after child-bearing is complete, and ideally, before the age of 35 years when ovarian cancer risk starts to increase markedly. The negative impact of BSO, including menopausal symptoms and effect on sexual function, must be discussed with the patient during consideration of BSO.

## What are the implications for the patient's family members including her sister, brother and niece?

Once a mutation has been discovered other family members can be tested for the same mutation; this is known as predictive testing. All those considering predictive testing must undergo genetic counselling to ensure they understand the implications of positive and negative results. This patient's brother and sister should be offered testing, as they each have a 50% chance of having inherited the BRCA1 mutation. If they have not inherited the mutation, then current guidelines make the assumption that their risk of developing breast cancer returns to population risk.[2] However, that view is challenged by a recent study, yet to be reproduced, suggesting that women from high-risk families who test negative for BRCA1/BRCA2 mutations still meet the criteria for 'moderate risk'[7]. Of note, male breast cancer is associated with BRCA2 not BRCA1 mutations (Table 39.1). However, if her brother is found not to have inherited the mutation then his daughter can be reassured in future that she cannot have inherited it. Even if he has the mutation, there is no indication for testing his 9-year-old daughter before she can provide informed consent as it will not affect her immediate management.

**Table 39.1** Comparison of the features of BRCA1 and BRCA2 mutations

| | BRCA1 | BRCA2 |
|---|---|---|
| Breast cancer risk | 65–85% | 40–85% |
| Ovarian cancer risk | 40–50% | 10–25% |
| Male breast cancer association | No | Yes |
| Other associated cancers | No | Pancreas |
| | | Prostate |
| | | Melanoma |
| Pathology of breast cancer | Often | No distinctive pathology |
| | ER negative (90%) | Often ER positive and associated with DCIS (which is unusual in BRCA1 associated cancers) |
| | High grade | |
| | Medullary appearance | |
| | HER-2 negative (90%) | |
| Molecular biology of mutated gene | Involved in recombination repair of double-stranded DNA breaks by controlling RAD51 | Involved in recombination repair of double-stranded DNA breaks by controlling RAD51 |

ER, oestrogen receptor; DCIS, ductal carcinoma *in situ*.

### How would the patient's management have changed if the germline BRCA1/2 mutation screen had not identified a mutation?

Even if a mutation in BRCA1/2 had not been found, the family history meets the criteria for high risk. The patient and her relatives must be aware that despite a mutation not being found on BRCA testing, there may still be an inherited risk of breast and/or ovarian cancer in the family. For example, there may be a mutation in another, as yet undescribed, gene or another known cancer gene (Table 39.2) may be involved. Therefore, even if no mutation is found the patient and her relatives should be counselled appropriately and still consider appropriate screening or risk-reducing surgery.

**Table 39.2** Some cancer genes implicated in breast cancer

| Syndrome | Gene | Features |
|---|---|---|
| Li Fraumeni | p53 | Very high breast cancer risk (especially <50 years) |
| | | Young sarcomas and gliomas |
| Cowden's syndrome | PTEN | Increased risk of breast cancer and thyroid tumours |
| | | Associated cutaneous manifestations |
| | ATM | Moderate breast cancer risk, no clinical testing as yet |
| | CHEK2 | Moderate breast cancer risk, no clinical testing as yet |

## Conclusion

This patient has a mutation of the BRCA1 gene. Her current cancer should be managed no differently from any other of similar stage and pathology. However, her risk of future primary cancers of the breast and ovary is increased and she should undergo appropriate screening and risk reduction measures. Her adult siblings should be offered testing for the BRCA1 mutation, with genetic counselling.

## Further Reading

1   Collaborative Group on Hormonal Factors in Breast Cancer. Familial breast cancer: collaborative reanalysis of individual data from 52 epidemiological studies including 58,209 women with breast cancer and 101,986 women without the disease. *Lancet* 2001; **358**: 1389–99.

2   National Institute for Clinical Excellence. Familial breast cancer: the classification and care of women at risk of familial breast cancer in primary, secondary and tertiary care. London: NICE, 2004.

3   Rijnsburger AJ, Essink-Bot ML, van Dooren S, Borsboom GJ, Seynaeve C, Bartels CC, Klijn JG, Tibben A, de Koning HJ. Impact of screening for breast cancer in high-risk women on health-related quality of life. *Br J Cancer* 2004; **91**: 69–76.

4   Leach MO, Boggis CR, Dixon AK, Easton DF, Eeles RA, Evans DG, Gilbert FJ, Griebsch I, Hoff RJ, Kessar P, Lakhani SR, Moss SM, Nerurkar A, Padhani AR, Pointon LJ, Thompson D, Warren RM; MARIBS study group. Screening with magnetic resonance imaging and mammography of a UK population at high familial risk of breast cancer: a prospective multicentre cohort study (MARIBS). *Lancet* 2005; **365**: 1769–78.

5   Rebbeck TR, Friebel T, Lynch HT, Neuhausen SL, van't Veer L, Garber JE, Evans GR, Narod SA, Isaacs C, Matloff E, Daly MB, Olopade OI, Weber BL. Bilateral prophylactic mastectomy reduces breast cancer risk in BRCA1 and BRCA2 mutation carriers: the PROSE Study Group. *J Clin Oncol* 2004; **22**: 1055–62.

6   Kauff ND, Satagopan JM, Robson ME, Scheuer L, Hensley M, Hudis CA, Ellis NA, Boyd J, Borgen PI, Barakat RR, Norton L, Castiel M, Nafa K, Offit K. Risk-reducing salpingo-oophorectomy in women with a BRCA1 or BRCA2 mutation. *N Engl J Med* 2002; **346**: 1609–15.

7   Smith A, Moran A, Boyd MC, Bulman M, Shenton A, Smith L, Iddenden R, Woodward ER, Lalloo F, Maher ER, Evans DG. Phenocopies in BRCA1 and BRCA2 families: evidence for modifier genes and implications for screening. *J Med Genetics* 2007; **44**: 10–15.

# 40 First-line Treatment of Ovarian Cancer

## Case History

A 56-year-old woman presents with a 3-month history of anorexia and abdominal swelling. The medical history is unremarkable. A computed tomography (CT) scan of abdomen shows an ovarian mass, ascites, extensive omental cake and liver surface deposits. The ascites contains malignant cells consistent with adenocarcinoma of ovarian origin.

**What evidence is there in favour of initial surgery rather than neoadjuvant chemotherapy?**

**What factors and/or further investigations will influence the decision to attempt surgery now?**

**What regimens are acceptable first-line treatments for ovarian carcinoma and on what evidence are they based?**

## Background

**What evidence is there in favour of initial surgery rather than neoadjuvant chemotherapy?**

For women with early-stage epithelial ovarian cancer (International Federation of Gynecology and Obstetrics [FIGO] stages I and II) the primary treatment is surgery. However, most women present with advanced disease (FIGO III or IV) – like our patient, who has at least FIGO stage IIIB disease. Optimal surgery in combination with platinum-based chemotherapy confers a survival advantage in women with ovarian cancer, which is largely related to the amount of postoperative residual bulk disease. Women with minimal residual disease, following optimal cytoreduction, i.e. residual disease less than 1 cm in greatest diameter, have the best prognosis.[1]

There is no definitive evidence from randomized controlled trials to support the optimal timing of surgery and chemotherapy. However, there is consensus that a 'maximal surgical effort', whatever the timing, is necessary. Primary surgery is useful for definitive staging and there are many plausible biological reasons why chemotherapy might be more effective after maximal debulking (all reviewed and further referenced by Thigpen[2]). Therefore primary surgery followed by chemotherapy remains the standard of care outside a clinical trial for a patient such as ours. A definitive answer for patients with advanced disease is awaited from a large prospective study (EORTC 55971) which finished recruitment in December 2006. This trial has randomized patients with IIIC and IV epithelial ovarian cancer to either neoadjuvant chemotherapy followed by surgery or primary surgery and postoperative chemotherapy.

### What factors and/or further investigations will influence the decision to attempt surgery now?

Cytoreductive surgery is beneficial for women in whom the planned surgical procedure is possible in the absence of excessive morbidity. There is substantial evidence that primary chemotherapy followed by interval debulking surgery is a valid alternative in a selected group of women with advanced ovarian cancer. Therefore women in whom optimal cytoreduction is not initially possible may be treated by primary administration of systemic chemotherapy, i.e. neoadjuvant treatment, followed by later cytoreductive surgery.

Uncountable peritoneal metastases (>100), large peritoneal metastatic plaques, large volume ascites and a performance status of 2 or 3 are all relative indications for neoadjuvant chemotherapy,[3–5] as are poor nutritional status or comorbidities which increase anaesthetic risk. If our patient is significantly cachectic or if full CT staging shows disease such as a large pleural effusion(s) or lung parenchymal disease which would not be debulked by surgery, this could lead to a decision to try neoadjuvant chemotherapy. Assuming that is not the case, however, the presence of liver surface deposits is not necessarily a contraindication to primary surgical treatment. The risk–benefit ratio for optimal cytoreduction must be carefully evaluated in all such cases, based on the bulk and location of liver disease.

## Discussion

### What regimens are acceptable first–line treatments for ovarian carcinoma and on what evidence are they based?

The standard of care for first-line chemotherapy is a regimen using a platinum/taxane combination. The National Institute of Health and Clinical Excellence (NICE) guidelines also state that first-line chemotherapy in ovarian cancer should include a platinum-based regimen with or without paclitaxel. Several studies and one meta-analysis have demonstrated equivalent therapeutic efficacy between cisplatin and carboplatin.[6,7] Cisplatin leads to more neurotoxicity, nephrotoxicity, ototoxicity, and gastrointestinal toxicity but is associated with less myelosuppression than carboplatin. Thrombocytopenia can be a concern with cumulative doses of carboplatin.

Many studies have evaluated the role of taxanes in the primary treatment of ovarian cancer. Although the ICON-3 trial concluded that single-agent carboplatin or cyclophosphamide, doxorubicin, and cisplatin are as effective as carboplatin/paclitaxel,[8] superior response rates and progression-free survival for carboplatin/paclitaxel have made it a generally accepted first-line approach. ICON 5, presented at American Society of Clinical Oncology meeting in 2006, showed that the addition/substitution of newer cytotoxic agents, e.g. gemcitabine, liposomal doxorubicin and topotecan for paclitaxel in sequential doublet or triplet combinations resulted in no significant difference in outcome.[9] The benefit of adding newer biological agents, e.g. antiangiogenic agents, to systemic chemotherapy is currently being evaluated in several large trials but is not yet standard treatment. Generally, therefore, outside a clinical trial, our patient would be offered systemic chemotherapy using the combination of carboplatin and paclitaxel.

The issue of intraperitoneal chemotherapy as part of primary treatment has been revisited lately. It is widely accepted that intraperitoneal chemotherapy is most effective in small-volume residual disease and that most treatments seem to work best in platinum-sensitive disease. Several trials have examined intraperitoneal treatment for patients who have had complete response to initial platinum-based systemic treatments. However, none has shown a disease-free or overall survival advantage when intraperitoneal chemotherapy is given as consolidation.

The recently published study by Armstrong *et al.*[10] has, for the first time, shown a survival advantage with the use of intraperitoneal treatment. This randomized study compared stage III patients, who had undergone optimally debulking surgery, treated with either six cycles (every 3 weeks) of intravenous cisplatin/paclitaxel or six cycles (every 3 weeks) of intravenous paclitaxel and intraperitoneal cisplatin/paclitaxel. Side effects were more common in the intraperitoneal group ($P \leq 0.001$), and only 42% completed six cycles of treatment. Median progression-free survival in the intravenous and intraperitoneal groups was 18.3 and 23.8 months, respectively ($P = 0.05$). Median overall survival in the stage IV group was 49.7 months and in the intraperitoneal group was 65.6 months ($P = 0.03$). This trial does indicate that intraperitoneal chemotherapy is valid, safe, and effective, and may have a role as a first-line treatment for stage III ovarian carcinoma, although, currently, international opinion remains divided over whether it is the standard of care.

## Conclusion

If it appears feasible that primary surgery will achieve maximal tumour debulking, then surgery followed by adjuvant chemotherapy is a rational approach. Adjuvant chemotherapy usually consists of intravenous platinum-based therapy, although intraperitoneal chemotherapy may be of value in selected patients.

## Further Reading

1 Bristow RE, Tomacruz RS, Armstrong DK, Trimble EL, Montz FJ. Survival effect of maximal cytoreductive surgery for advanced ovarian carcinoma during the platinum era: a meta-analysis. *J Clin Oncol* 2002; **20**: 1248–54.

2 Thigpen T. The if and when of surgical debulking for ovarian carcinoma. *N Engl J Med* 2004; **351**: 2544–6.

3 Vergote IB, De Wever I, Decloedt J, Tjalma W, Van Gramberen M, van Dam P. Neoadjuvant chemotherapy versus primary debulking surgery in advanced ovarian cancer. *Semin Oncol* 2000; **27**: 31–7.

4 van der Burg ME, van Lent M, Buyse M, Kobierska A, Colombo N, Favalli G, Lacave AJ, Nardi M, Renard J, Pecorelli S. The effect of debulking surgery after induction chemotherapy on the prognosis in advanced epithelial ovarian cancer. *N Engl J Med* 1995; **332**: 629–34.

5 Rose PG, Nerenstone S, Brady MF, Clarke-Pearson D, Olt G, Rubin SC, Moore DH, Small JM; Gynecologic Oncology Group. Secondary surgical cytoreduction for advanced ovarian cancer. *N Engl J Med* 2004; **351**: 2489–95.

6 Ozols RF, Bundy BN, Greer BE, Fowler JM, Clarke-Pearson D, Burger RA, Mannel RS, DeGeest K, Hartenbach EM, Baergen R; Gynecologic Oncology Group. Phase III trial of carboplatin and paclitaxel compared with cisplatin paclitaxel in patients with optimally resected stage III ovarian cancer. A Gynaecologic Oncology Group study. *J Clin Oncol* 2003; **21**: 3194–201.

7  Aabo K, Adams M, Adnitt P, Alberts DS, Athanazziou A, Barley V, Bell DR, Bianchi U, Bolis G, Brady MF, Brodovsky HS, Bruckner H, Buyse M, Canetta R, Chylak V, Cohen CJ, Colombo N, Conte PF, Crowther D, Edmonson JH, Gennatas C, Gilbey E, Gore M, Guthrie D, Yeap BY, *et al.* Chemotherapy in advanced ovarian cancer: four systemic meta-analyses of individual patient's data from 37 randomised trials. Advanced Ovarian Trialists' Group. *Br J Cancer* 1998; **78**: 1478–85.

8  Paclitaxel plus carboplatin versus standard chemotherapy with either single agent carboplatin or cyclophosphamide, doxorubicin, and cisplatin in women with ovarian cancer, the ICON 3 randomised trial. *Lancet* 2002; **360**: 505–11.

9  Bookman MA, for the GCIG through the GOG GOG0182-ICON5: 5-arm phase III randomized trial of paclitaxel and carboplatin vs combinations with gemcitabine, PEG-liposomal doxorubicin, or topotecan in patients with advanced-stage epithelial ovarian or primary peritoneal carcinoma. *J Clin Oncol* 2006; **24**(18Suppl) (abstract 5002).

10 Armstrong DK, Bundy B, Wenzel L, Huang HQ, Baergen R, Lele S, Copeland LJ, Walker JL, Burger RA; Gynecologic Oncology Group. Phase III randomised trial of intravenous cisplatin and paclitaxel versus an intensive regimen of intravenous paclitaxel, intraperitoneal cisplatin, and intraperitoneal paclitaxel in stage III ovarian cancer: A Gynecologic Oncology Group Study. *N Engl J Med* 2006; **354**: 34–43.

## PROBLEM

# 41  Chemotherapy for Relapsed Ovarian Cancer

## Case History

A 58-year-old woman has completed six cycles of carboplatin and paclitaxel chemotherapy for a papillary serous carcinoma of the ovary that has been previously optimally debulked. At the end of treatment she is asymptomatic, there is no residual disease and her CA125 levels are within normal limits.

**What follow-up will you recommend now? In particular, discuss the utility of measuring the CA125 during follow-up, and how it might direct your future actions.**

Eight months following completion of carboplatin and paclitaxel chemotherapy the patient returns complaining of abdominal fullness. A computed tomography (CT) scan reveals a small amount of recurrent ascites and some diffuse omental disease.

**What is the standard treatment option at this point, and on what evidence is it based?**

**Discuss the role of non–platinum–based treatment in relapsed ovarian cancer, and the evidence which supports choosing this treatment.**

## Background

**What follow-up will you recommend now? In particular, discuss the utility of measuring the CA125 during follow-up, and how it might direct your future actions**

Unfortunately, despite initial good responses, most women with ovarian cancer usually have a relapse. There are retrospective data suggesting that response rates to second-line chemotherapy are improved with reduced tumour bulk (<5 cm versus ≥5 cm) and better performance status.[1] This shows the importance of follow-up so that recurrent disease can be identified and treated at the optimum time; not too early when treatment toxicity outweighs its benefit, but not too late when there is a reduced chance of responding, and poorer reserves to cope with treatment. The results of two trials, OV05 and EORTC55955, are currently awaited to know whether there are survival differences between starting chemotherapy when CA125 increases in the absence of symptoms or starting chemotherapy when symptoms develop.

Most women with ovarian cancer show a rise in serum concentration of CA125 at diagnosis and relapse. There is evidence that nadir CA125 level attained and CA125 half-life are of prognostic value in ovarian cancer.[2] In women with a raised CA125 at diagnosis, CA125 is a more sensitive marker of relapse than radiological monitoring. The recommended follow-up for ovarian cancer is therefore regular outpatient visits with CA125 levels checked each time. Radiological imaging is not routinely done outside the clinical trial setting unless there is clinical, or CA125, suspicion of progression. The exception may be the monitoring of the 10–20% of women who do not have raised CA125 at initial diagnosis, or those presenting with very early stage disease.

## Discussion

**What is the standard treatment option at this point, and on what evidence is it based?**

The treatment of ovarian cancer that has recurred is palliative, and therefore the primary aims of management are to prolong life, relieve symptoms attributable to the disease and maintain quality of life. Active drugs include platinum, taxanes, pegylated liposomal doxorubicin, topotecan and gemcitabine.

An important factor when considering second-line treatment is the time since completion of the platinum-based chemotherapy. The response to re-challenge platinum is strongly correlated to the platinum-free interval (Table 41.1). Women with platinum-sensitive disease show higher rates of response to second-line treatments, both platinum-based (22–59%) and non-platinum-based treatments (10–30%), compared with women with platinum-resistant or platinum-refractory disease. The longer the platinum-free interval, the higher the chance of responding to re-challenge platinum-based therapy.[3]

The ICON4 trial[4] showed for the first time an overall survival benefit for combination chemotherapy (carboplatin plus paclitaxel) over single-agent carboplatin in the second-line setting (hazard ratio [HR] 0.82, $P = 0.02$). There was also an improvement in median progression-free survival of 3 months (10 versus 13 months) in favour of the combination arm. A third of patients in the control arm, however, did not receive a taxane at any

**Table 41.1** Definitions of ovarian cancer that has recurred

| Disease | Definition |
| --- | --- |
| Platinum-sensitive disease | Disease that responds to platinum-based therapy but relapses 12 months or more after completion of this |
| Partially platinum-sensitive disease | Disease that responds to platinum-based therapy but relapses between 6 and 12 months after completion of this |
| Platinum-resistant disease | Disease that responds to platinum-based therapy but relapses less than 6 months after completion of this |
| Platinum-refractory disease | Disease that does not respond to platinum-based therapy |

time during their illness, and there was a high rate of neurotoxicity (20% grade $\geq 2$) even though only 45% of patients in the trial had received a prior taxane agent. Another randomized phase III trial, AGO-OVAR 2.5, compared combination therapy with carboplatin and gemcitabine with carboplatin alone, and also showed an improvement in progression-free survival (8.6 months versus 5.8 months, $P = 0.003$, HR 0.72). More patients in this study than in the ICON4 study had already received a taxane in first-line therapy. This trial was not powered to detect a difference in overall survival.[5]

No prospective studies have shown a clear survival benefit for secondary surgical cytoreductive surgery. However, one group reported that successful optimal secondary surgical cytoreduction was the most important variable affecting overall survival, assessed by multivariate analysis.[6] Secondary surgical cytoreduction is not currently considered standard practice. Surgery may have a role in specific cases to ameliorate symptoms, especially in patients with slowly progressing localized disease. The role of intraperitoneal treatment in this population of patients is also unclear and should only be carried out in the setting of a clinical trial.

This patient, according to current evidence, should be considered for treatment with carboplatin and paclitaxel, assuming no contraindication, for example, major residual neurotoxicity. However, in presence of previous neurotoxicity or clinical reasons for fearing it, gemcitabine and carboplatin or single-agent carboplatin, should be considered. She should also be informed that combination treatments, although demonstrating slight improvements in progression-free survival and/or overall survival, do also increase toxicity.

### Discuss the role of non–platinum-based treatment in relapsed ovarian cancer, and the evidence which supports choosing this treatment

If platinum-based treatment was unsuitable for this patient, or if she subsequently has a relapse and her disease is resistant to platinum or is refractory, there is the option of using single-agent paclitaxel or pegylated liposomal doxorubicin. Topotecan is another alternative but it is only recommended if the other drugs mentioned are unsuitable, due to its increased toxicity and dosing inconvenience. Tamoxifen may also be used in the second-line treatment of ovarian cancer, with responses of up to 18%,[7] however, this is more often used in asymptomatic patients with minimal or no radiological evidence of disease, rather than the scenario described here.

There is current interest in the use of molecular-targeted treatments in ovarian cancer, some of which have already shown promise in phase II trials. Drugs currently under study include erlotinib and ZD2171 (tyrosine kinase inhibitors) and bevacizumab and VEGF-TRAP (vascular endothelial growth factor inhibitors). Patients should be offered the option of entry into clinical trials available locally to establish whether these novel drugs will have a role in the treatment of ovarian cancer recurred in the future.

## Conclusion

This patient has partially platinum-sensitive ovarian cancer. Depending on whether or not she experienced neurotoxicity during her first treatment, and her other risk factors for toxicity, she can be considered for treatment with carboplatin/paclitaxel, carboplatin/gemcitabine or single-agent carboplatin.

## Further Reading

1   Eisenhauer EA, Vermorken JB, van Glabbeke M. Predictors of response to subsequent chemotherapy in platinum pretreated ovarian cancer: a multivariate analysis of 704 patients [see comments]. *Ann Oncol* 1997; **8**: 963–8.

2   Riedinger JM, Wafflart J, Ricolleau G, Eche N, Larbre H, Basuyau JP, Dalifard I, Hacene K, Pichon MF. Ca 125 half-life and Ca 125 nadir during induction chemotherapy are independent predictors of epithelial ovarian cancer outcome: results of a French multicentric study. *Ann Oncol* 2006; **17**: 1234–8.

3   Markman M, Rothman R, Hakes T, Reichman B, Hoskins W, Rubin S, Jones W, Almadrones L, Lewis JL Jr. Second-line platinum therapy in patients with ovarian cancer previously treated with cisplatin. *J Clin Oncol* 1991; **9**: 389–93.

4   Parmar MK, Ledermann JA, Colombo N, du Bois A, Delaloye JF, Kristensen GB, Wheeler S, Swart AM, Qian W, Torri V, Floriani I, Jayson G, Lamont A, Trope C; ICON and AGO Collaborators. Paclitaxel plus platinum-based chemotherapy versus conventional platinum-based chemotherapy in women with relapsed ovarian cancer: the ICON4/AGO-OVAR-2.2 trial. *Lancet* 2003; **361**: 2099–106.

5   Pfisterer J, Plante M, Vergote I, du Bois A, Hirte H, Lacave AJ, Wagner U, Stahle A, Stuart G, Kimmig R, Olbricht S, Le T, Emerich J, Kuhn W, Bentley J, Jackisch C, Luck HJ, Rochon J, Zimmermann AH, Eisenhauer E; AGO-OVAR; NCIC CTG; EORTC GCG. Gemcitabine plus carboplatin compared with carboplatin in patients with platinum-sensitive recurrent ovarian cancer: an intergroup trial of the AGO-OVAR, the NCIC CTG, and the EORTC GCG. *J Clin Oncol* 2006; **24**: 4699–707.

6   Hoskins WJ, Rubin SC, Dulaney E, Chapman D, Almadrones L, Saigo P, Markman M, Hakes T, Reichman B, Jones WB, *et al.* Influence of secondary cytoreduction at the time of second-look laparotomy on the survival of patients with epithelial ovarian carcinoma. *Gynecol Oncol* 1989; **34**: 365–71.

7   Hatch KD, Beecham JB, Blessing JA, Creasman WT. Responsiveness of patients with advanced ovarian carcinoma to tamoxifen. A Gynecologic Oncology Group study of second-line therapy in 105 patients. *Cancer* 1991; **68**: 269–71.

# 42 Chemoradiotherapy for Cervical Cancer

## Case History

A 38-year-old woman, para 2 + 0, presents with post-coital bleeding. Colposcopy shows a cervical lesion, which on biopsy is a mixed adeno-squamous carcinoma. Examination under anaesthesia suggests right parametrial involvement. Radiological staging confirms this and suggests the presence of a single, enlarged left iliac lymph node but no disease elsewhere and no hydronephrosis.

**What is the stage of this tumour?**

**What is the standard treatment? Discuss the evidence to support the use of chemotherapy in this scenario.**

**Discuss the factors that most strongly predict the prognosis in this patient. What implications does that have for management?**

## Background

### What is the stage of this tumour?

The stage is IIB. The International Federation of Gynecology and Obstetrics (FIGO) staging (Table 42.1) of cervical cancer is based on clinical evaluation, which, preferably, should be carried out by an experienced examiner and under anaesthesia. When it is uncertain which the stage a particular case should be allocated, the earlier stage is mandatory. Staging may involve palpation, inspection, colposcopy, endocervical curettage, hysteroscopy, cystoscopy, proctoscopy, intravenous urography and radiographic examination of the lungs and skeleton. Confirm involvement of the bladder or rectum with a biopsy.

There are some drawbacks of the FIGO classification. Lymph node involvement is one of the most important negative prognostic factors in cervical cancer, other than metastasis, but this is not included in the current FIGO staging classification. In addition, staging does not depend on the contemporary radiological imaging techniques (e.g. computed tomography [CT], magnetic resonance imaging and positron emission tomography) that are commonly used in developed countries. If surgery is done, it may reveal that the cancer is more advanced than initially thought. Although this new information may alter the treatment plan, it does not change the patient's FIGO stage. The American Joint Committee on Cancer's TNM nomenclature should be used for this purpose.

| Table 42.1 | Staging guidelines from the International Federation of Gynecology and Obstetrics (FIGO) | |
| --- | --- | --- |
| Stage 0 | | Carcinoma *in situ* |
| Stage I | | Limited to the cervix |
| IA | | Invasive carcinoma diagnosed by microscopy |
| | IA1 | <3 mm deep and <7 mm wide |
| | IA2 | 3–5 mm deep and <7 mm wide |
| IB | | Visible tumour or by microscopy >5 mm deep and 7 mm wide |
| | IB1 | Visible tumour <40 mm |
| | IB2 | Visible tumour >40 mm |
| Stage II | | Beyond uterus but not onto pelvic wall |
| IIA | | Upper two-thirds of vagina |
| IIB | | Parametrial tissues |
| Stage III | | Lower vagina or extension onto the pelvic sidewall |
| IIIA | | Lower third of vagina but no extension into pelvic wall |
| IIIB | | Pelvic wall and/or hydronephrosis |
| Stage IV | | Spread to adjacent or distant organs |
| IVA | | Rectum or bladder |
| IVB | | Distant organs including lungs or liver |

# Discussion

## What is the standard treatment? Discuss the evidence to support the use of chemotherapy in this scenario

Standard primary treatment for locally advanced cervical cancer is irradiation, given as a combination of external radiation and intracavity brachytherapy, with concurrent platinum chemotherapy (Figure 42.1). Previously, radiation had been the main modality but three meta-analyses have confirmed that cisplatin-based chemoradiation adds an absolute 12% benefit in 5-year survival over radical radiation alone in women with locally advanced cervical cancer (stages IB2–IIIB).[1] Cisplatin is given weekly during the external beam therapy at a dose of 40 mg/m$^2$. Extended field radiation should be considered for women with positive common iliac or para-aortic nodes. The toxic effects are greater than with pelvic radiation alone, but they are mostly confined to women who have previously undergone abdominopelvic surgery.

Five randomized phase III trials, published almost simultaneously around 1999, formed the basis for adopting cisplatin-based chemotherapy concurrent with radiation therapy as the standard of care for women with locally advanced cervical cancer.[2–6] The patient populations in these studies included women with FIGO stages IB2–IVA cervical cancer treated with primary radiation therapy and stages I–IIA with poor prognostic factors (metastatic disease in pelvic lymph nodes, parametrial disease, or positive surgical margins) at the time of primary surgery. Although there was wide variation in terms of

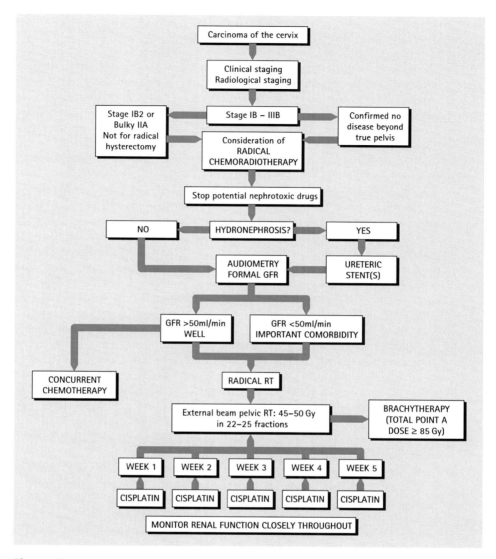

**Figure 42.1** Algorithm for the management of cervical cancer. RT, radiotherapy; GFR, glomerular filtration rate.

inclusion criteria, treatment specifics and control treatments, the trials demonstrated a marked survival benefit for this combined modality approach. The risk of death from cervical cancer was decreased by 30% to 50% with the use of concurrent chemoradiation therapy. However, acute haematological and gastrointestinal toxicity markedly increased in the concomitant chemoradiation group.

The GOG85 study, reported by Whitney *et al.*, compared concurrent radiation, cisplatin and fluorouracil (5-FU) with concurrent radiation and hydroxyurea in women with locally advanced cervical cancer.[2] The inclusion of hydroxyurea in the control arm is considered a relative weakness of this trial as it may have resulted in inferior results in the control group. Three years from the time of diagnosis, 67% of women receiving radiation with cisplatin and 5-FU were alive compared with 57% in the control arm. The Radiation Therapy Oncology Group 9001 study, reported by Morris *et al.* was similar, but used radiation therapy alone as the control arm.[3] Three-year survival rates were 75% in the radiation, cisplatin and 5-FU group compared with 63% in the control arm. This study was the only one that prescribed concurrent chemotherapy with the brachytherapy portion of treatment. This approach seems attractive as 50% of the central dose of radiation is usually given during this part of the treatment.

The GOG120 study, reported by Rose *et al.*, had three arms: weekly cisplatin plus radiation versus cisplatin, 5-FU, hydroxyurea and radiation versus hydroxyurea plus radiation.[4] In both groups receiving cisplatin, the 3-year survival rate was 65% compared with 47% in the hydroxyurea and radiation arm. Treatment with cisplatin alone was less toxic than treatment with the three-drug regimen. The SWOG8797 study, reported by Peters *et al.*, compared radiation plus 5-FU and cisplatin with radiation alone in early-stage, high-risk women with cervical carcinoma.[5] Three-year survival rates were 87% and 77%, respectively. In this trial, adenocarcinomas and adeno-squamous carcinomas had a poorer prognosis in patients with at least one other poor prognostic factor. Importantly, the addition of chemotherapy seemed to improve disease-free survival in this subgroup of poor-prognosis patients. The GOG123 trial, reported by Keys *et al.*, compared radiation with weekly cisplatin versus radiation alone in patients with stage IB bulky tumours.[6] The combined-therapy group had fewer relapses in the pelvic region.

A later trial reported by Pearcey *et al.* in 2002 did not find any benefit from radiotherapy plus weekly cisplatin versus radiation alone. However, critics suggest that this may reflect the smaller size of that trial.[7] The GOG165 trial failed to show any benefit of protracted intravenous infusion of 5-FU over weekly cisplatin. On the basis of these results, strong consideration should be given to the incorporation of concurrent cisplatin-based chemotherapy with radiation therapy in women who require radiation therapy for treatment of cervical cancer.

To date, there is no established role for neoadjuvant chemotherapy outside the setting of a clinical trial. A phase III randomized Japanese study compared neoadjuvant chemotherapy (bleomycin, vincristine, mitomycin, cisplatin) followed by radical hysterectomy versus radical hysterectomy alone in women with bulky stage I or II cervical cancer. A planned interim analysis revealed a markedly inferior overall survival associated with the neoadjuvant arm.[8]

## Discuss the factors that most strongly predict the prognosis in this patient. What implications does that have for management?

As with many other cancers, the major prognostic factors are stage, volume and grade of tumour, histologic type, lymphatic spread, and vascular invasion. The 5-year survival of women treated with chemoradiation ranges from 80% in bulky IB tumours to only 25% in stage IVA disease. Larger tumours appear to be less radiosensitive. In a retrospective study of women with stage IIB cervical cancer, treated with irradiation alone, tumour extension into the lateral versus medial parametrium was associated with markedly increased pelvic failure rates (30% versus 17%).[9] Survival and local control are better with unilateral rather than bilateral parametrial involvement. There are conflicting reports regarding the effect of adeno-squamous cell type on prognosis. One report suggested that approximately 25% of apparent squamous tumours have demonstrable mucin production and behave more aggressively than their pure squamous counterparts suggesting that any adenomatous differentiation may confer a negative prognosis. However, other reports suggest that the decreased survival is mainly due to more advanced stage and higher grade rather than the specific cell type.[10]

Anaemia is correlated with decreased patient survival and seems to be one of the most powerful prognostic factors after clinical stage and tumour size. Hypoxia can increase resistance to radiation and chemotherapy, and lead to the development of a more aggressive tumour phenotype. In addition, anaemia may affect the patient's quality of life and compliance with treatment. Despite a randomized trial demonstrating that red cell transfusions improve local control and survival, many patients are not given transfusion due to toxicity concerns.[11]

Recombinant human erythropoietin (rHuEPO) is a therapeutic option for women with haemoglobin levels 100–120 g/l. SWOG demonstrated a gradual increase in haemoglobin following the administration of rHuEPO and oral iron in women with advanced cervical carcinoma undergoing chemoradiation.[12] The target haemoglobin of 125 g/l was achieved in 40% of women by the midpoint of chemoradiation from a baseline of 104 g/l. Survival was strongly associated with the haemoglobin level at the end of treatment, but not with the baseline haemoglobin levels. However, there was an appreciable occurrence of deep vein thrombosis (7.5%) requiring discontinuation of the rHuEPO. Unsurprisingly, smoking, associated with increased tissue hypoxia, also predicts worse overall survival in women with locally advanced cervical carcinoma treated with chemoradiation and all women should be helped to stop smoking.[13]

## Conclusion

For this patient, the treatment of choice is external beam radiation with weekly concurrent cisplatin therapy followed by brachytherapy.

## Further Reading

1 Green JA, Kirwan JM, Tierney JF, Symonds P, Fresco L, Collingwood M, Williams CJ. Survival and recurrence after concomitant chemotherapy and radiotherapy for cancer of the uterine cervix: a systematic review and meta-analysis. *Lancet* 2001; **358**: 781–6.

2 Whitney CW, Sause W, Bundy BN, Malfetano JH, Hannigan EV, Fowler WC Jr, Clarke-Pearson DL, Liao SY. Randomized comparison of fluorouracil plus cisplatin versus hydroxyurea on an adjuvant to radiation therapy in stage IIB-IVA carcinoma of the cervix with negative para-aortic lymph nodes: A Gynecologic Oncology Group and Southwest Oncology Group study. *J Clin Oncol* 1999; **17**: 1339–48.

3 Morris M, Eifel PJ, Lu J, Grigsby PW, Levenback C, Stevens RE, Rotman M, Gershenson DM, Mutch DG. Pelvic radiation with concurrent chemotherapy compared with pelvic and para-aortic radiation for high-risk cervical cancer. *N Engl J Med* 1999; **340**: 1137–43.

4 Rose PG, Bundy BN, Watkins EB, Thigpen JT, Deppe G, Maiman MA, Clarke-Pearson DL, Insalaco S. Concurrent cisplatin-based radiotherapy and chemotherapy for locally advanced cervical cancer. *N Engl J Med* 1999; **340**: 1144–53.

5   Peters WA 3rd, Liu PY, Barrett RJ, Stock RJ, Monk BJ, Berek JS, Souhami L, Grigsby P, Gordon W, Alberts DS. Cisplatin and 5-fluorouracil plus radiation therapy are superior to radiation therapy as adjunctive in high-risk early stage carcinoma of the cervix after radical hysterectomy and pelvic lymphadenectomy: Report of a phase III intergroup study. *J Clin Oncol* 2000; **18**: 1606–13.

6   Keys HM, Bundy BM, Stehman FB, Muderspach LI, Chafe WE, Suggs CL, Walker JL, Gersell D. A comparison of weekly cisplatin during radiation therapy versus irradiation alone each followed by adjuvant hysterectomy in bulky stage IB cervical carcinoma: a randomized trial of the Gynecologic Oncology Group. *N Engl J Med* 1999; **340**: 1154–61.

7   Pearcey R, Brundage M, Drouin P, Jeffrey J, Johnston D, Lukka H, MacLean G, Souhami L, Stuart G, Tu D. Phase III trial comparing radical radiotherapy with and without cisplatin chemotherapy in patients with advanced squamous cell cancer of the cervix. *J Clin Oncol* 2002; **20**: 996–1072.

8   Katsumata N, Yoshikawa H, Hirakawa T, *et al.* Phase III randomised trial of neoadjuvant chemotherapy followed by radical hysterectomy for bulky stage I/II cervical cancer: JCOG 0102. *Proc Am Soc Clin Oncol* 2006; **24**: 259s (abstract 5013).

9   Perez CA, Grigsby PW, Nene SM, Camel HM, Galakatos A, Kao MS, Lockett MA. Effect of tumor size on the prognosis of carcinoma of the uterine cervix treated with irradiation alone. *Cancer* 1992; **69**: 2796–806.

10  Farley JH, Hickey KW, Carlson JW, Rose GS, Kost ER, Harrison TA. Adenosquamous histology predicts a poor outcome for patients with advanced-stage, but not early-stage, cervical carcinoma. *Cancer* 2003; **97**: 2196–202.

11  Kapp KS, Poschauko J, Geyer E, Berghold A, Oechs AC, Petru E, Lahousen M, Kapp DS. Evaluation of the effect of routine packed red blood cell transfusion in anemic cervix cancer patients treated with radical radiotherapy. *Int J Radiat Oncol Biol Phys* 2002; **54**: 58–66.

12  Lavey RS, Liu PY, Greer BE, Robinson WR 3rd, Chang PC, Wynn RB, Conrad ME, Jiang C, Markman M, Alberts DS. Recombinant human erythropoietin as an adjunct to radiation therapy and cisplatin for stage IIB-IVA carcinoma of the cervix. *Gynecol Oncol* 2004; **95**: 145–51.

13  Waggoner SE, Darcy KM, Fuhrman B, Parham G, Lucci J 3rd, Monk BJ, Moore DH; Gynecologic Oncology Group. Association between cigarette smoking and prognosis in locally advanced cervical carcinoma treated with chemoradiation: A Gynecologic Oncology Group study. *Gynecol Oncol* 2006; **103**: 853–8.

# Uncommon Cancers

**PROBLEM**

# 43 Gastrointestinal Stromal Tumours: Selection of Patients for Imatinib Treatment

## Case History

A 45-year-old woman presents to your general surgical colleague with vague abdominal symptoms and a computed tomography (CT) scan shows a large mass involving the stomach, spleen and left kidney. The surgeon has arranged a percutaneous Tru-cut biopsy and the report indicates a gastrointestinal stromal sarcoma. The surgeon discusses the patient with you and asks if she should attempt to resect this mass.

**What are gastrointestinal stromal tumours (GISTs)?**

**How are they diagnosed?**

**How should patients with GIST be managed?**

# Background

### What are gastrointestinal stromal tumours (GIST)?

GISTs are soft tissue sarcomas of mesenchymal origin arising in the gastrointestinal tract and account for 5% of soft tissue sarcomas overall. Historically these tumours were thought to be of smooth muscle origin and were regarded as leiomyomas or leiomyosarcomas. However, with advances in electron microscopy and immunohistochemical techniques, it was seen that they lacked the features of smooth muscle differentiation typical of leiomyomas occurring elsewhere in the body. It was later identified that these tumours specifically express CD34 and KIT (CD117) establishing the group as a separate entity.

KIT, the product of the proto-oncogene c-KIT, is a tyrosine kinase growth factor receptor. It is expressed on interstitial cells of Cajal (ICC) which act as pacemaker cells for intestinal motility and GISTs probably develop from ICC precursors. The receptor is activated by stem cell factor leading to homodimerization of adjacent receptors and activation of the intracellular KIT kinase domain. This ultimately activates the cell-signalling cascades involved in tumorigenesis – cell proliferation, adhesion and differentiation. Mutations of the c-KIT gene occur in up to 90% GISTs resulting in gain of function activation of the KIT receptor and unopposed cellular proliferation.[1]

In the UK the incidence of GIST is in the region of 15/100 100 which equates to approximately 900 new cases per year.[2] The median age at diagnosis is 60 years and they are rare before the age of 40. They can occur anywhere in the gastrointestinal tract from the oesophagus to the rectum but up to 90% occur in the stomach or small intestine. The size of tumour can vary from ≤2 cm to over 20 cm. Smaller tumours are often identified incidentally on upper gastrointestinal imaging whereas larger tumours can present with gastrointestinal bleeding, abdominal pain, obstruction or non-specific vague symptoms as in this case.

### How are they diagnosed?

GISTs can be difficult to diagnose and the pathology sample should always be reviewed by a pathologist experienced in the tumour type. If a tumour is resectable the diagnosis should be made after surgery. Biopsy should not be attempted in such circumstances due to a risk of tumour rupture or seeding, unless there is a possibility of an alternative diagnosis, such as lymphoma or germ cell tumour, the management of which would be entirely different. In unresectable disease a biopsy should be done to confirm the diagnosis.

The typical appearance of a large GIST on a CT scan is of a mass arising from the gastrointestinal tract wall with mucosal ulceration, central necrosis and cavitation and heterogeneous enhancement. Smaller tumours tend to be well defined, smooth walled and homogeneous, and they are often better defined by endoscopic ultrasound if confined to oesophagus, stomach or duodenum. Staging CT should be done in all cases and will confirm the presence or absence of liver metastases, which is the most common site of metastatic disease. Histologically, GIST can be defined as spindle cell type (70% cases), epithelioid type (20% cases) or mixed.[3] Positive CD117 staining as part of an immunohistochemistry panel in a spindle cell or epithelioid tumour of the gastrointestinal tract confirms the diagnosis of GIST when morphological and clinical features of the tumour are consistent with GIST. Approximately 95% GISTs are positive for KIT (CD117).[4] Other supporting immunohistochemistry includes immunopositivity for CD34

| Table 43.1 | Consensus approach of assessing aggressiveness of gastrointestinal stromal tumour[3] | |
|---|---|---|
| | Size | Mitotic count/50 HPF |
| Very low risk | <2 cm | <5 |
| Low risk | 2–5 cm | <5 |
| Intermediate risk | <5 cm | 6–10 |
| | 5–10 cm | <5 |
| High risk | >5 cm | >5 |
| | >10 cm | Any rate |
| | Any size | >10 |

HPF, high power field.

(60–70% cases) and smooth muscle actin (SMA) (30–40% cases). They are rarely positive for desmin or S-100.

Any GIST has the potential to behave in a malignant fashion but they have different degrees of aggressiveness. Several studies have attempted to identify prognostic features that can predict biological behaviour. The most widely accepted prediction is based on size of tumour and mitotic activity (Table 43.1).[3]

In general, oesophageal tumours are thought to have the most favourable prognosis and small intestinal tumours the worst.[5] More recently specific c-KIT point mutations have also been shown to correlate with poor prognosis.[6]

# Discussion

### How should patients with GIST be managed?

It is accepted that GISTs should be managed by a multidisciplinary team with experience in the disease. Surgical resection is the mainstay of treatment and should be carried out by a surgeon familiar with radical cancer resection in the appropriate organ. A wide local excision is recommended and *en-bloc* resection is not required unless there is direct invasion of adjacent organs.[7] In the index patient, the surgeon must decide whether resection is feasible, given there is invasion of the spleen and left kidney, and may need to work with other relevant surgical teams. Even with complete surgical resection, 5-year survival rates are 35–65%.[7] Median time to recurrence is 18–24 months.

GISTs are resistant to conventional cytotoxic chemotherapy with a response rate in the region of 5%[8] and there is limited role for radiotherapy. However, the recent development of imatinib (Glivec, Novartis Pharma AG, Basel, Switzerland) has revolutionized the management of these patients. Imatinib is an example of a molecular targeted therapy functioning by tyrosine kinase inhibition. It inhibits c-ABL, bcr-ABL, platelet-derived growth factor receptor (PDGFR) and c-KIT leading to inhibition of downstream signalling and reduced cellular proliferation. An early study using imatinib 400 mg or

600 mg in patients with KIT positive GISTs reported a partial response rate of 53.7% (decrease in at least 50% size of tumour) and stable disease in a further 27.9%.[9] Two phase III trials comparing 400 mg/day with 800 mg/day are still accumulating data, but the European trial reported interim results showing similar response rates at both doses (47% partial response, 32% stable disease and 5% complete response). There was a longer time to progression with higher dose but at expense of increased toxicity.[10] The standard dose of treatment currently recommended is 400 mg/day. The 2-year survival of patients with metastatic disease is now reported as 70%[7] compared with a previous median survival of 10–20 months.

The role of adjuvant or neoadjuvant therapy with imatinib remains unclear and at the current time such treatment is not advocated unless in the context of a clinical trial. Several studies are underway to investigate the role of such treatments.[11]

There is a group of patients with initially unresectable locally advanced or metastatic disease who become operable following a good response to imatinib therapy. Surgical resection should always remain an option in these circumstances and evidence is accumulating that such intervention improves prognosis.[12] All patients will develop resistance to imatinib at some stage during their treatment and therefore timing of surgery under these circumstances is crucial. Similarly, there is no consensus on the appropriate timing of further imatinib if resection margins are positive following surgery. Some advocate the use of early treatment to delay the time to progression whereas others wait for the occurrence of progressive disease. There are currently no clinical trial data to support improved overall survival with either of these approaches and hence decisions should be made on an individual basis until further data become available.

## Conclusion

The extent of the GIST in this patient should be determined by imaging on CT scan, including liver scanning to check for metastases. A multidisciplinary team of surgeons then need to decide if the tumour is resectable. If not, it may be possible to shrink the tumour using imatinib therapy, and resect at a later date.

## Further Reading

1 Rubin BP, Singer S, Tsao C, Duensing A, Lux ML, Ruiz R, Hibbard MK, Chen CJ, Xiao S, Tuveson DA, Demetri GD, Fletcher CD, Fletcher JA. KIT activation is a ubiquitous feature of gastrointestinal stromal tumors. *Cancer Res* 2001; **61**: 8118–21.

2 Nilsson B, Bumming P, Meis-Kindblom JM, Oden A, Dortok A, Gustavsson B, Sablinska K, Kindblom LG. Gastrointestinal stromal tumors: the incidence, prevalence, clinical course, and prognostication in the preimatinib mesylate era: a population-based study in western Sweden. *Cancer* 2005; **103**: 821–9.

3 Fletcher CD, Berman JJ, Corless C, Gorstein F, Lasota J, Longley BJ, Miettinen M, O'Leary TJ, Remotti H, Rubin BP, Shmookler B, Sobin LH, Weiss SW. Diagnosis of gastrointestinal stromal tumors: a consensus approach. *Hum Pathol* 2002; **33**: 459–65.

4 Miettinen M, Majidi M, Lasota J. Pathology and diagnostic criteria of gastrointestinal stromal tumors (GISTs): a review. *Eur J Cancer* 2002; **38**(Suppl 5): S39–51.

5  Emory TS, Sobin LH, Lukes L, Lee DH, O'Leary TJ. Prognosis of gastrointestinal smooth-muscle (stromal) tumors: dependence on anatomic site. *Am J Surg Pathol* 1999; **23**: 82–7.

6  Andersson J, Bumming P, Meis-Kindblom JM, Sihto H, Nupponen N, Joensuu H, Oden A, Gustavsson B, Kindblom LG, Nilsson B. Gastrointestinal stromal tumors with KIT exon 11 deletions are associated with poor prognosis. *Gastroenterology* 2006; **130**: 1573–81.

7  DeMatteo RP, Lewis JJ, Leung D, Mudan SS, Woodruff JM, Brennan MF. Two hundred gastrointestinal stromal tumors: recurrence patterns and prognostic factors for survival. *Ann Surg* 2000; **231**: 51–8.

8  Dematteo RP, Heinrich MC, El-Rifai WM, Demetri G. Clinical management of gastrointestinal stromal tumors: before and after STI-571. *Hum Pathol* 2002; **33**: 466–77.

9  Demetri GD, von Mehren M, Blanke CD, Van den Abbeele AD, Eisenberg B, Roberts PJ, Heinrich MC, Tuveson DA, Singer S, Janicek M, Fletcher JA, Silverman SG, Silberman SL, Capdeville R, Kiese B, Peng B, Dimitrijevic S, Druker BJ, Corless C, Fletcher CD, Joensuu H. Efficacy and safety of imatinib mesylate in advanced gastrointestinal stromal tumors. *N Engl J Med* 2002; **347**: 472–80.

10  Verweij J, Casali PG, Zalcberg J, LeCesne A, Reichardt P, Blay JY, Issels R, van Oosterom A, Hogendoorn PC, Van Glabbeke M, Bertulli R, Judson I. Progression-free survival in gastrointestinal stromal tumours with high-dose imatinib: randomised trial. *Lancet* 2004; **364**: 1127–34.

11  van der Zwan SM, DeMatteo RP. Gastrointestinal stromal tumor: 5 years later. *Cancer* 2005; **104**: 1781–8.

12  Raut CP, Posner M, Desai J, Morgan JA, George S, Zahrieh D, Fletcher CD, Demetri GD, Bertagnolli MM. Surgical management of advanced gastrointestinal stromal tumors after treatment with targeted systemic therapy using kinase inhibitors. *J Clin Oncol* 2006; **24**: 2325–31.

PROBLEM

# 44 Chemoradiotherapy in Head and Neck Cancer

## Case History

A 55-year old English patient has been diagnosed with T3 N1 M0 nasopharyngeal carcinoma.

**What is the treatment in this case?**

**What additional evaluations and supportive measures should be considered before and during his treatment?**

**Is the approach you have recommended for this patient applicable worldwide?**

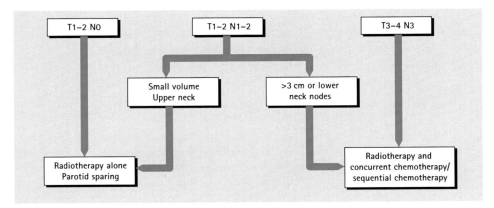

**Figure 44.1** Algorithm for the management of nasopharyngeal carcinoma.

# Background

## What is the treatment in this case?

Current best practice requires a multidisciplinary team approach in managing nasopharyngeal carcinoma (NPC). This patient's tumour has invaded the bony structures and/or paranasal sinuses with unilateral metastasis of lymph node(s), and is <6 cm in greatest dimension above the supraclavicular fossa. This falls into American Joint Committee of Cancer (AJCC) stage III. NPC is a disease that is sensitive to radiotherapy and chemotherapy. Unlike other cancers of the head and neck region where surgery is preferred, early stage NPC is mainly treated with radiotherapy (Figure 44.1). For stage III and locally confined stage IV disease, 50–80% of patients develop recurrent or metastatic disease within 5 years of treatment with radiotherapy alone. Although chemotherapy was used only for palliation of metastatic disease in the past, it has now become an integral part of the treatment of locally advanced NPC.

Chemotherapy in the concurrent setting is aimed at enhancing and complementing radiation by exploiting the radiosensitizing properties of cisplatin and/or 5-fluorouracil (5-FU). The activity of cisplatin in squamous cell cancer in the head and neck led to several landmark trials in the 1980s and 1990s that showed improved loco-regional control and overall survival. The Intergroup trial 0099 compared standard radiotherapy alone with radiotherapy plus cisplatin followed by adjuvant cisplatin and 5-FU for stage III and IV NPC. Marked reduction in loco-regional recurrence and distant metastases was noted. The rate of 3-year progression-free survival (PFS) was 24% and 69% in the radiotherapy and chemoradiotherapy arm, respectively. The 3-year survival rate was 46% in the radiotherapy arm compared with 76% in the chemoradiotherapy arm.[1] Other trials also confirmed benefit, though less dramatic and greater in locally advanced than in early-stage disease.[2,3] A recent meta-analysis confirmed the overall survival benefit of chemotherapy concomitant with radiotherapy.[4] Standard radiotherapy treatment delivers around 70 Gy in 2 Gy fractions to tumour and gross lymphadenopathy and 50 Gy to lower-risk neck nodal stations.[5] Although in other squamous cell cancers of the head and neck, concurrent cisplatin and 5-FU may be preferred, published guidelines for NPC recommend the Intergroup regimen of concurrent single-agent cisplatin 100 mg/m$^2$ every 21 days followed by adjuvant cisplatin and 5-FU.[5] The improved results with chemotherapy do come, however, with increased toxicity.

Recently, use of concomitant cetuximab rather than platinum in head and neck cancer has been considered with the publication of a trial showing that it too improves overall survival and progression-free survival when administered with radiotherapy.[6] However, it has not been compared directly with cisplatin, which remains the usual standard of care. The addition of agents increasing hypoxic cell killing (e.g. tirapazamine) to radiotherapy and/or chemoradiotherapy is currently under investigation. Optimization of radiotherapy through accelerated fractionation and intensity-modulated radiation therapy (IMRT) is also under research.[7] The Radiation Therapy Oncology Group (RTOG) recently completed a phase II trial of IMRT with standard concomitant cisplatin and adjuvant cisplatin and 5-FU in NPC.

# Discussion

### What additional evaluations and supportive measures should be considered before and during his treatment?

Supportive care during and after radiotherapy is vital to deal with toxicities, from early acute problems such as mucositis and myelosuppression to late effects such as xerostomia and thyroid dysfunction.[8] Oral hygiene is one of the most important aspects during treatment, as oral mucositis is inevitable, and, if severe, can lead to nutritional deficiency and/or delays in treatment. Eliminating all secondary sources of irritation such as alcohol and smoking can decrease the severity of oral mucositis. All patients should be referred to a dentist (preferably a specialist oncological dentist) for a thorough radiographic and oral/dental examination. Teeth with poor prognosis should be extracted before treatment. Reducing sites of infection decreases the chances of osteoradionecrosis in patients undergoing irradiation and infectious episodes in patients who receive chemotherapy. Post-treatment follow-up by an oncological dentist for at least a year after treatment is mandatory.

If nutritional status is inadequate prior to treatment and/or if radiotherapy fields indicate a high probability of swallowing complications during treatment, dietician assessment and elective insertion of a percutaneous endoscopic gastrostomy tube and enteral feeding should be considered. There is a relatively high level of alcohol consumption and smoking in patients with head and neck carcinoma. Management of alcohol intake and anticipation of potential withdrawal symptoms is also important. Appropriate counselling and rehabilitation should be offered to minimize complications and improve compliance during treatment.

Creatinine clearance should be measured prior to commencement of chemotherapy. If baseline renal function is abnormal, dose modification of cisplatin treatment may be required. Even if treatment can proceed, creatinine clearance should be monitored frequently during treatment.

### Is the approach you have recommended for this patient applicable worldwide?

NPC incidence is higher in the Chinese and Tunisian population. In very young patients, NPC is more common in African Americans. Therefore treatment strategies in the UK and USA may not yield the same results in endemic areas. Also, the association with the Epstein–Barr virus may also play a part in response to standard treatment. However, one of the randomized trials mentioned above did confirm improved local control of NPC with chemoradiotherapy in an endemic area.[2] Economic and social restraints may limit appropriate treatment delivery in some countries. The inability of patients to afford the cost of relevant healthcare service due to serious poverty and/or the absence of effective supportive care will also limit access to and use of available treatments. As radiotherapy is the main form of treatment in locally advanced NPC, it may be appropriate to offer single-modality radiotherapy where there are financial implications in delivering chemoradiotherapy, or where serious risks are posed by the lack of facilities necessary to manage its major additional toxicities.

## Conclusion

This patient's cancer cannot be resected and will be treated using a combination of radiotherapy and chemotherapy, which increases the radiosensitivity of the tumour cells. Early and late toxicities can be minimised by a systematic, pro-active approach to dentition, nutrition and renal function.

## Further Reading

1   Al-Sarraf M, LeBlanc M, Giri PG, Fu KK, Cooper J, Vuong T, Forastiere AA, Adams G, Sakr WA, Schuller DE, Ensley JF. Chemoradiotherapy versus radiotherapy in patients with nasopharyngeal cancer: phase III randomised Intergroup study 0099. *J Clin Oncol* 1998; **16**: 1310–17.

2   Chan AT, Teo PM, Ngan RK, Leung TW, Lau WH, Zee B, Leung SF, Cheung FY, Yeo W, Yiu HH, Yu KH, Chiu KW, Chan DT, Mok T, Yuen KT, Mo F, Lai M, Kwan WH, Choi P, Johnson PJ. Concurrent chemotherapy-radiotherapy compared with radiotherapy alone in loco-regionally advanced nasopharyngeal carcinoma. Progression-free survival analysis of a phase III randomised trial. *J Clin Oncol* 2002; **20**: 2038–44.

3   Wendt TG, Grabenbauer GG, Rodel CM, Thiel HJ, Aydin H, Rohloff R, Wustrow TP, Iro H, Popella C, Schalhorn A. Simultaneous radiochemotherapy versus radiotherapy alone in advanced head and neck cancer: a randomised multi-centre study. *J Clin Oncol* 1998; **16**: 1318–24.

4   Langendijk JA, Leemans CR, Buter J, Berkhof J, Slotman BJ. The additional value of chemotherapy to radiotherapy in locally advanced nasopharyngeal carcinoma: a meta analysis of published literature. *J Clin Oncol* 2004; **22**: 4604–12.

5   National Comprehensive Cancer Network Practice Guidelines in Oncology; Head and Neck Cancer v.1.2006. Available at: www.nccn.org.

6   Bonner JA, Harari PM, Giralt J, Azarnia N, Shin DM, Cohen RB, Jones CU, Sur R, Raben D, Jassem J, Ove R, Kies MS, Baselga J, Youssoufian H, Amellal N, Rowinsky EK, Ang KK. Radiotherapy plus cetuximab for squamous-cell carcinoma of the head and neck. *N Engl J Med* 2006; **354**; 567–78.

7   Huguenin P, Beer KT, Allal A, Rufibach K, Friedli C, Davis JB, Pestalozzi B, Schmid S, Thoni A, Ozsahin M, Bernier J, Topfer M, Kann R, Meier UR, Thum P, Bieri S, Notter M, Lombriser N, Glanzmann C. Concomitant cisplatin significantly improves loco-regional control in advanced head and neck cancers treated with hyper fractionated radiotherapy. *J Clin Oncol* 2004; **22**: 4665–73.

8   Harrison LB, Sessions RB, Hong WK. *Head and Neck Cancer – A Multidisciplinary Approach*, 2nd edn. Philadelphia: Lippincott Williams & Wilkins, 2003.

**PROBLEM**

# 45  Choriocarcinoma

## Case History

A 30-year-old woman, 2 months pregnant, presented with vaginal bleeding. Examination of the uterus suggests a 4-month pregnancy. Her human chorionic gonadotrophin (hCG) levels are markedly elevated and there are no fetal heart sounds. Abdominal ultrasound suggests the diagnosis of a molar pregnancy.

**How should the condition be managed?**

**What are the most common sites of metastatic disease?**

**What forms of chemotherapy are available for choriocarcinoma?**

**What is the outcome and how should patients be monitored?**

## Background

Gestational trophoblastic neoplasia (GTN) comprises a spectrum of neoplastic conditions that arise from placental trophoblastic tissue after abnormal fertilization.[1,2] These disorders are uncommon and can be classified into three distinct groups:

- Hydatidiform mole (complete or partial) – pre-malignant, can metastasize if become persistent.

- Choriocarcinoma – malignant.

- Placental site trophoblastic tumour (PSTT) – malignant, very rare.

These tumours are generally chemosensitive (except PSTT), can be monitored with a tumour-specific, semiquantitative marker, β-hCG, and have a cure rate of over 90%, making them almost unique in the world of oncology.[3] Most molar pregnancies resolve spontaneously, but about 10–20% of women develop persistent GTN.[1] This can become metastatic and often requires further treatment – either chemotherapy or surgery.

In northern Europe and USA, the incidence of hydatidiform mole is around 1 in 1500–2000 pregnancies and of choriocarcinoma is 0.7/1000 pregnancies.[2] The incidence is higher in Chinese, Malays, Indonesians and Native Alaskans, and lowest in Caucasians.

Classic symptoms of GTN include hyperemesis gravidarum, excessive uterine enlargement, early severe pre-eclampsia and hyperthyroidism. However, with the advent of high-resolution ultrasonography, GTN is now being diagnosed at a much earlier stage (8.5–9.5 weeks' versus 16–18 weeks' gestation) and therefore, in the developed world, the women are usually treated before these classic symptoms develop.[4] Women with GTN usually present with vaginal bleeding between 6 and 12 weeks into the pregnancy. They may also be large-for-dates and have more nausea and vomiting compared with a normal pregnancy, possibly due to high levels of hCG. GTN can also be an incidental finding either on ultrasound scanning in early pregnancy or on histological examination of products of conception of spontaneously passed tissue or after a therapeutic termination of pregnancy.[2,5] In women with no known antecedent pregnancy or term pregnancy, it can be more difficult to detect and may present with abnormal vaginal bleeding, postpartum haemorrhage or symptoms secondary to metastatic disease. Persistent GTN should be suspected in any pregnancy or in any woman of reproductive age where the woman represents with persistent abnormal vaginal bleeding, or develops new and acute respiratory or neurological symptoms.

## Discussion

### How should the condition be managed?

The initial management of this patient includes suction uterine evacuation to remove tumour, confirm the diagnosis histologically, and aid in controlling vaginal bleeding.[4–6] Other methods of uterine evacuation are not recommended as they can increase uterine blood loss and incidence of malignant sequelae.[2,4] Histological diagnosis is helpful for prognostic reasons – the risk of persistent GTN after a partial mole is 0.5%, and after a complete mole it is 15%. Choriocarcinoma is a malignant disease and will require further treatment (see below).

In the UK, the patient should be referred to a specialist trophoblastic screening centre for follow-up either in London, Sheffield or Dundee – where monitoring with serial urinary hCG measurements is undertaken and advice on necessary treatment given. Persistent GTN is most easily detected by a rising or plateauing hCG level.[5] In Sheffield only 5–6% of women on the screening programme receive chemotherapy.

The need for treatment in GTN is determined by the criteria given below (by definition, women fulfilling any of these criteria have persistent GTN):

● β-hCG levels greater than 20 000 IU/l after one or two uterine evacuations – the hCG is a semiquantitative estimate of the amount of trophoblastic tissue in the patient, thus a high level confers risk of uterine perforation or major haemorrhage.

● Static or rising β-hCG levels after one or two uterine evacuations.

| Table 45.1 | International Federation of Gynecology and Obstetrics 2000 prognostic risk assessment | | | |
|---|---|---|---|---|
| | Score | | | |
| | 0 | 1 | 2 | 4 |
| Age | ≤39 | >39 | – | – |
| Antecedent pregnancy | Hydatidiform mole | Abortion | Term pregnancy | – |
| Interval months from index pregnancy | <4 | 4–6 | 7–12 | >12 |
| Pretreatment hCG (IU/ml) | $<10^3$ | $10^3$–$10^4$ | $10^4$–$10^5$ | $>10^5$ |
| Largest tumour size including uterus | <3 cm | 3–4 cm | ≥5 cm | – |
| Site of metastases | None | Spleen, kidney | Gastrointestinal tract | Brain |
| Number of metastases identified | 0 | 1–4 | 5–8 | >8 |
| Previous failed chemotherapy | – | – | Single drug | Two or more drugs |

● Persistent βhCG elevation 6 months post-uterine evacuation – due to increasing likelihood of developing drug-resistant disease.

● Persistent uterine haemorrhage with raised β-hCG levels.

● Pulmonary metastases with static or rising β-hCG levels (some pulmonary metastases will regress spontaneously).

● Evidence of metastases in liver, brain or gastrointestinal tract.

● Histological diagnosis of choriocarcinoma – choriocarcinoma is a malignant disease and will therefore not regress spontaneously.

If the patient has any of the above features she will be invited to her local trophoblastic centre for investigations (β-hCG level, chest radiograph, ultrasound of abdomen and pelvis, computed tomography [CT] scan of the chest and, in high-risk women, CT or magnetic resonance imaging (MRI) of brain and lumbar puncture). The treatment depends on the score. The most commonly used scoring system in the UK is the International Federation of Gynecology and Obstetrics (FIGO) 2000 prognostic risk assessment, which contains multiple weighted prognostic factors (Table 45.1).

## What are the most common sites of metastatic disease?

Metastases in GTN are uncommon. The most common sites of metastases are lung (80%), vagina (30%), brain (10%), liver (10%), gastrointestinal tract and kidney (<10% each).[2,6,7]

## What forms of chemotherapy are available for choriocarcinoma?

On prognostic risk scoring, a score of less than 7 indicates low-risk disease and the patient is treated with single-agent chemotherapy, most commonly intramuscular methotrexate or intravenous dactinomycin. Rates of remission for each of these approach 70–80%.[7] The advantages of using single-agent methotrexate are that it is easier to administer, does not cause alopecia and causes less nausea, myelosuppression and mucositis than dactinomycin.[8] If treatment resistance develops patients can be changed to combination treatment or single-agent dactinomycin (if β-hCG level is low and methotrexate was used first).

A score of 7 or greater indicates high risk disease and these women should be treated initially with combination chemotherapy as several studies have demonstrated a better prognosis if the first-line treatment is combination rather than single-agent treatment. The most widely used regimen is etoposide, methotrexate, dactinomycin, cyclophosphamide and vincristine (EMA/CO) with a cumulative survival rate of around 80%. Patients developing resistance to the EMA/CO regimen are switched to etoposide, cisplatin, methotrexate and dactinomycin (EP/EMA). An alternative is methotrexate, etoposide and dactinomycin (MEA) chemotherapy which has a similar response rate to EMA/CO. Some centres offer prophylactic intrathecal chemotherapy to all high-risk women.[7]

### What is the outcome and how should patients be monitored?

Cure rates of GTN in the UK are around 98%–100% for low-risk disease and 80–90% for high-risk disease.[1,5,8] Persistent GTN following a non-molar pregnancy has a worse prognosis probably due to a delay in diagnosis and referral to the specialist centre. Long-term risks of chemotherapy include the rare but appreciable risk of second malignancies (usually acute myelocytic leukaemia) when using etoposide chemotherapy. Fertility is usually preserved but earlier menopause can occur.[7]

Patients should be monitored as per the trophoblastic centre's follow-up protocol. This involves computerized postal monitoring of urinary hCG. Women are advised to avoid the oestrogen-containing contraception pill until hCG levels are normalized and to avoid coil contraception until normal menstrual cycle recommences. A woman should avoid getting pregnant for minimum of 6 months after hCG levels return to normal, or 12 months from finishing treatment if she had chemotherapy. Urine sample for hCG is required at 6 weeks after delivery following all subsequent pregnancies to exclude reactivation of dormant trophoblastic tissue.[5]

## Conclusion

Following removal of the tumour, by suction uterine evacuation, the patient should be monitored by a specialist trophoblast screening centre, who will decide if chemotherapy is appropriate. The prognosis and long-term survival are generally good.

## Further Reading

1   Kudelka AP, Freedman RS, Kavanagh JJ. Gestational trophoblastic tumours. In: Pazdur R, Coia LR, Hoskins WJ, Wagman LD, editors. *Cancer Management. A Multidisciplinary Approach*. F.A. Davis: Philadelphia; 499–508.

2   Soper JT, Mutch DG, Schink JC. Diagnosis and management of gestational trophoblastic disease: ACOG practice bulletin no. 53. *Gynecol Oncol* 2004; **93**: 575–85.

3   Lurain JR. Treatment of gestational trophoblastic tumours. *Curr Treat Opin Oncol* 2002; **3**: 113–24.

4   Hurteau JA. Gestational trophoblastic disease: management of hydatidiform mole. *Clin Obstet Gynecol* 2003; **46**: 557–69.

5  Tidy JA, Hancock BW, Newlands ES. *The Management of Gestational Trophoblastic Neoplasia.* The Royal College of Obstetricians and Gynaecologists: Guideline No. 38.

6  Newlands ES. Presentation and management of persistent trophoblastic disease and gestational trophoblastic tumours in the UK. In: Hancock BW, Newlands ES, Berkowitz RS, Cole LA. *Gestational Trophoblastic Diseases,* 2nd edn. Sheffield: International Society for the Study of Trophoblastic Diseases, 2003. (www.isstd.org/gtd/index.html).

7  Ng TY, Wong LC. Diagnosis and management of gestational trophoblastic neoplasia. *Best Pract Res Clin Obst Gynaecol* 2003; **17**: 893–903.

8  Carney ME. Treatment of low risk gestational trophoblastic disease. *Clin Obstet Gynecol* 2003; **46**: 579–92.

PROBLEM

# 46  Merkel's Cell Tumour

## Case History

A 78-year-old woman presents with a 6-month history of a red nodule on her forearm which has enlarged to >2 cm in diameter. Excision biopsy reveals Merkel's cell tumour with <2 mm excision margins.

**How should this patient be further assessed?**

**How should the primary site be managed?**

**What adjuvant treatment should be considered?**

**What is the prognosis?**

**How should recurrent disease be managed?**

## Background

### How should this patient be further assessed?

The patient needs to be further assessed to determine the extent of the disease. There is no widely accepted staging system for Merkel's cell carcinoma or a standardized classification based on prognosis. Either the American Joint Committee on Cancer[1] staging system for cancer or the TNM staging (see Table 46.1) can be used for staging purposes. However, it is commonly staged according to clinical presentation as follows:[2]

| Table 46.1 | TNM staging for Merkel's cell carcinoma |
|---|---|
| T1 | Primary tumour <2 cm |
| T2 | Primary tumour ≥2 cm |
| N0 | Negative regional lymph nodes |
| N1 | Positive regional lymph nodes |
| M0 | No evidence of distant metastatic disease |
| M1 | Distant metastatic disease present |
| *Stage* | *Criteria* |
| I | T1 N0 M0 |
| II | T2 N0 M0 |
| III | Any T N1 M0 |
| IV | Any T Any N M1 |

● Stage IA: Primary tumour <2 cm with no evidence of spread to lymph nodes or distant sites.

● Stage IB: Primary tumour ≥2 cm with no evidence of spread to lymph nodes or distant sites.

● Stage II: Regional node involvement but no evidence of distant metastases.

● Stage III: Presence of systemic metastases beyond the regional lymph nodes.

Further assessment includes investigations to determine whether there is lymph node involvement. Identification of disease in the sentinel lymph node basin will provide information about prognosis and also identifies the draining lymph node bed for surgery and any adjuvant radiotherapy.

The sentinel lymph node is the hypothetical first lymph node reached by micro metasta-sizing cancer cells from a primary tumour. Sentinel lymph node biopsy is carried out by injecting blue dye and a harmless radioactive substance around the primary tumour several hours prior to the biopsy. During the biopsy, the surgeon inspects the lymph nodes for staining and uses a Geiger counter (which detects $\alpha$ and $\beta$ radiation) to assess which lymph nodes have taken up the radioactive substance. The node(s) which take up the dye are des-ignated the sentinel lymph node(s) and the surgeon can then remove these for histopatho-logical examination. Often a frozen section will be carried out to detect neoplasia, and if positive further lymph node dissection may be done. The advantage of sentinel lymph node biopsy is that it can avoid the need for large lymph node dissections, thus reducing the risk of lymphoedema. In Merkel's cell carcinoma, sentinel lymph node biopsy has been shown to be beneficial for both prognosis and decision regarding further management.[3]

Other investigations include computed tomography (CT) to help demonstrate the presence of regional lymph node involvement or systemic metastases in the liver, lungs and other sites. Ultrasonography has also been used; it shows hypoechoic nodules arising from the dermis.

It is also possible to evaluate loco-regional disease and distant metastases with somatostatin-receptor scintigraphy based on the neuroendocrine characteristics of Merkel's cell carcinoma.[4]

# Discussion

### How should the primary site be managed?

Assuming further investigation reveals no spread to the lymph nodes or distant metastases, this patient has stage IB disease. No prospective controlled trials have looked at the best excision margins in Merkel's cell carcinoma. It is generally accepted that margins of 2–3 cm wide and 2 cm deep are adequate. Earlier series recommended margins of ≥3 cm and some studies have shown reduction in local recurrence with margins ≥3 cm.[4]

The case study patient has had surgery with an inadequate margin and requires further wide local excision of the primary site. This can be done by either conventional surgical wide local excision or by Mohs' micrographic surgery, which is a tissue-sparing technique that allows the surgeon to keep removing thin layers of skin following resection of the primary tumour until there is no microscopic disease left in the sample removed. This technique has been considered as the best method of wide local excision for Merkel's cell carcinoma. However, although its use has been previously evaluated, none of the controlled clinical trials comparing it with traditional wide local excision have shown it to be beneficial.[4]

### What adjuvant treatment should be considered?

Assuming the patient had sentinel lymph node biopsy as part of her initial staging investigations and this was found to be negative, she would not require a prophylactic lymph node dissection as part of her standard management. However, adjuvant radiotherapy should be considered.

It is known that Merkel's cell carcinoma is an aggressive subcutaneous malignancy with a high risk of recurrence despite treatment. Recently published data suggest that combination treatment with adequate surgery followed by adjuvant radiotherapy may greatly reduce the risk of local recurrence. It has also been suggested that the rate of progression from stage I to stage II disease is markedly lower following combination treatment compared with surgery alone. Overall survival and cause-specific survival advantages have been shown among patients with stage I disease treated with combination treatment.[5]

Several studies have looked at adjuvant radiotherapy following surgery for Merkel's cell carcinomas, with conflicting results about its use in this setting.[4] Also, there are no convincing data from prospective trials, however, even then radiotherapy is being advocated in the adjuvant setting. Currently it is generally used in patients with large tumours, tumours with lymphatic invasion, tumours approaching the surgical resection margins and locally unresectable tumours.

Studies suggest the appropriate total dose of radiotherapy is approximately 50 Gy to the surgical bed and the draining regional lymph nodes, delivered in 2 Gy fractions. Higher doses have been recommended in unresectable tumours or those with microscopic evidence of spread beyond resected margins.[6,7]

## What is the prognosis?

Most patients present with localized disease (approximately 70–80%), like the index patient. Five-year survival rates in stage I disease have been reported to be up to 64%. However, despite adequate local excision, local recurrence rates are high and risk of regional lymph node metastases are even higher and usually occur within 2 years of primary diagnosis. Distant metastases can occur in up to half of these patients and this is usually what causes patients with Merkel's cell carcinomas to die. The common sites of recurrence and distant metastases are liver, lung, bone, brain or distant lymph nodes.

Prognosis seems to be better in patients who present with no obvious primary tumour.[4,8]

## How should recurrent disease be managed?

Management of recurrent disease depends largely on the site of recurrence. If the patient develops local recurrence then treatment can include regional lymph node dissection with or without adjuvant radiotherapy depending on the management the patient received at presentation of the primary tumour. If the patient presents with recurrent unresectable tumours or for those patients who have received their maximum radiation dose previously, chemotherapy can be considered.

The most commonly used regimens are similar to those used in small cell lung cancer due to the morphological and immunohistochemical similarities. They include cisplatin and etoposide, and cyclophosphamide, doxorubicin and vincristine. Merkel's cell carcinomas tend to respond initially to chemotherapy, but responses tend to be short-lived and the impact of chemotherapy on survival is uncertain.[9–11]

# Conclusion

The initial surgery had inadequate excision margins and so further surgery must now be performed, as these tumours have a high rate of local recurrence. Sentinel lymph node biopsy is also advisable in this patient, as it helps to determine the prognosis. There is inadequate evidence to advocate adjuvant therapy.

# Further Reading

1 American Joint Committee on Cancer. *AJCC Cancer Staging Manual.* Springer, New York, 2002.

2 Aasi SZ, Leffell DJ. Cancer of the skin. In: De Vita VT Jr, Hellman S, Rosenberg SA, eds. *Cancer: Principles and Practice of Oncology*, 7th edn. Lippincott Williams & Wilkins, Philadelphia, 2005: 1717–44.

3 Gupta SG, Wang LC, Penas PF, Gellenthin M, Lee SJ, Nghiem P. Sentinel lymph node biopsy for evaluation and treatment of patients with Merkel cell carcinoma: the Dana-Farber experience and meta-analysis of the literature. *Arch Dermatol* 2006; **142**: 685–90.

4 Pectasides D, Pectasides M, Economopoulos T. Merkel cell cancer of the skin. *Ann Oncol* 2006: 17: 1489–95.

5 Lewis KG, Weinstock MA, Weaver AL, Otley CC. Adjuvant local irradiation for Merkel call carcinoma. *Arch Dermatol* 2006; **142**: 693–700.

6  Goessling W, McKee PH, Mayer RJ. Merkel cell carcinoma. *J Clin Oncol* 2002; **20**: 588–98.

7  Marks ME, Kim RY, Salter MM. Radiotherapy as an adjunct in the management of Merkel cell carcinoma. *Cancer* 1990; **65**: 60–4.

8  Allen PJ, Bowne WB, Jaques DP, Brennan MF, Busam K, Coit DG. Merkel cell carcinoma: prognosis and treatment of patients from a single institution. *J Clin Oncol* 2005; **23**: 2300–09.

9  Tai PT, Yu E, Winquist E, Hammond A, Stitt L, Tonita J, Gilchrist J. Chemotherapy in neuroendocrine/Merkel cell carcinoma of the skin: case series and review of 204 cases. *J Clin Oncol* 2000; **18**: 2493–9.

10  Feun LG, Savaraj N, Legha SS, Silva EG, Benjamin RS, Burgess MA. Chemotherapy for metastatic Merkel cell carcinoma. Review of the M.D. Anderson Hospital's experience. *Cancer* 1988; **62**: 683–5.

11  Voog E, Biron P, Martin JP, Blay JY. Chemotherapy for patients with locally advanced or metastatic Merkel cell carcinoma. *Cancer* 1999; **85**: 2589–95.

**PROBLEM**

# 47  Brain Tumours

## Case History

A 62-year-old man presents with a short history of headaches and unsteadiness. He had no neurological signs. A computed tomography (CT) scan demonstrated a rim-enhancing lesion in his left parietal lobe and magnetic resonance imaging (MRI) (Figure 47.1) showed strong enhancement with gadolinium, with appearances typical of a glioblastoma multiforme. His symptoms reduce with corticosteroids.

**What are the important prognostic features and likely outcome?**

**What is the role of surgery?**

**Is there any benefit for radiotherapy (Figure 47.2 – *see inside back cover*)?**

**Is chemotherapy beneficial?**

**Are any treatments available for relapse?**

**What experimental approaches are being explored?**

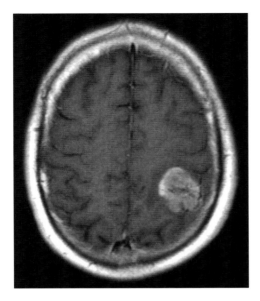

**Figure 47.1** Axial T1-weighted MRI with gadolinium showing enhancing left parietal lesion.

## Background

### What are the important prognostic features and likely outcome?

High-grade gliomas (HGGs) are locally invasive, incurable and have a poor prognosis in terms of survival, quality of life and social functioning. HGGs include grade IV glioma or glioblastoma multiforme with a median survival of about 6–12 months, and the less common grade III or anaplastic gliomas which have a median survival of 2–3 years. Increasing age and reduced performance status (PS) are key poor prognostic factors in the Medical Research Council (MRC) and Radiation Therapy Oncology Group (RTOG) trials, and this patient's age (over 60) is not in his favour. Other prognostic factors include a history of fits (patients with >3 months history of fits do better), mental status and extent of surgery.

## Discussion

### What is the role of surgery?

Resection as opposed to biopsy allows complete histological examination and grading, which is important for the selection of postoperative treatment. Debulking can also provide rapid symptom improvement. However, tumour infiltrates well beyond the enhancing rim seen on cross-sectional imaging and because of this surgical resection is not curative. Although maximal cytoreductive surgery would usually be the preferred option for this patient if he is fit and the tumour does not involve a critical structure, there is little randomized trial evidence for a survival benefit. In patients with poorer prognosis, a biopsy may be preferred or it may even be most appropriate to accept a clinical and radiological diagnosis and adopt a best supportive approach.

## Is there any benefit for radiotherapy?

HGGs are relatively radioresistant, and dose is limited by the sensitivity of surrounding brain tissue. Early trials of radical radiotherapy suggested an improved outcome, with survival of about 3 months with supportive care, and 9 months with radiotherapy.[1] Survival benefit can be inferred from dose fractionation studies. In an MRC trial[2] 60 Gy in 30 fractions was associated with longer median survival compared with 45 Gy in 20 fractions (12 months versus 9 months). Recurrence is inevitable following radiotherapy, and is predominantly in-field. Attempts to improve outcome using accelerated, hyperfractionated or dose-escalated regimens have to date not been generally successful.

Age and performance status are the main prognostic factors that are used to select patients most likely to benefit from radiotherapy.[3] Conventionally fractionated radical regimens over 6 weeks are associated with optimal survival and would be appropriate if this patient's postoperative World Health Organization (WHO) performance status is 0/1. However, if his performance status has deteriorated, his likely survival is short, and radiotherapy of this type would occupy much of remaining survival with major acute toxicity including nausea, lethargy and alopecia, along with multiple hospital visits. Many patients do not live long enough to develop late toxicity from radiotherapy, which can include impaired cognitive function and memory. Shorter hypofractionated schedules, such as 30 Gy in 6–10 fractions over 2 weeks, offer a more palliative approach, with functional improvement in over a third of patients.[3,4]

## Is chemotherapy beneficial?

Until recently, chemotherapy had been of minimal benefit, as the blood–brain barrier limits drug access to the brain. Meta-analysis of adjuvant chemotherapy had shown only a small survival benefit[5] and toxic effects were felt by many to outweigh any minimal benefit. A randomized trial by the European Organisation for Research and Treatment of Cancer (EORTC)/National Cancer Institute of Canada has now shown substantially improved survival with the addition of an alkylating agent, temozolomide, to radiotherapy.[6] A total of 573 patients with glioblastoma multiforme, <70 years of age, with WHO performance status 0–2 were randomized to standard radiotherapy alone (60 Gy in 30 fractions) and the same radiotherapy with concurrent daily temozolomide 75 mg/m$^2$, followed by up to six maintenance cycles 150–200 mg/m$^2$ daily for 5 days every 4 weeks. Median survival was 15 months and 12 months, and 2-year survival was 26% and 10%, favouring temozolomide. It is not possible to distinguish the relative benefit of the concomitant and adjuvant components. The benefit was not significant in the minority of patients who had undergone only a diagnostic biopsy, and patients with a gross total resection derived more benefit than those with an incomplete resection, suggesting maximal tumour removal may be important for the efficacy of combination adjuvant treatment. WHO performance status 2 patients did not show any benefit. Molecular analysis showed an increased benefit of temozolomide in the presence of a methylated promoter for the DNA repair gene methylguanine methyltransferase (MGMT). This biomarker offers the potential to identify patients most likely to benefit from combined modality treatment and, in future, concurrent chemoradiotherapy will probably be considered as standard practice in suitable patients.

To circumvent the problem of access via the blood–brain barrier, biodegradable carmustine-containing polymers (Gliadel® wafers) have been tested after deposition into the surgical cavity both at the time of initial surgery and after surgery for recurrence. Although small survival benefits were seen, benefits are at best limited.

Treatment decisions for this patient are guided by his fitness. If he is fit for radical radiotherapy, on the basis of the trial evidence, concurrent and adjuvant temozolomide could be considered if his WHO performance status is 0 or 1.

### Are any treatments available for relapse?

Trial evidence is limited.[7] Further resection may improve quality of life and possibly survival. Re-irradiation is rarely employed due to the risk of exceeding normal brain tolerance. Palliative chemotherapy regimens include procarbazine, lomustine and vincristine (PCV), and single-agent lomustine or temozolomide. Benefit is limited with response rates less than 10%, and progression-free survival rates at 6 months of approximately double the response rate. A current UK National Cancer Research Institute trial is comparing temozolomide with PCV.

### What experimental approaches are being explored?

Many novel approaches are now being tested to improve outcomes for HGGs.[7] Molecular profiling is ongoing to identify prognostic and predictive markers to allow individualization of treatment. There is some evidence for limited activity for targeted therapies, including anti-epidermal growth factor receptor and anti-angiogenic agents. Other research is exploring oncolytic viruses, gene therapy and immunotherapy approaches.

## Conclusion

Surgical excision or debulking may help to alleviate symptoms, but will not necessarily increase survival and therefore needs to be discussed with the patient. Radiotherapy and chemotherapy are of limited use, and toxicity can be a problem, especially given the short life-expectancy, but options can be discussed with the individual patient.

## Further Reading

1   Walker MD, Alexander E Jr, Hunt WE, MacCarty CS, Mahaley MS Jr, Mealey J Jr, Norrell HA, Owens G, Ransohoff J, Wilson CB, Gehan EA, Strike TA. Evaluation of BCNU and/or radiotherapy in the treatment of anaplastic gliomas. A cooperative clinical trial. *J Neurosurg* 1978; **49**: 333–43.

2   Bleehan NM, Stennin SP. A Medical Research Council trial of two radiotherapy doses in the treatment of grades 3 and 4 astrocytomas. *Br J Cancer* 1991; **64**: 769–74.

3   Laperriere N, Zuraw L, Cairncross G; Cancer Care Ontario Practice Guidelines Initiative Neuro-Oncology Disease Site Group. Radiotherapy for newly diagnosed malignant glioma in adults: a systematic review. *Radiother Oncol* 2002; **64**: 259–73.

4   Thomas R, James N, Guerrero D, Ashley S, Gregor A, Brada M. Hypofractionated radiotherapy as a palliative treatment in poor prognosis patients with high grade glioma. *Radiother Oncol* 1994; **33**: 113–16.

5   Stewart LA. Chemotherapy in adult high grade glioma: a systematic review and meta-analysis of individual patient data from 12 randomised trials. *Lancet* 2002; **23**: 1011–18.

6   Stupp R, Mason WP, van den Bent MJ, Weller M, Fisher B, Taphoorn MJ, Belanger K, Brandes AA, Marosi C, Bogdahn U, Curschmann J, Janzer RC, Ludwin SK, Gorlia T, Allgeier A, Lacombe D, Cairncross JG, Eisenhauer E, Mirimanoff RO; European Organisation for Research and Treatment of Cancer Brain Tumor and Radiotherapy Groups; National Cancer Institute of Canada Clinical Trials Group. Radiotherapy plus concomitant and adjuvant temozolomide for glioblastoma. *N Eng J Med* 2005; **352**: 987–96.

7   Stupp R, Hegi ME, van den Bent MJ, Mason WP, Weller M, Mirimanoff RO, Cairncross JG; European Organisation for Research and Treatment of Cancer Brain Tumor and Radiotherapy Groups; National Cancer Institute of Canada Clinical Trials Group. Changing paradigms: an update on the multidisciplinary management of malignant glioma. *Oncologist* 2006; **11**: 165–180.

PROBLEM

# 48  Thymoma

## Case History

A 55-year-old man complains of aching central chest pain, slowly progressive over the past 6 months. There are no abnormal findings on examination. A chest radiograph and a computed tomography (CT) scan reveal an anterior mediastinal mass with extension of the tumour around the pleura and pericardium. A biopsy confirms a thymoma.

**What is the stage of the thymoma?**

**What is the place of surgical resection?**

**In the presence of residual or recurrent disease what are the treatment options?**

**What is the patient's prognosis?**

## Background

### What is the stage of the thymoma?

Thymomas are a rare form of cancer, accounting for 0.2–1.5% of all malignancies. However, they represent the most common tumours of the anterior mediastinum, where most thymomas (90%) occur. The rest arise in the neck or other areas of the medi-astinum. They are indolent tumours, and are typically discovered as an incidental finding on chest radiograph. Of those patients with symptoms, 40% have local symptoms of chest pain, cough, or dyspnoea related to tumour compression or invasion, and 30% pre-sent with systemic symptoms. Parathymic syndromes, in particular myasthenia gravis, hypogammaglobulinaemia and pure red cell aplasia, may develop.

Although thymomas are often encapsulated and non-invasive at the time of presenta-tion, approximately 50% of tumours invade through their own capsules, extending into surrounding structures. Transdiaphragmatic extension into the abdomen and metastasis into the ipsilateral pleura and pericardium can occur. Rarely, there is haematogenous/lymphogenous spread with metastases to the liver and bone.

The most widely used staging system for thymomas is the system proposed by Masaoka *et al.* in 1981.[1] Based on the extent of either microscopic or macroscopic invasion into mediastinal structures, patients can be grouped into four main stages (Table 48.1).

| Table 48.1 Thymoma staging system of Masaoka | |
| --- | --- |
| Stage | Description |
| I | Macroscopically completely encapsulated and no microscopic capsular invasion |
| II | Macroscopic invasion into surrounding fatty tissue or mediastinal pleura or microscopic invasion into capsule |
| III | Macroscopic invasion into neighbouring organs (pericardium, great vessels, lung) |
| IVA | Pleural or pericardial dissemination |
| IVB | Lymphogenous or haematogenous metastasis |

At presentation, approximately 40% of thymomas are stage I, 25% each are stage II or III, 10% are stage IVA and only 1% or 2% are stage IVB.[2] This patient presents with a classic history of slow-onset chest pain and the finding of pleural and pericardial involve-ment on CT scan makes this stage IVA disease.

## What is the place of surgical resection?

Surgery is the treatment of choice for localized thymomas. Patients with stage I disease who undergo a complete resection have 5-year survival rates of over 90%. In patients with more advanced disease, radical surgery aimed at complete resection should also be considered, since completeness of surgical resection is a highly important prognostic fac-tor in thymoma. In one large series, total resection was achieved in 85% and 42% of patients with stage III and IV disease, respectively.[3] Ten-year survival in patients who undergo complete resection is approximately 76% compared with 28% in patients with incomplete resection or biopsy only.[4]

For those patients in whom a complete resection is not achievable, the role of debulk-ing surgery or subtotal resection remains controversial. Studies comparing patients undergoing subtotal resection versus biopsy have had inconsistent results, with some series suggesting a small benefit with surgery and others not. The role of surgery in this setting therefore remains unclear, and the management of such patients should take into account the other treatment modalities.

# Discussion

### In the presence of residual or recurrent disease what are the treatment options?

Overall, between 10% and 30% of patients will have a relapse following resection of their thymoma. Most of these recurrences occur in the intra-thoracic cavity. Treatment options to be considered would include one or more of radiotherapy, chemotherapy and further surgery. As above, firm treatment recommendations are difficult to make given a lack of evidence from randomized clinical trials, a reflection of the rarity of these tumours. The literature instead consists of numerous case reports and prospective studies, usually involving small (<50) numbers of patients.

Thymomas are radiosensitive tumours. Although the role of adjuvant radiotherapy in completely resected disease remains controversial, there is a general consensus that post-operative radiotherapy is beneficial following a subtotal resection. Doses of 50–60 Gy are typically used, in 20–30 fractions, with reduced rates of recurrence consistently reported in such patients.[5,6]

Chemotherapy is an effective treatment modality in the management of thymomas and it has been used to treat patients with metastatic disease, as well as in a neoadjuvant and adjuvant setting. The most effective regimen reported to date uses a combination of cisplatin, doxorubicin and cyclophosphamide. Combined complete remission and partial remission rates in patients vary between 50% and 92% using this combination.[7,8] In one study looking specifically at patients with metastatic or recurrent disease, the overall response rate was 50%, with a median duration of response of 11.8 months and median survival of 37.7 months.[7] Other agents that have been used include corticosteroids (thought to act on the lymphocytic component of the tumour) and ifosfamide. In chemorefractory tumours, somatostatin analogues have shown promising early results.[9]

For recurrent disease that is confined to the thoracic cavity, an aggressive surgical approach is advocated by many authors. The data seem to support this. The 10-year survival of patients who undergo a complete re-resection is between 53% and 72%, compared with 0% to 11% in those who undergo incomplete resection.[2] Ultimately, many patients are likely to derive most benefit from a combined modality approach. For example, patients with primary unresectable disease have shown long-term survival using a combination of primary chemotherapy, followed by surgery and postoperative radiotherapy.

### What is the patient's prognosis?

The most important factors in determining prognosis in patients with thymoma are the Masaoka stage at presentation and the completeness of surgical resection. For many years, myasthenia gravis was considered to be an adverse prognostic factor but not any more because of improvements in perioperative care.

The overall 5-year survival rates of stage I, II, III and IV thymomas are approximately 93–100%, 70–98%, 50–89% and 50–62%, respectively.[1,3,4] The prognosis for this patient would, in part, be determined by the completeness of surgery he undergoes. In one series, among patients with stage III and IV disease who undergo a complete resection, 5-year survival was 93% compared with 64% in those undergoing a partial resection.[3] Similarly, a 5-year survival of 64% (total resection) compared with 34% (partial) in stage IV disease was reported by Regnard *et al.*, although the difference was not statistically significant due to the small numbers of patients.[10] Finally, long-term follow-up is required in all patients with thymoma, as they have been known to have a relapse many years (>25 years in some cases) after initial surgery.

## Conclusion

Surgical excision of the thymoma is crucial to improve this patient's prognosis. Even if the tumour cannot be completely excised, they are generally radio- and chemotherapy sensitive. A combined modality approach may be the optimal strategy.

## Further Reading

1  Masaoka A, Monden Y, Nakahara K, Tanioka T. Follow-up study of thymomas with special reference to their clinical stages. *Cancer* 1981; **48**: 2485–92.

2  Detterbeck FC, Parsons AM. Thymic tumours. *Ann Thorac Surg* 2004; **77**: 1860–9.

3  Kondo K, Monden Y. Therapy for thymic epithelial tumors: a clinical study of 1,320 patients from Japan. *Ann Thorac Surg* 2003; **76**: 878–85.

4  Blumberg D, Port JL, Weksler B, Delgado R, Rosai J, Bains MS, Ginsberg RJ, Martini N, McCormack PM, Rusch V, *et al.* Thymoma: a multivariate analysis of factors predicting survival. *Ann Thorac Surg* 1995; **60**: 908–14.

5  Pollack A, Komaki R, Cox JD, Ro JY, Oswald MJ, Shin DM, Putnam JB Jr. Thymoma: treatment and prognosis. *Int J Radiat Oncol Biol Phys* 1992; **23**: 1037–43.

6  Gripp S, Hilgers K, Wurm R. Thymoma: prognostic factors and treatment outcomes. *Cancer* 1998; **83**: 1495–503.

7  Loehrer PJ Sr, Kim K, Aisner SC, Livingston R, Einhorn LH, Johnson D, Blum R. Cisplatin plus doxorubicin plus cyclophosphamide in metastatic or recurrent thymoma: final results of an intergroup trial. The Eastern Cooperative Oncology Group, Southwest Oncology Group, and Southeastern Cancer Study Group. *J Clin Oncol* 1994; **12**: 1164–8.

8  Fornasiero A, Daniele O, Ghiotto C. Chemotherapy for invasive thymoma. A 13-year experience. *Cancer* 1991; **68**: 30–3.

9  Palmieri G, Montella L, Martignetti A, Muto P, Di Vizio D, De Chiara A, Lastoria S. Somatostatin analogs and prednisone in advanced refractory thymic tumors. *Cancer* 2002; **94**: 1414–20.

10  Regnard JF, Magdeleinat P, Dromer C, Dulmet E, de Montpreville V, Levi JF, Levasseur P. Prognostic factors and long-term results after thymoma resection: a series of 307 patients. *J Thorac Cardiovasc Surg* 1996; **112**: 376–84.

# 49 Adrenocortical Cancer: Medical Care

## Case History

A 55-year-old woman has been diagnosed with metastatic adrenocortical carcinoma. She is unwell and cushingoid.

**What should be the medical care? What treatments are available for her?**

**What is the role of mitotane?**

**What is the management of adrenal suppression and replacement?**

**Is there a role for chemotherapy?**

**How do you control Cushing's syndrome?**

## Background

**What should be the medical care? What treatments are available for her?**

Adrenal cortical carcinoma (ACC) is an uncommon tumour which occurs at all ages and in both sexes, accounting for approximately 0.02% of all cancer.[1] The average age at presentation ranges from approximately 40 to 50 years and it occurs equally frequently in men and women (1:1). Most cases represent non-functioning tumours.[2] About two-thirds of all patients with ACC have tumours that hypersecrete glucocorticoids and or androgens, and one-third of patients have classic Cushing's syndrome. In addition to symptoms of hormonal excess, patients with ACC commonly present with an abdominal mass, weight loss and other constitutional symptoms.

The mainstay of current treatment for ACC is complete surgical excision at the time of initial evaluation.[3] If metastatic disease is limited, there remains an apparent benefit of surgery aimed at rendering the patient free of measurable disease. The role of radiotherapy in ACC has not been well defined and is usually regarded as of limited benefit.[4] However, palliative radiotherapy for metastatic disease has been shown to be effective in a considerable proportion of patients, and it is the treatment choice for bone metastases (30–40 Gy). More importantly, adjuvant postoperative radiation therapy may have a role in patients at high risk for local recurrence.

Medical treatment aims to control hormone hypersecretion and – more importantly – partial or complete remission of tumour spread (Figure 49.1).

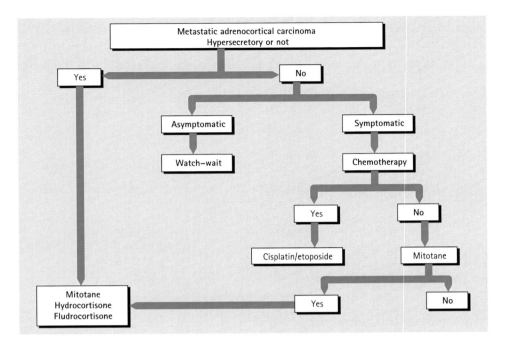

**Figure 49.1** Algorithm of management of metastatic adrenal cortical carcinoma.

# Discussion

### What is the role of mitotane?

Mitotane is the only adrenal-specific agent available for the treatment of ACC. Mitotane (1,1 dichloro-2(O-chlorophenyl)-2-(p-chloro-phenyl) ethane) is an isomer of the insecticide p,p'-DDD and a chemical congener of the insecticide DDT. It is an adrenolytic compound with specific activity on the adrenal cortex.[5] Mitotane's therapeutic effects depend on intra-adrenal metabolic transformation, and its clinical efficacy remains disputed. Response rate of 35% has been reported, with mostly partial and transient responses and only an occasional complete remission. More recent series have reported lower response rates.[6] The role of mitotane as adjuvant therapy after complete surgical removal of ACC remains a matter of debate.

Mitotane is either given as tablets (Lysodren, Bristol Myers Squibb, Princeton, USA) usually at a dose of >3 g/day or as capsules of micronized mitotane mixed with cellulose acetylphthalate, with a lower absorption rate, but, possibly, a better gastrointestinal tolerance.[6] Drug monitoring is important. It has been found that drug levels >14 mg/l are required to induce tumour regression. Objective response rates range between 31% and 80%[8] of patients achieving this level, whereas no response was seen in patients with a lower serum concentration. Side effects are mainly gastrointestinal (diarrhoea, nausea, anorexia) or related to the central nervous system (lethargy, somnolence, ataxia, dizziness, confusion).

Due to its adrenolytic activity long-term mitotane treatment induces adrenal insufficiency. Glucocorticoid deficiency precedes mineralocorticoid deficiency. Inadequately treated adrenal insufficiency enhances mitotane-induced side effects and reduces mitotane tolerance.[7]

## What is the management of adrenal suppression and replacement?

The patient needs glucocorticoid replacement. Hydrocortisone is the treatment of choice and the glucocorticoid replacement is monitored best with careful clinical assessment and measurements of plasma adrenocorticotropic hormone (ACTH) levels, which should not be raised. A daily dose of 50 mg hydrocortisone (20 mg, 20 mg, 10 mg) or more may be needed. Fludrocortisone may also be given depending on blood pressure, serum potassium levels and plasma renin activity.[8]

## Is there a role for chemotherapy?

In patients with advanced local or metastatic disease not amenable to surgical resection cytotoxic chemotherapy has been investigated. Several cytotoxic agents have been used as single drugs or in combination to treat patients with advanced ACC including cisplatin, doxorubicin, etoposide, vincristine, 5-fluorouracil and streptozocin.[9]

Although the results are variable, there is evidence that cisplatin alone or in combination with etoposide has some activity in advanced ACC.[10] Bonacci et al. treated patients with etoposide and cisplatin every 4 weeks and maintenance mitotane therapy with an overall response of 33%.[10] Burgess et al.,[11] using the same drugs without mitotane, reported a response rate of 46%. The highest response rate so far has been observed in a phase II multicentre trial from Italy, which used the combination of etoposide (100 mg/m$^2$/day on days 5–7), doxorubicin (20 mg/m$^2$/day on days 1 and 8) and cisplatin (40 mg/m$^2$/day on days 1 and 9) every 4 weeks (three to eight cycles) given together with continuous mitotane (planned dose 4 g/day).[12] According to the World Health Organization (WHO) criteria, an overall response rate of 53.5% was achieved (two complete and 13 partial responses in 28 patients). Due to mitotane's side effects, a reduced mitotane dose (2–3 g/day) was given to most of these patients. Recently, Khan et al. evaluated the efficacy of streptozocin plus mitotane in ACC. Oral mitotane (1–4 g/day) was given together with intravenous streptozocin (1 g/day for 5 days, thereafter 2 g once every 3 weeks). Complete or partial responses were obtained in 36.4% (8/22) of patients with measurable disease.[13]

## How do you control Cushing's syndrome?

As hormone excess (in particular hypercortisolism) is associated with a decreased of quality of life and an increased risk of complications, it is essential that patients do not develop Cushing's syndrome. Adrenostatic drugs other than mitotane may be needed to control endocrine activity. Metyrapone, ketoconazole, etomidate and aminoglutethimide inhibit P450 steroidogenic enzymes such as 11β-hydroxylase and side-chain cleavage enzyme. Ketoconazole (400–1200 mg/day) is most frequently used and may even possess antiproliferative activity in some patients with ACC.[14,15]

Prognosis in ACC is poor, with an overall and median 5-year survival rate of 14 months and 24%. Most studies conclude that early diagnosis and treatment by radical surgery offer the best odds for long-term survival. The development of small molecule inhibitors that can target generalized tumour pathways (e.g. angiogenesis) or ACC-specific signalling pathways suggests the possibility of new hope for patients with metastatic ACC.

## Conclusion

This patient's Cushing' symptoms need to be addressed and subsequent surgical, mitotane and adjuvant treatments discussed.

## Further Reading

1 Samaan NA, Hickey RC. Adrenal cortical carcinoma. *Semin Oncol* 1987; **14**: 292–6.

2 Mansmann G, Lau J, Balk E, Rothberg M, Miyachi Y, Bornstein SR. The clinically inapparent adrenal mass: update in diagnosis and management. *Endocr Rev* 2004; **25**: 309–40.

3 Dackiw AP, Lee JE, Gagel RF, Evans DB. Adrenal cortical carcinoma. *World J Surg* 2001; **25**: 914–26.

4 Schulick RD, Brennan MF. Long-term survival after complete resection and repeat resection in patients with adrenocortical carcinoma. *Ann Surg Oncol* 1999; **6**: 719–26.

5 Schteingart DE. Conventional and novel strategies in the treatment of adrenocortical cancer. *Brazilian J Med Biol Res* 2000; **33**: 1197–200.

6 Wooten MD, King DK. Adrenal cortical carcinoma. Epidemiology and treatment with mitotane and a review of the literature. *Cancer* 1993; **72**: 3145–55.

7 Robinson BG, Hales IB, Henniker AJ, Ho K, Luttrell BM, Smee IR, Stiel JN. The effect of o,p.'-DDD on adrenal steroid replacement therapy requirements. *Clin Endocrinol* 1987; **27**: 437–44.

8 Hahner BAS, Weismann D, Fassnacht M. Management of adrenocortical carcinoma. *Clin Endocrinol* 2004; **60**: 273.

9 Ahlman H, Khorram-Manesh A, Jansson S, Wangberg B, Nilsson O, Jacobsson CE, Lindstedt S. Cytotoxic treatment of adrenocortical carcinoma. *World J Surg* 2001; **25**: 927–33.

10 Bonacci R, Gigliotti A, Baudin E, Wion-Barbot N, Emy P, Bonnay M, Cailleux AF, Nakib I, Schlumberger M. Cytotoxic therapy with etoposide and cisplatin in advanced adrenocortical carcinoma. Reseau Comete INSERM. *Br J Cancer* 1998; **78**: 546–9.

11 Burgess MA, Legha SS, Sellin RV. Chemotherapy with cisplatinum and etoposide (UP16) for patients with advanced adrenal cortical carcinoma (ACC). *Proc Ann Soc Clin Oncol* 1993; **12**: 188.

12 Berruti A, Terzolo M, Sperone P, Pia A, Casa SD, Gross DJ, Carnaghi C, Casali P, Porpiglia F, Mantero F, Reimondo G, Angeli A, Dogliotti l. Etoposide, doxorubicin and cisplatin plus mitotane in the treatment of advanced adrenocortical carcinoma: a large prospective phase II trial. *Endocr Relat Cancer* 2005; **12**: 657–66.

13 Khan TS, Imam H, Juhlin C, Skogseid B, Grondal S, Tibblin S, Wilander E, Oberg K, Eriksson B. Streptozocin and o,p'DDD in the treatment of adrenocortical cancer patients: long-term survival in its adjuvant use. *Ann Oncol* 2000; **11**: 1281–7.

14 Luton JP, Cerdas S, Billaud L, Thomas G, Guilhaume B, Bertagna X, Laudat MH, Louvel A, Chapuis Y, Blondeau P, Bonnin A, Bricaire H. Clinical features of adrenocortical carcinoma, prognostic factors, and the effect of mitotane therapy. *N Engl J Med* 1990; **322**: 1195–201.

15 Contreras P, Rojas A, Biagini L, Gonzalez P, Massardo T. Regression of metastatic adrenal carcinoma during palliative ketoconazole treatment. *Lancet* 1985; **2**: 151–2.

# Psychosocial Issues and Symptom Control

## 50  Approach to Psychological Aspects of Cancer Care

## Case History

A 42-year-old woman with a recent diagnosis of breast cancer is referred for assessment. She has been crying persistently since diagnosis, unable to manage at home and is tearful during most of her recent consultations. Her husband thinks she is depressed and is concerned about her. Past history includes an episode of depression 20 years ago.

**How do you make a distinction between 'appropriate' distress and a markedly depressed mood?**

**Are there any risk factors that may predispose to depression?**

**When should you treat depression?**

**How should you treat depression?**

# Background

**How do you make a distinction between 'appropriate' distress and a markedly depressed mood?**

Many patients with cancer develop distress. For most patients this is transient, often appropriate and adaptive to what is extremely distressing news. For some patients, however, this develops into a major depression. Prevalence rates in the literature vary widely between 20% and 35% for depression in patients with cancer, depending on the studies reviewed. Although there are notable problems with some of these studies, there is no doubt that a large subgroup of patients with cancer become depressed. Distinguishing depression from distress is particularly difficult in patients with cancer as many of the so-called 'biological' depressive symptoms and signs are unhelpful. Thus, many patients with cancer have anorexia, weight loss, insomnia and poor concentration for reasons related directly to their cancer. One must rely therefore on other aspects of depression to make the diagnosis. These include the following:

- With depression the low mood/distress is pervasive, persisting throughout all or most of the day with no appreciable alleviation. It permeates all aspects of the patient's life. Sometimes there is diurnal mood variation, with the mood being worse in the morning and improving as the day goes on.

- Patients show reduced interest and motivation. This has to be assessed within the confines of physical disability. Patients, however, are usually clear that their lack of interest and motivation is not just due to physical constraints. But one can ask about activities that do not require much physical exertion, for example reading, watching TV, or following their favourite football team.

- Reduced enjoyment is another key feature of low mood. Patients describe how nothing can lift their mood, not even, for example, visits from friends or close family.

- Patients are often pessimistic and hopeless, feeling things will never get better.

- Rarely a patient may feel life is not worth going on with, even possibly considering suicide.

- Symptoms are present for a large part of the time, at least a 2-week period.

### Are there any risk factors that may predispose to depression?

In general, patients with a previous episode of depression are at increased risk of a further episode. It is important, however, to clarify whether this patient did, indeed, have an episode of depression, and whether it required treatment, responded to treatment and whether it recurred. Should patients need to be given steroids as part of their chemotherapy regimen, this will also increase the risk of affective disturbance (mania or depression). Family history of depression is also associated with an increased risk of depressive illness.

# Discussion

### When should you treat depression?

If a patient has marked depression they require active intervention. By definition, to have depression, in addition to having the above symptoms, their depressed mood should be interfering with their everyday functioning – work, family, social or leisure. Patients can quite readily give this information if asked. Treatment should be started immediately and titrated according to response.

### How should you treat depression?

Social, psychological and pharmacological interventions need to be considered. Adverse social circumstances need to be assessed and addressed where possible. Thus, for example, patients living on their own, with poor social supports, or major housing problems will need help targeted at these areas. Psychological interventions are diverse. These may include intervening with spouse, siblings or children for advice and support. A variety of psychological treatments are available. The most studied treatment is cognitive-behaviour therapy (CBT).

CBT is a brief, problem-orientated intervention that focuses on a collaborative approach with the patient. It is goal-directed, focused on the 'here-and-now'. Patients generate goals of treatment and work towards achieving them. Treatment includes behavioural components, for example, graded activity scheduling. Cognitive components include the recognition of 'thinking errors' which are often very relevant to the patient with cancer. These include 'catastrophization' – automatically assuming the worst; 'all or nothing thinking' – viewing all events as though there are only two possibilities 'complete disaster' or 'complete success'. When people are distressed, these thinking errors are magnified, and contribute appreciably to further distress and functional impairment. Cognitive therapy helps patients recognize these thinking strategies. It gives them a sense of control over their own behaviour and emotions which is helpful in dealing with future crises. CBT is effective in a variety of settings and is particularly useful in depression. Patients do need to be able to engage in treatment and motivated to attend. Thus, some patients with severe depression or psychotic depression will not be able to engage initially. For these patients, a combined approach using psychotropic medication is the preferred option. Equally, patients with major cognitive impairment will not be able to engage in comprehensive CBT. Nonetheless, selected approaches may be helpful, for example, simple behavioural components may be used. CBT should be administered by individuals with appropriate training in mental health and in CBT techniques, such as clinical psychologists, psychiatrists, and mental health nurses with specific training in CBT.

Anti-depressant therapies include serotonin-specific reuptake inhibitors (SSRIs); serotonergic-noradrenergic reuptake inhibitors (SNRIs); tricyclic anti-depressants (TCADs). The SSRIs/SNRIs are the most commonly used currently. In general, they are better tolerated than the more traditional TCADs – being less sedative, with fewer anticholinergic side effects. They are less likely to aggravate underlying medical conditions, interact with other medicines and are safer in overdose. The most common side effects with SSRIs are gastrointestinal – nausea, anorexia, vomiting. All of the anti-depressants, but particularly the SSRIs, may cause hyponatraemia. The TCADs cause significant anticholinergic side effects and are much less well tolerated in medically compromised patients.

## Conclusion

 It is important to determine whether this patient is actually suffering from depression or if her symptoms are totally attributable to distress caused by the cancer diagnosis, bearing in mind her past history. If depression is apparent, the appropriate social, psychological and/or pharmacological interventions should be selected, tailored to the individual's needs.

## Further Reading

1   Holland J, Greenberg D, Hughes MK. *Quick Reference for Oncology Clinicians: The Psychiatric and Psychological Dimensions of Cancer Symptom Management.* IPOS Press.

2   Distress management – clinical practice guidelines. JNCCN 2003; **1**: 344–74.

3   National Institute for Health and Clinical Excellence. *Supportive and Palliative Care for Adults with Cancer – Clinical Guidelines.* NICE, London.

**PROBLEM**

# 51  Breaking Bad News

## Case History

 A 38-year-old woman accompanied by her partner attends her first appointment after completion of adjuvant chemoradiotherapy for breast cancer. She mentions vague nausea and abdominal pain, which she ascribes to residual side effects of treatment. Investigations in clinic reveal liver and lung metastases. Her treatment had delayed her wedding to her long-term partner, at which their daughters (4 and 6) were to be bridesmaids. Her partner does not get on with her parents, and has always wanted to protect her from bad news, seeing a positive approach as vital to her success in battling her cancer.

**How will you approach the patient?**

**What should be the approach with the adult relatives?**

**How should the news be communicated to the patient's children?**

**How should the question of unfinished business be handled – how to maintain hope when time is limited?**

# Background

Breaking bad news is a complex communication task. It involves more than simply providing information to patient and relatives and requires other important skills. Some of the tasks the doctor will face are: responding to patients' emotional reactions; involving the patient in decision making; dealing with multiple family members; and the difficulty of maintaining hope in a situation with a bad prognosis.

How bad news is discussed can affect the patient's understanding of information and psychological adjustment. Poor communication can result in patients being unaware of their diagnosis, prognosis and the intent of any treatment.[1] In an informal survey conducted at the 1998 annual meeting of the American Society of Clinical Oncology (ASCO) 55% of the participants identified 'being honest with the patient without destroying hope' as their most important difficulty when breaking bad news, followed by 'dealing with the patient's emotions' (25%). Only 26% of the participants had a consistent strategy when conveying bad news, 52% followed several techniques but no overall plan.[2]

# Discussion

## How will you approach the patient?

Undoubtedly this news will be a severe shock to the patient, as she is not prepared and attributes her symptoms to her recent chemotherapy. The necessary transition from adjuvant treatment aiming for cure to a limited prognosis and treatment with palliative intent can become overwhelming for both patient and doctor. Strong patient emotions often provoke equally strong feelings of sympathy, anxiety, guilt and failure in the doctor, who in response might give false hope, provide premature reassurance or prescribe unnecessary treatments.[3] To avoid these pitfalls, doctors may find it helpful to reflect on their own feelings and work with 'guidelines' such as SPIKES (Table 51.1).[4] This six step protocol for delivering bad news incorporates key communication techniques in a stepwise plan to achieve the four essential goals of disclosing bad news:

1. determine the patient's understanding, expectations and readiness for the news by gathering information from the patient

2. provide information according to patient's requirements and wishes

3. provide support to reduce the emotional impact experienced by the patient

4. formalize a treatment plan in cooperation with the patient.

Critics suggest that all strategies for delivering bad news should only be seen as guidance, as the actual doctor–patient/family interactions are likely to be much more complex and often arise without warning: communication training should help doctors to flexibly respond to changing informational and emotional needs of all participants at all stages of care.[5]

## What should be the approach with the adult relatives?

After analysing interactions between oncologists, patients and companions in oncology outpatients clinics Eggly *et al.*[5] challenged the assumption that the bad news interaction is

**Table 51.1** SPIKES, a six-step protocol for delivering bad news[4]

| | | Helpful questions/remarks |
|---|---|---|
| S – *setting up* the interview | This includes mental rehearsal, arranging for the physical setting of the interview including privacy, involvement of significant others (relatives, nurses), allowing sufficient time and trying to establish rapport with the patient | |
| P – Assessing the patient's *perception* | By following the axiom 'before you tell, ask' the doctor can establish how the patient perceives the medical situation, correct misinformation and tailor the news to what the patients understands | 'What is your understanding about your medical situation?' |
| I – Obtaining the patient's *invitation* | Asking the patient about how much and how detailed information he or she wants gives the doctor the opportunity to further plan the delivery of the bad news | 'How would you like me to give you information about test results, would you like to know them in detail or rather sketched out?' |
| K – Giving *knowledge* and information | Before giving the medical facts in non-technical words, starting at the level of comprehension and vocabulary of the patient, it is useful to warn the patient that bad news is coming. It is also important to give information in small amounts and to check the patient's understanding, allowing the patient to reflect and ask clarifying questions. Avoid excessively blunt language | 'I'm afraid I have some bad news to tell you.' |
| E – Addressing *emotions* with empathic responses | Be observant for any sign of emotion, try to identify and name it. Ask in an open question if you are not sure about the patient's emotion or the reason for it. Give the patient time to take the information in and express feelings. Also let the patient know that you connected the emotion with the reason for it | 'I can see how upsetting this must be for you' |
| S – *strategy* and summary | A clear plan for the future helps the patient to feel less anxious and uncertain. After summarizing the information given so far and checking with the patient if he or she is ready to engage in planning further treatment options the doctor should discuss available treatment possibilities and include the patient as much as possible in the decision making. It is important to take goals and priorities specific for the patient into account | |

limited to the dyad between patient and physician. They found that companions played an active part in the conversation and actually asked many more questions than the patients (62% versus 38%, respectively).

Different family members are likely to introduce different levels into the interaction, which might distract doctor and patient from finding a strategy to deal with the current problem. However, family members can be a valuable resource of information as they often are main carers for the patient and have a key role in the patient's support. Thus the doctor should be aware of strategies to manage interactions with multiple participants.[6] One of the core elements of a three-party consultation is to acknowledge the importance of the relative's presence and concerns[7] in the context of the patient's concerns without taking sides.

In the case study consultation the doctor should appreciate the partner's concerns, but the patient needs to continue to be the focus of attention and confidentiality needs to be preserved. The doctor might have to clarify with the patient's partner that all information will be discussed to the extent of her wishes and in her pace. As her partner does not get on with the her parents, another level of complexity is added to the problem: if the patient also appreciates the issues between her partner and her parents then it could be useful to arrange for a family meeting. This could be a forum for the healthcare team to explain the treatment goals, let the family state their wishes for care, give everyone the opportunity to express their feelings and clarify caregiving tasks.[8]

### How should the news be communicated to the patient's children?

Confrontation with a parent's cancer can be very threatening for children and may result in the development of psychosocial problems, such as anxiety, confusion, sadness, anger, and feelings of uncertainty with respect to the outcome of the illness. They may face many changes in daily family routines due to repeated hospital admissions, hospital visits and care of the parent when at home.[9] When trying to protect their children many patients might decide not to tell them about a potentially life-threatening illness. It is, however, known that children are aware of and sensitive to (unexplained) changes in the atmosphere at home and that their potential to understand illness is actually higher than expected by adults. Research suggests that effective communication between parents and children about their parent's diagnosis improves their psychological adjustment and reduces anxiety.[9]

In a qualitative interview study of communication between parents and children about maternal breast cancer it became apparent that many mothers experienced helpful discussions with a doctor about their disease, but only few were offered support with talking to children; many would have liked to consult a health professional with experience in child development for guidance on ways to communicate difficult news to their children effectively.[10]

For the case scenario above it again is important for the doctor to find out how much the children know and understand. The parents might have decided that they did not want their children to know about their mother's illness because they thought that after completion of adjuvant treatment everything would return to normal. It is important to appreciate the parent's approach to the mother's cancer without judging and patronizing them. However, it might be helpful to explain that children are likely to cope better with a threatening situation if this is shared with them – in a way appropriate to their age.

The doctor should elicit how the parents prefer to inform the children about their mother's cancer and offer support on different levels. This can include a health professional informing the girls as well as providing the family with contact details for support organizations (e.g. Macmillan team) or information material (websites, leaflets, booklets). Pointing out that it is not a sign of failure to accept help might support the family through such a difficult time.

### How should the question of unfinished business be handled – how to maintain hope when time is limited?

Time is an important issue for the patient and her family. Especially in her situation where there is not only herself to think about, time becomes even more precious. The patient needs time to adjust to the implications of the limited prognosis for her, her family and her children. There is the incredibly painful thought of not being there to see her daughters grow up and the equally painful knowledge of not being around to support them along the way. Practical matters in the daily family life and arrangements about, e.g. childcare, now and later, need to be discussed and put into practise. Realization of long-standing plans like the wedding and starting memory boxes for her daughters also need to be seen in the context of limited time. To be able to deal with these issues the patient needs to have a realistic perspective of her outlook, so prognosis has to be discussed with her at some point. How proactively should the doctor act in this matter?

Most patients with metastatic cancer want detailed prognostic information but prefer to negotiate the extent, format and timing of the information they receive from their oncologist.[11] Rather than actively pushing for a conversation about prognosis it seems more important for the doctor to listen and respond to any cues given by the patient.

Helft[12] sees 'necessary collusion' as an ethical strategy of prognosis communication and describes it as 'a style of communication that allows patients to dictate most of the flow of prognostic information or to avoid it'. This collusion preserves hope by allowing information to emerge over time. It, however, needs to be taken into account that the illness might progress faster than expected, therefore the treating team has a responsibility to help the patient to make informed decisions by providing information adjusted to her pace of coping.

## Conclusion

The complexity of the case scenario mirrors the complexity of real life and only a few issues arising have been touched on rather than discussed in detail. The situation described cannot be addressed in one single visit and consultation. It should rather be seen as the beginning of a journey for the cancer patient and her family accompanied by a multidisciplinary medical team.

## Further Reading

1 Fallowfield L, Jenkins V. Communicating sad, bad, and difficult news in medicine. *Lancet* 2004; **363**: 312–19.

2 Baile W, Buckman R, Lenzi R, *et al.* Breaking Bad News Symposium, ASCO, 1998, presented in part at the annual meeting of the American Society of Clinical Oncology, 2000.

3 Maguire P, Pitceathly C. Key communication skills and how to acquire them. *BMJ* 2002; **325**: 697–700.

4 Baile WF, Buckman R, Lenzi R, Glober G, Beale EA, Kudelka AP. SPIKES: a six-step protocol for delivering bad news: application to the patient with cancer. *Oncologist* 2000; **5**: 302–11.

5 Eggly S, Penner L, Albrecht TL, Cline RJ, Foster T, Naughton M, Peterson A, Ruckdeschel JC. Discussing bad news in the outpatient oncology clinic: rethinking current guidelines. *J Clin Oncol* 2006; **24**: 716–19.

6 Lang F, Marvel K, Sanders D, Waxman D, Beine KL, Pfaffly C, McCord E. Interviewing when family members are present. *Am Fam Physician* 2002; **65**: 1351–4.

7 Delvaux N, Merckaert I, Marchal S, Libert Y, Conradt S, Boniver J, Etienne AM, Fontaine O, Janne P, Klastersky J, Melot C, Reynaert C, Scalliet P, Slachmuylder JL, Razavi D. Physician's communication with a cancer patient and a relative: a randomized study assessing the efficacy of a consolidation workshop. *Cancer* 2005; **103**: 2397–411.

8 National Cancer Institute. www.cancer.gov/cancertopics/When-Someone-You-Love-Is-Treated/

9 Visser A, Huizinga GA, van der Graaf WT, Hoekstra HJ, Hoekstra-Weebers JE. The impact of parental cancer on children and the family: a review of the literature. *Cancer Treat Rev* 2004; **30**: 683–94.

10 Barnes J, Kroll L, Burke O, Lee J, Jones A, Stein A. Qualitative interview study of communication between parents and children about maternal breast cancer. *BMJ* 2000; **321**: 479–82.

11 Hagerty RG, Butow PN, Ellis PA, Lobb EA, Pendlebury S, Leighl N, Goldstein D, Lo SK, Tattersall MH. Cancer patient preferences for communication of prognosis in the metastatic setting. *J Clin Oncol* 2004; **22**: 1721–30.

12 Helft P. Necessary collusion: prognostic communication with advanced cancer patients. *J Clin Oncol* 2005; **23**: 3146–50.

## PROBLEM

# 52  Social Issues in Cancer Patients

## Case History

A 69-year-old woman attends clinic to discuss the management of her recently diagnosed early-stage breast cancer. Her husband, who has mild dementia, accompanies her. A neighbour has brought them but she has to be back in time to collect her children from school. The patient expresses doubt whether she will be able to attend for treatment.

**How would you assess how the patient is currently managing?**

**How should review treatment alternatives be evaluated bearing in mind their social impact?**

**What are the options for support?**

**Should the social issues be monitored over time?**

## Background

Patients come from diverse backgrounds and with varied social responsibilities. Cancer and cancer treatments disrupt the everyday life of patients and their families. How people cope with the disruption depends on a number of inter-related complex factors including the type of cancer, individual characteristics and available support.[1] Although the type of cancer will inform the treatment plan, the social situation of the patient may have a major bearing on any decisions made.

# Discussion

### How would you assess how the patient is currently managing?

When a cancer patient is the main caregiver for a dependent, not only will they have to cope with their illness but also find ways of managing their ongoing responsibilities even though their time and energy are limited. Caring for dependants (children and older frail dependants) is a common concern of cancer patients. A quarter of patients surveyed expressed concern about providing care for their partner.[2] Thirty-five per cent of carers of cancer patients report a long-standing illness or disability of their own.[3] Running a home is hard for patients with newly diagnosed cancer and increasingly burdensome for those with advanced disease.[4] Patients' carers usually step in to take over these chores with 70% reporting increased activity in this area.[2] When the patient's partner is dependent this option is not available, although it may be possible to call on assistance from others within their close network.[3] Buying in additional support may be another option but only possible if the patient has the resources to do this. Older patients tend to be more financially secure than younger patients as they are likely to have a stable income from a pension, paid off mortgages and not have employment worries.[4] However, some will be reliant on a set limited income with very little in the way of savings. Add to this the additional costs of travel, special diets, heating and telephone bills, prescription charges (for those under retirement age) and 'baby-sitting' and the load may become considerable.[5] Eighty-five per cent of patients and carers who had incurred additional expense due to cancer received no financial support from any source for this.[2]

Evaluation of the case study patient should include assessment of her husband's level of dependency, what her usual roles and responsibilities are within the household, how she copes with problems, what support she has access to and whether she has the means to obtain any additional support (stage 1, Figure 52.1).

### How should review treatment alternatives be evaluated bearing in mind their social impact?

Once cancer staging is complete treatment options need to be considered. The primary treatment plan will be based on clinical evidence. However, when several options are available these should be discussed with the patient in the light of the social difficulties reported. Issues that need to be covered include:

- duration of the treatment plan
- where the treatment will be administered
- time taken for each treatment (inpatient, outpatient, day patient)
- the number of treatments
- intensity and side effects of treatment (fatigue, nausea etc.)
- recovery time.

The pros and cons of each option, in the light of the type of cancer, its prognosis and its social impact, should be discussed bearing in mind both short- and long-term outcomes (stage 2, Figure 52.1).

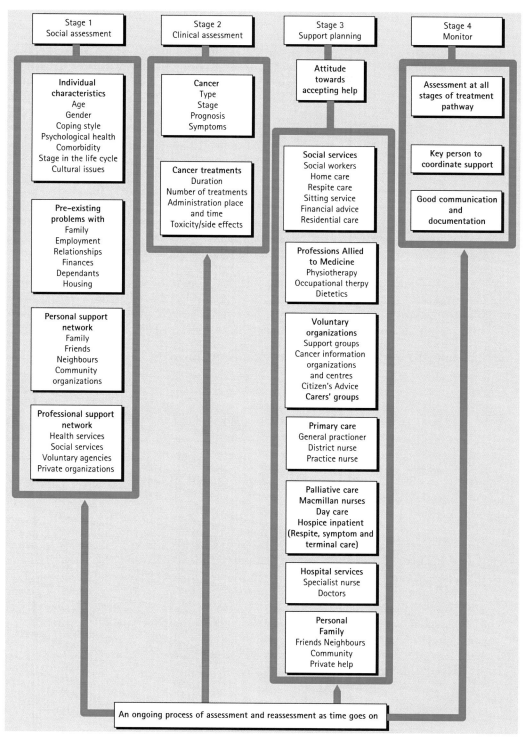

**Figure 52.1** A model for managing social issues in oncology clinical practice.

### What are the options for support?

Family members undertake the majority of caring for cancer patients.[3] The more advanced the cancer the greater the burden of care. Providing care may have a negative impact on everyday life in terms of problems with time off work and finances, restrictions in social activities, increased stress and isolation.[6] If family support is limited or not available then other sources of help may need to be found. There is great variability in the provision of and access to local support services across cancer networks.[7] However, usually there are some basic services that may be called on and members of the wider clinical team may be able to advise on these (stage 3, Figure 52.1). Patients may be eligible for financial support from the Benefits Agency (i.e. Income Support, Disability Living Allowance) or grants from, for example, Macmillan Cancer Relief that may allow them the means to 'buy in' private help.

Support may be planned only if our patient agrees she wants to go ahead with it. She may be influenced by previous experiences of supportive care or her husband's attitude to a different care arrangement. Her feelings on accepting help must be assessed and time given to her to consider various options and to discuss them with her family or friends. Once the treatment is agreed and support planned then coordination of both may be arranged. This is likely to be undertaken by several people working in together, including our patient, her family, members of the clinical team, and by community health, social and voluntary services. Depending on the level of support indicated the arrangement may be formal, through social or health services, or informal using unofficial networks.

### Should the social issues be monitored over time?

Dementia is a progressive disease. Over time the condition of our patient's husband is likely to deteriorate. The course of cancer is uncertain. In the National Institute for Health and Clinical Excellence guidance on *Improving Supportive and Palliative Care for Adults with Cancer* emphasis is placed on the importance of coordination of care: 'services need to work closely together to ensure that the patients' and carers' needs are addressed with no loss of continuity' and this should be undertaken: 'at all stages of the patient pathway'.[2]

## Conclusion

It is important to set in place an effective method of monitoring how our patient manages over time. This is likely to be a joint effort of those involved in the support of both our patient and her husband. The ongoing assessment will rely on good communication between the patient, her family and the support services. If there are several people involved then it may be that one person will take the responsibility for being the key person in monitoring how things are going. This may be our patient, someone in her family or a professional from the agencies involved. If formal assessments are undertaken then these should be shared between agreed parties so that there is not a duplication of assessment (stage 4, Figure 52.1).

# Further Reading

1   Corrado M, Worcester R for Ipsos MORI. The social impact of cancer: research study conducted for CANCER relief Macmillan Fund. Cancer Relief Macmillan Fund, London, 1992.

2   National Institute for Clinical Excellence. Guidance on cancer services. *Improving Supportive and Palliative Care for Adults with Cancer. The Manual.* NICE, London, 2004.

3   Payne S, Smith P, Dean S. Identifying the concerns of informal carers in palliative care. *Palliat Med* 1999; **13**: 37–44.

4   Pearce S, Kelly D, Stevens W. 'More than just money' – widening the understanding of the costs involved in cancer care. *J Adv Nurs* 2001; **33**: 371–9.

5   Thomas C, Morris SM, Harman JC. Companions through cancer: the care given by informal carers in cancer contexts. *Soc Sci Med* 2002; **54**: 529–44.

6   Wells NL, Turney ME. Common issues facing adults with cancer. In: Lauria MM, Clark EJ, Hermann JF, Stearns NM, eds. *Social Work in Oncology.* Atlanta: American Cancer Society 2001: 27–43.

7   Wright EP, Kiely MA, Lynch P, Cull A, Selby PJ. Social problems in oncology. *Br J Cancer* 2002; **87**:1099–104.

**PROBLEM**

# 53  Pain: A General Approach

# Case History

You are seeing a 76-year-old man who was diagnosed with non-small cell lung cancer 4 months ago. He had lung metastases and small-volume liver metastases at the time of diagnosis. He was initially treated with three cycles of chemotherapy, which was stopped due to a lack of clinical response. He now presents to the oncology clinic with moderate right-sided chest pain, which is present most of the time despite regular paracetamol.

**What approach would you use for the treatment of his pain?**

**What do you need to do if the pain does not respond to this initial approach?**

**If investigations confirm bone metastases what other treatments should be considered?**

# Background

## What approach would you use for the treatment of his pain?

Pain occurs in approximately 70% of patients with advanced cancer, but can be controlled in about 80% using the simple stepwise approach of the World Health Organization (WHO) analgesic ladder (Figure 53.1).[1] The first step in assessment of pain is always to take an accurate pain history including site, severity, nature and radiation of pain, any exacerbating or relieving factors and any psychosocial or spiritual factors which may be affecting the pain. It is important to know which analgesics have been tried, their effect on the pain and any adverse effects they have caused. Many patients have a fear of opioids, which may need to be explored further before starting treatment.

The three-step WHO analgesic ladder is the mainstay of the approach to analgesia. The severity of pain and previous analgesic exposure dictate the strength of analgesia to be used. Analgesia should always be given regularly (*by the clock*), orally if possible (*by the mouth*) and using the logical stepwise approach (*by the ladder*). At each step of the ladder, co-analgesics can be added depending on the nature and pathophysiology of the pain. Non-steroidal anti-inflammatory drugs (NSAIDs) and steroids can be helpful in cancer pain, especially pain associated with bone metastases and soft tissue inflammation, although the risk of serious adverse effects needs to be considered. The addition of paracetamol to weak or strong opioids may give additional benefit, but this needs to be weighed against the tablet burden. Neuropathic pain and its treatment are discussed in Chapter 54.

This patient has already tried regular paracetamol without effect, so needs to move up to step 2 of the ladder. Codeine is usually the weak opioid of choice and can be used in combination with paracetamol as co-codamol (30/500), two tablets four times a day, without increasing the tablet burden. At this dose the patient will be taking 240 g of codeine a day. Above this dose there are more undesirable effects such as nausea, vomit-

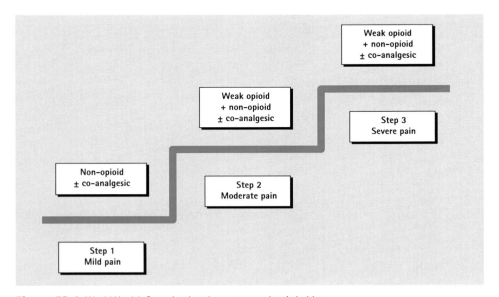

**Figure 53.1** World Health Organization three-step analgesic ladder.

ing and constipation, which outweigh any additional analgesic effect. He will also need analgesia available for breakthrough pain, which should be an immediate-release strong opioid equivalent to one-sixth of his daily dose of codeine (e.g. Oramorph 5 mg). Information on equivalence tables can be found in the *British National Formulary* and palliative care textbooks.

If the patient's pain is still uncontrolled after 48 hours on this regimen he should progress to step 3 of the ladder. The weak opioid should be stopped and switched to a strong opioid; an alternative weak opioid will not offer additional analgesic benefit. Morphine, which is approximately ten times more potent than codeine, is generally the strong opioid of choice, with other strong opioids being reserved for patients who cannot tolerate morphine or require a non-oral route. When calculating the dose of morphine to be used it is important to include any breakthrough doses that have been given over the previous 24 hours (Box 53.1).

---

**Box 53.1 Example calculation**

Codeine 60 mg four times daily = 240 mg daily ≡ 24 mg oral morphine
Plus PRN Oramorph 4 × 5 g = 20 mg oral morphine
Total in past 24 hours ≡ 44 mg oral morphine
Commence immediate-release oral morphine
7.5 mg 4 hourly and PRN

---

After 24–48 hours the daily requirements should be reassessed and adjusted as necessary. For convenience, the patient may be switched to a controlled release formulation given twice daily once a steady state is reached.

Strong and weak opioids all cause constipation and may cause nausea and vomiting. Any patient prescribed opioids should also be prescribed a regular laxative, ideally with stimulant and softening properties, such as co-danthramer. They should also have an antiemetic available, although the incidence of nausea and vomiting is lower (30%), so it is reasonable to prescribe this as required.[2] They need to be warned about the risk of drowsiness and told not to drive if affected when the drugs are first started or after a dose increase. However, once they are on a regular dose without central side effects driving is not a problem.[3] If these potential side effects are not dealt with when opioids are commenced many patients will not tolerate them and will be reluctant to try opioids again. This deprives them of the mainstay of treatment of cancer-related pain.

## Discussion

**What do you need to do if the pain does not respond to this initial approach?**

If pain control is not achieved it is important to repeat the assessment carefully. The problem may be related to the pain:

● Is it a new pain?

● What is the pathophysiology?

- Are co-analgesics required?
- Are further investigations needed?

Or it may be related to the patient:

- Is he depressed?
- Are there psychosocial factors influencing his perception of pain?
- Is he taking the prescribed analgesia?

Or it may also be possible that there is a problem with the prescription:

- Does the dose simply need increasing?
- Is it possible that the patient is not absorbing the drug?

The patient should be given a clear explanation of the likely cause of pain; this can reduce fear, which in turn will reduce pain levels.

### If investigations confirm bone metastases what other treatments should be considered?

Bone pain is often only partially opioid responsive, but may respond well to other interventions.

### NSAIDs

The addition of diclofenac or another NSAID, in the absence of contraindications, would be a possibility if bone metastases were suspected or confirmed. Patients on palliative care often need gastric protection with a proton pump inhibitor and renal function should be checked before and 1 week after starting an NSAID. The drug should be stopped if renal function deteriorates markedly. If NSAIDs are contraindicated or ineffective the daily opioid dose could be increased by a third in the absence of opioid-related toxicity.

### Radiotherapy

In patients with good enough performance status, pain from bone metastasis often responds well to radiotherapy. Following radiotherapy there may be a flare-up of pain before things improve and it takes 1–2 weeks before any notable improvement is seen. Patients therefore need to have a minimum prognosis of several weeks to benefit from radiotherapy.[4]

### Bisphosphonates

Bisphosphonates may be effective in malignant bone pain and can be used in patients with a shorter prognosis. Following either treatment with bisphosphonates or radiotherapy pain may improve dramatically, sometimes allowing a reduction in the doses of regular analgesia.[5]

Any patient taking opioids should be monitored for signs of toxicity. This may present as confusion, drowsiness, myoclonic jerks, agitation, vivid dreams, hallucinations or shadows at the periphery of the visual field. Respiratory depression is rare in patients on long-term opioids and pinpoint pupils are **not** a reliable measure of toxicity. Deterioration in renal function, addition of a co-analgesic or interventional treatment for pain can all precipitate toxicity. This can be a frightening and life-threatening experience for patients but is usually reversible if diagnosed early.

## Conclusion

Optimum pain control can only be achieved when a thorough evaluation has been carried out. Analgesia should be given regularly and a breakthrough dose should always be available. Patients need an explanation of the likely cause of pain and side effects of treatment that need to be anticipated and prevented. If good analgesia is not achieved the pain, the patient and the prescription all need to be reassessed.

## Further Reading

1   World Health Organization. *Cancer Pain Relief: with a guide to opioid availability.* WHO, Geneva, 1996.

2   Campora E, Merlini L, Pace M, Bruzzone M, Luzzani M, Gottlieb A, Rosso R.  The incidence of narcotic-induced emesis. *J Pain Symptom Manage* 1991; **6**: 428–30.

3   Drivers Medical Group, DVLA. *At a Glance.* Guide to Current Medical Standards of Fitness to Drive. DVLA, Swansea, 2006. Available at: www.dvla.gov.uk/medical/ataglance.aspx (accessed 13 May 2007).

4   Hoegler D. Radiotherapy for palliation of symptoms in incurable cancer. *Curr Prob Cancer* 1997; **21**: 129–83.

5   Mannix K, Ahmedzai SH, Anderson H, Bennett M, Lloyd-Williams M, Wilcock A. Using bisphosphonates to control the pain of bone metastases: evidence-based guidelines for palliative care. *Palliat Med* 2000; **14**: 455–61.

## Additional Further Reading

Management of pain. In: Doyle D, Hanks GWC, MacDonald N, eds. *Oxford Textbook of Palliative Medicine*, 2nd edn. Oxford University Press, Oxford, 1998: 231–487.

Twycross R, Wilcock A. Pain relief. In: *Symptom Management in Advanced Cancer*, 3rd edn. Radcliffe Medical Press, Oxford, 2001: 17–68.

Stannard C, Booth S. *Churchill's Pocketbook of Pain.* Churchill Livingstone, Edinburgh, 2004.

Twycross R, Wilcox A, Thorp S. *Palliative Care Formulary*, 2nd edn. Radcliffe Medical Press, Oxford, 2002.

# 54 Pain Relief: A Special Problem

## Case History

You are asked to see a 60-year-old man who has widespread bone metastases from prostate cancer, which is no longer responding to hormone treatment. He lives alone and was completely independent until a few days ago. He has been admitted to hospital because he has become unable to care for himself. When you see him, he complains of pain around his trunk, which he finds difficult to describe. The ward nurse thinks he is exaggerating the pain, because he cries out even when the bed sheets touch his abdomen or legs.

**What could this pain represent?**

**What must be done next?**

**What is the initial approach to his pain?**

**If systemic drugs have been exhausted, what other options exist for treating this pain?**

## Background

### What could this pain represent?

Band-like trunk pain in patients with cancer can represent malignant spinal cord compression. Such pain is often dermatomal, roughly corresponding to the level of compression. Patients may also have pain in dermatomes below this sensory level (e.g. radiating down the legs). Bone pain at the level of spinal metastases is common in cord compression, but its absence does not exclude the diagnosis.[1]

Pain caused by nerve compression or injury is called *neuropathic* pain. This is in contrast to *nociceptive* pain, which is due to physiological activation of pain fibres by noxious stimuli, e.g. tissue damage. It is often difficult for patients to describe the quality of neuropathic pain. Damaged *peripheral* nerves may cause burning or scalding pain in a dermatomal distribution. A classic example is post-herpetic neuralgia. The distribution of pain from damaged *central* nerves is more likely to extend beyond the dermatomes and can be aching or stabbing in nature. In our clinical case, the leg pain is caused by compression of the central nervous system (CNS) sensory fibres in the spinal cord.[2]

When sensory nerves are damaged, pain fibres can be activated by non-noxious stimuli. This is called *allodynia*. In this patient, gently brushing the affected dermatome with bed sheets is causing pain. It occurs because the damaged nerves are hyper-excitable, and sometimes activate spontaneously. Over time, neuropathic pain causes chemical and physiological changes in the spinal cord, resulting in 'central sensitization'. Once central sensitization is established, pain becomes less responsive to opioids. Therefore, it is important to treat neuropathic pain sooner rather than later.[2]

### What must be done next?

In this case, urgent action is required. The attending doctor must:

- take a thorough history including any change in limb and sphincter function

- conduct a thorough neurological examination, palpate the abdomen for evidence of urinary retention, and examine the rectum to assess anal tone

- consider an urgent (same day) magnetic resonance scan of the *whole* spine as cord compression can occur at multiple levels simultaneously.[3]

It is vital to remember that *early cord compression can occur in the absence of neurological signs.* Further more, the earlier spinal cord compression is treated, the better the results. Once neurological function is lost, radiotherapy usually serves to delay progression, rather than reverse weakness. However, if a patient is unfit for treatment of spinal cord compression, magnetic resonance imaging (MRI) should be avoided, as it is unlikely to change management.[3]

If there is a suspicion of spinal cord compression, the patient should be given high-dose corticosteroids (usually dexamethasone 16 mg) while waiting for an urgent MRI.[4] In addition to their neuroprotective effects, steroids have an analgesic effect. This is mediated by reducing inflammation and oedema around spinal metastases, thus decompressing the affected nerves. High-dose dexamethasone can cause insomnia and agitation. It should be given as a once-daily dose in the *morning*, to minimize the impact of these side effects.[5] If spinal cord compression is confirmed, dexamethasone should not be stopped abruptly, even if there is no improvement in pain.

Demonstration of spinal cord compression on MRI should prompt an urgent referral for radiotherapy or spinal surgery. As discussed in Chapter 53, radiotherapy can cause a temporary worsening in pain. However, if successful, radiotherapy can relieve pain by reducing the mass effect of a tumour and its surrounding oedema.

In some cases, steroids are used to treat neuropathic pain even though nerve function is not at risk, for example, pain due to invasion of intra-abdominal nerves by pancreatic cancer. The starting dose of dexamethasone is usually 8–10 mg given in the morning. If the pain does not improve within 3–5 days of commencing treatment, the steroids should be stopped immediately to minimize side effects.[2] Patients are at risk of adrenal suppression once they have been on steroids for 3 weeks, or sooner if the dose is high.[6]

## Discussion

### What is the initial approach to his pain?

Whether or not the patient receives radiotherapy, pharmacological treatments should be considered. In addition to steroids, opioids are used in the initial management of severe neuropathic pain. The principles and pitfalls of opioid use have been described in Chapter 53. Some neuropathic pain is inadequately treated by opioids, either because the pain is not entirely opioid-responsive, or because side effects limit the dose. In these cases, co-analgesic drugs such as antidepressants (e.g. amitriptyline) or anticonvulsants (e.g. gabapentin) should be considered. Both can cause CNS side effects, in particular sedation. They are started at low doses (amitriptyline 10–25 mg nocte, gabapentin 100–300 mg at night) and titrated upwards. They can be used alone or in combination with each other. In practice, they are sometimes used before opioids, particularly if there is no obvious nociceptive pain. In deciding which of these to use, it is important to consider the patient's comorbidities. For example, patients with a history of dysrhythmias should avoid amitriptyline, whereas gabapentin doses need adjusting in renal impairment.[2]

Antidepressants and anticonvulsants work by:

● directly inhibiting ascending pain pathways, and

● stimulating descending nerves that inhibit pain pathways.

The evidence (Table 54.1) supporting their use is based on studies involving patients with post-herpetic neuralgia and diabetic peripheral neuropathy.[7]

| Table 54.1 | Evidence for the use of antidepressants and anticonvulsants in the treatment of neuropathic pain | | | |
|---|---|---|---|---|
| | Number needed to harm (NNH) | 95% CI | Number needed to treat (NNT) | 95% CI |
| Antidepressants | Minor adverse effect: 2.7 | 2.1 to 3.9 | Diabetic peripheral neuropathy: 3.4 | 2.6 to 4.7 |
| | Major adverse effect: 17 | 10 to 43 | Post-herpetic neuralgia: 2.1 | 1.7 to 3.0 |
| Anticonvulsants | Minor adverse effect: 2.7 | 2.2 to 3.4 | Diabetic peripheral neuropathy: 2.7 | 2.2 to 3.8 |
| | Major adverse effect: N/A | | Post-herpetic neuralgia: 3.2 | 2.4 to 5.0 |

Pregabalin is a new anticonvulsant related to gabapentin. It may be less sedating than gabapentin and can be tried if side effects limit the use of gabapentin. Note that amitriptyline is not licensed for treatment of neuropathic pain, whereas gabapentin and pregabalin are.[6] Non-steroidal anti-inflammatory drugs (NSAIDs) are often used as a first- or second-line adjuvant to opioids. In the clinical case above, the use of corticosteroids compounds the risk of peptic ulceration. As such, NSAIDs might be reserved in case other drugs are ineffective. The risk–benefit ratio must be considered individually for each patient.

If pain is uncontrolled despite the above, or if there are unacceptable side effects, specialist advice from the palliative care team or chronic pain team is indicated. The following drugs can be used under specialist supervision:

● benzodiazepines which act via activation of γ-aminobutyric acid (GABA) inhibitory systems in the dorsal horn of the spinal cord

● ketamine which acts via N-methyl-D-aspartate (NMDA) receptor-channel blockade in the spinal cord

● methadone which acts via NMDA-receptor-channel blockade, and opioid receptors

● systemic lidocaine or other local anaesthetics, which act via blockade of sodium-dependent ion channels in peripheral nerves.[2]

## If systemic drugs have been exhausted, what other options exist for treating this pain?

In addition to the above, transcutaneous electrical nerve stimulation (TENS) can be used. A small portable generator box and electrode pads are used to stimulate large diameter sensory fibres that inhibit transmission in pain pathways. Its success is partially user dependent. Patients must be able to understand how and when to adjust the simple controls, and they must be physically capable of doing so. The patient should be educated by someone familiar with the use of TENS.[8]

Neuropathic pain is sometimes amenable to neurolytic therapy and paravertebral blocks may be considered in this patient. Intrathecal analgesia delivers opioids and co-analgesics such as clonidine and bupivacaine directly to the spinal cord, and is usually highly effective. However, it is invasive, and is only useful when pain is confined distally. The presence of spinal metastases adds specific risks to the use of intrathecal analgesia. In particular,

- when inserting the catheter into the intrathecal space, there is a risk of trauma to tumour tissue, possibly resulting in local haemorrhage, epidural haematoma and further cord compression

- there is an increased risk of cerebrospinal fluid (CSF) obstruction and local sequestration of intrathecal drugs.[4]

## Conclusion

Neuropathic pain is a common problem in cancer patients. Although it is often controlled by first-line drugs, a specialist palliative care team or chronic pain team can advise on more specialist medication and interventions.

## Further Reading

1   Twycross R, Wilcock A. Neurological symptoms. In: *Symptom Management in Advanced Cancer*, 3rd edn. Radcliffe Medical Press, Oxford, 2001: 259–81.

2   Twycross R, Wilcock A. Pain relief. In: *Symptom Management in Advanced Cancer*, 3rd edn. Radcliffe Medical Press, Oxford, 2001: 17–68.

3   Spinal cord compression. In: Cassidy J, Bissett D, Spence RAJ, eds. *Oxford Handbook of Oncology*. Oxford University Press, Oxford, 2002; 573–82.

4   Caraceni A, Cinzia M, Simonetti F. Neurological problems in advanced cancer. In: Doyle D, Hanks G, Cherney N, Calman K, eds. *Oxford Textbook of Palliative Medicine*, 3rd edn. Oxford University Press, New York, 2005: 702–26.

5   Twycross R, Wilcock A, Charlesworth S. Endocrine system and immunomodulation. In: Twycross R, Wilcox A, Charlesworth S, Dickman A, eds. *Palliative Care Formulary*, 2nd edn. Radcliffe Medical Press, Oxford, 2002; 215–40.

6   Mehta D. Withdrawal of corticosteroids. In: *British National Formulary* 51. British Medical Association and Royal Pharmaceutical Society of Great Britain, London, March 2006.

7   Moore A, Edwards J, Barden J, *et al.* Chronic pain. In: *Bandolier's Little Book of Pain (An Evidence-based Guide to Treatments)*. Oxford University Press, Oxford 2003: 218–38.

8   Bercovitch M, Waller A. Transcutaneous electrical nerve stimulation (TENS). In: Doyle D, Hanks G, Cherney N, Calman K, eds. *Oxford Textbook of Palliative Medicine*, 3rd edn. Oxford University Press, New York, 2005: 405–10.

## Additional Further Reading

Hicks F, Simpson KH. *Nerve Blocks in Palliative Care*. Oxford University Press, Oxford, 2004.

Twycross R. *Introducing Palliative Care*. Radcliffe Medical Press, Oxford, 2002.

Twycross R, Wilcock A, Charlesworth S, Dickman A. *Palliative Care Formulary*, 2nd edn. Radcliffe Medical Press, Oxford, 2002.

# Index